One Beat at a Time

One Beat at a Time

Living with Sudden Cardiac Death

An Autobiography

Matthew D. Noble

Foreword by: Leonard Ganz, M.D.

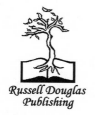

Russell Douglas
Publishing

13097 Golfside Ct. Suite 103
Clio, MI 48420
www.russell-douglas.com

©2005 by Matthew D. Noble

Printed and bound in the United States of America. All rights reserved.
No part of this book may be reproduced or transmitted in any form or by
any means, electronic or mechanical, including photocopying, recording,
or by an information storage and retrieval system-except by a reviewer
who may quote brief passages in a review to be printed in a magazine,
newspaper, or on the Web-without permission in writing from the
publisher. For information please contact Russell Douglas Publishing,
13097 Golfside Ct., Suite 103, Clio, MI 48420. Phone: 810-686-7005
Fax: 810-686-4973 www.Russell-Douglas.com

ISBN-0-9769436-0-3

Library of Congress Control Number: 2005907694

First Printing

Although the author and publisher have made every effort to ensure
the accuracy and completeness of information contained in this book,
we assume no responsibility for errors, inaccuracies, omissions, or any
inconsistency herein. Any slights of people, places, or organizations are
unintentional. Some of the names in this story have been changed to
protect anonymity.

In this book you will find many stories of the author's medical struggles.
Do not use these stories to draw any conclusions about your heart or
other health issues. Each person is unique, as is each heart, and the
author is in no way the norm. If you have any questions about your
health or what you should or should not be doing, contact your
physician.

1 2 3 4 5 6 7 8 9 10   12 11 10 09 08 07 06 05

Edited by: Karen Chernyaev
Cover design by: David Spohn
Interior design by: Lisa Beck
Front Cover Photo: Tina Timmons
Back cover photo of Matt and his sister compliments of the Noble Family.
All photographs contained within this book are compliments of the
Noble family unless otherwise noted.

Contents

Acknowledgments

I have so many people to thank for their involvement in this project, and in my life. **Aunt Jan and Uncle Don:** Stacy and I have always known that we were your favorites. Just so you know, the feeling is mutual. **Aaron Emmendorfer:** Thanks for taking care of my lil' sister and for climbing up those press boxes back in the day. **My extended family:** Thank you for your support throughout the years. I know that what I've been through has caused some chaos in each of your lives. Thank you for caring. **Zac Lloyd:** Those years in the zoo were the best, thanks for everything. **Chris White:** I really miss having you around man, and "No," I don't care what Dan said. **Joe Heystek:** Thanks for pulling my butt out of the pool, throwing that pitch in Little League, and being a great friend.—Bless you Boys '84 **Tim Hobson:** Thank you for showing me how it's supposed to be done, living this life I mean. Also, thank you for passing on your guitar knowledge. I've used it the best I know how. **Paul Filan:** Thanks for being a real friend Paul, and thank you for your work on my website. **Rob Cannon:** You have been more passionate about this project than anyone, even me at times. I can't thank you enough for your direct impact on this book, and on my life. **The Team at the U:** To Dr. Dick, Pete, Ian, Sarah, and everyone else who's ever gotten their hands on me, thanks for caring more than most. **Tony Annese:** Thanks for the motivation; I don't think you realize how much it's helped get me through. **Mary Jane:** Thank you for the prayers, showing Mom the way, and thank you for panicking that day. It saved my life. **That emergency medical something or other:** Thanks for not worrying about getting sued. **Jeff Mullen:** Thanks for being a friend and taking me under your wing, I have learned so much from you, the least of which has to do with pacemakers. **Sally Williams, Scott Berens, Todd Moore, and Malcolm Miyasato:** You guys make my day job great. Thank you so much. **Bob Olson:** Thank you for convincing me that I could write this on my own. I wouldn't have done it without your encouragement. **Karen Chernyaev:** Thank you so much Karen for all your work. Your edits have turned this little story of mine into an actual book. **Janet Helin, Anita Marzoni, and Darrin Edelman:** Thank you for your help on this project. **Jamie Avram:** I wasn't too sure about this book until I saw the look in your eyes when reading it. Thank you. **Bob Koch and everyone at the LOGF:** Thank you for always being there throughout the years. **Rick Warren:** Thank you for showing us all how to be purpose driven. It's really the way to live. **Rob Bell, Jr., and Joel Osteen:** Even though I've never seen either of you in person, I learn from you nearly every week. Thank You. **Seinfeld:** Thank you Jerry Seinfeld and the cast and crew of *Seinfeld*. You brought a lot of laughter into my life. **All of the people who have prayed for me:** I would like to start this book out with a very special thank you to everyone who has ever uttered a prayer for me. Throughout all of my struggles, I know that I've had hundreds and hundreds of people remember me in their prayers. For that, I am humbled and completely grateful.

Foreword

Since entering the field of cardiac electrophysiology in the early 1990s, I have encountered thousands of patients with implantable cardioverter defibrillators (ICDs). As you will learn, an ICD is a device implanted under the skin that continuously monitors the heart, and in case of cardiac arrest, delivers an electric shock to convert the dangerous heart rhythm back to the normal heart rhythm. These patients have been old and young, cardiac arrest survivors, as well as many who receive an ICD for preventative reasons. I have learned from each of my patients but have heard few stories as compelling as Matt Noble's. Matt is not my patient; I first met him at a corporate function sponsored by a medical device manufacturer in July 2005. I was struck with his poise, confidence, eloquence, and intelligence as he recounted the exciting, emotional, and gripping story that has been his life. I was particularly amazed with the absence of self-pity in his words.

Living with an ICD is not easy. Many patients struggle with fear of dying, fear of getting a painful shock from the device, and related issues. Although an ICD shock can be life-saving, it can induce serious emotional trauma. Even before the device is implanted, most patients have at some level anxiety and fear about what getting a shock will be like. Once a patient experiences a first shock, many are fearful about the possibility of a future shock. Patients who receive repeated or multiple shocks are at risk for serious psychological trauma.

Young patients find these issues particularly challenging. As young ICD patients are relatively uncommon, physicians, nurses, and other health care professionals are less equipped to provide appropriate and relevant support and counseling. Young people in general tend to believe in the "immortality of youth," a feeling the ICD may foster, and may not want to limit their lifestyles in the ways that their heart disease and ICD dictate. Moreover, desires to "fit in" with their peers may limit whom young patients tell about their ICD, which of course limits who can provide support regarding day-to-day "living with an ICD" issues, as well as the specific issues that arise when a shock occurs.

Though I encounter ICD patients on a daily basis, my response to hearing Matt's story was the same as most other people; I said, "You should write a book." As it turned out, Matt had, and I was flattered when he asked me to read it for medical accuracy. I can assure you that the book is accurate from a medical and scientific perspective. Although the style of the book is not overtly technical, Matt and his colleagues assist patients, physicians, and nurses on a daily basis with respect to the implantation and follow-up of ICDs, so his technical expertise is extensive. Matt is thus an invaluable resource to patients and their families, as well as physicians, nurses, and colleagues in the industry, given his unique perspective as a patient and allied professional.

Matt's medical issues have been cardiovascular; he was born with an unusual congenital anomaly and had to undergo a number of corrective cardiac surgeries. As a result, his heart is prone to life-threatening rhythm disturbances. While Matt's reason for needing an ICD is relatively unusual, sudden cardiac death (SCD) is the leading cause of death in the United States (*see* More About ICD's and Sudden Cardiac Death at the end of the book). Matt had survived multiple cardiac arrests prior to receiving an ICD, and his ICDs have subsequently saved his life on a number of occasions. Though his medical history is filled with surprises, complications, and disappointments, his personal story is one of courage, fulfillment, and self-realization and can be readily generalized to other medical, and even non-medical, struggles.

I am sure you will enjoy and learn from Matt Noble's story.

Leonard Ganz, M.D., F.A.C.C.
Temple University School of Medicine
The Western Pennsylvania Hospital
Pittsburgh, PA
August 2005

"The glory of God is man fully alive."

—St. Irenaeus

Prologue

My life at times has been as normal as that of any middle-class kid named Matthew in any small town in Michigan. At other times it has been so abnormal and miraculous that it could make even the most devout atheist question his views. Like everyone, I've had struggles; the difference is that my tough times have been quite stunning, even worthy of telling in a book. Like a Fourth of July fireworks display, those times in my life when I've escaped sudden cardiac death look amazing from the outside and are so powerful as to shake me to the core.

Each and every person on this planet has had or will have at least one moment, most of us many more, where we find ourselves crying out "Why God?" from deep inside. We cry out until we remember that we aren't even sure we believe God exists. My life seems to have been filled with those moments, one after another. Yet each and every time I have managed to come out on the other side with at least a smile, and usually a laugh.

This book is the story of my fireworks display and how I've made it through. The story will be told along with my reactions, my reasons, my thoughts, and my prayers. For some, the story alone will be enough. For others, the story won't be so impressive, for they've got one of their own. For them, the help may come through seeing a different way of thinking, of reacting, and of living.

As I sit here today, I am prepared to tell my story like I've never told it before. I plan on opening up completely for the very first time, as I have come to realize that when you open up beyond what feels comfortable, that's when people are touched.

One wintry Michigan night back in college, I was out with some fairly new friends. We had just spent hours at the library studying when we decided to walk across campus to a local gathering place to sit fireside and chat. As we talked, they knew nothing of my past or my current struggles; I was just a guy they were getting to know.

I don't know what it was about that night, maybe the lateness of the evening, the warmth of the fire, or the look of acceptance in Lauren's eyes, but I revealed much more of myself than I normally would have at that point in a friendship. I opened up. For some reason, I not only told the amazing details of what had happened to me, but also let them see the fears I faced at the time. I told the story like I'd never told it before. I also got a response like never before. I don't even remember the words they used, but the looks on their faces said it all. It touched them in a way I never expected.

So as I sit here prepared to tell my story, I am going to tell it as I did that night, sitting in a large overstuffed leather chair by the fire, late into a cold night, opening up more than ever before. I'm not going back to look up dates, making sure to get every detail perfectly right. This isn't intended to be a record of history. This is my story the way it sits in my mind, all true, the way I and those closest to me remember it.

So as the fire crackles in the background and you forget about the lateness of the hour, relax, enjoy, and picture this . . .

Chapter One

Let the Fireworks Begin

Some people are born on third base and go
through life thinking they hit a triple.

—Barry Switzer

It was a cold day late in February of 1976 as she sat lean-ing out of her second-story bedroom window, willing to put up with the cold just to get the high. It was a good cold though, the kind of day that makes the slush-filled gray Michigan winters worthwhile. The sky was as blue, and the sun as bright, as any summer day. The air was so crisp it made her want to breathe in deep, just to feel the sting in her lungs.

She sat there in a marijuana-induced mode of con-templation thinking about how weird it was leaning out of the bedroom window that just a few years before belonged to her parents. She was married now, living in the house that held all of her childhood memories. The house was in the small autoworkers town of Montrose, just outside of Flint, the kind of town where everyone knows everybody. Yet no one really knew her. She thought about her marriage, her job, and her friends. She thought about everything as she sat there resting heavy in her insecurities; she thought about everything but the consequences.

Just a month later she gave birth to me, and man, was I cute, in a weird sort of way. Like a baby monkey, my ears were all folded in on themselves, and I had entirely too much hair, but other than that things were pretty normal. In order to correct the slight oddities of appearance, my mom, a second-generation hairdresser, used hair tape to set my ears back and quickly gave me a haircut. She trimmed off about an inch of that jet-black, arrow-straight hair that would not cooperate with any amount of hair spray that was commercially available in 1976. Yes, life was grand for me then.

Life was great for my mom, Sue, as well. She was a young mother worrying about her baby just like any other. She worried about the little things—a cold, a runny nose, and at times what seemed to be my inability to sleep—but never about what was actually to come. She never once found herself imagining what it would be like to hold on to her lifeless son while crying out to God for help. Yet in the years to come that is exactly where she would find herself, more than once. For a twenty-five-year-old party girl, anything that serious was inconceivable. Even when thoughts of doom and fear (of a much lesser variety) did crowd her mind, she would simply smoke them away. She wasn't the type to let herself get down. She was about having fun. Enjoying life.

These days my mom says that if she had known what she would go through over the first twenty-eight years of my life, the thought alone probably would have killed her. It's funny how this life only lets us see just enough ahead to take a step, and no more.

I don't mean to leave out my dad. He was around then too; he's always been around. I guess I just don't know as much about who he was back then. For as long as I can remember, he has been the type to not say too much. He usually only jumps into a conversation with a funny one-liner or a priceless piece of wisdom. Rarely does he sit back in his chair and talk about his younger days.

I do know, however, that he was starting his career as a teacher in the local school. That is how he and my mom met. Dad (Doug to everyone but my younger sister and me) had my mom's kid sister in class. She set them up, and the next thing you knew, they were buying Grandpa Vette's house from him after his four kids were gone and his wife lost her battle with cancer.

I never knew Grandma Vette, but on all accounts she was a lot like Mom is now—a fun-loving hairdresser who enjoys life while focusing on her family. She was always willing to share a story but never too busy to listen.

Dad came from a much different kind of family than Mom. Whereas Grandpa Vette was a shop worker, making cars in nearby Flint, Grandpa Noble owned his own business. It was a small sporting goods shop. Almost every story that I've heard my dad recount (with a smile) of his childhood was related to the shop in one way or another. The top-of-the-line fishing gear that he and Grandpa would get to use on fishing trips easily comes to mind. But the biggest smiles usually came when talking about the time he and Grandpa spent together, no

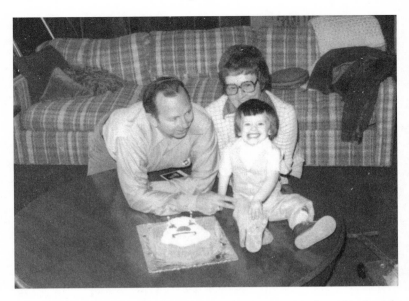

Grandpa Vette and Grandma Donna (my step-grandmother) with me on the table

matter what they were doing. I guess it's a lot like the smile-inducing stories of my childhood, more about the man in the hospital room with me than about the toys that he brought. But that's the kind of guy Grandpa Noble was and that Dad is now. You smile just thinking about being with them, let alone actually spending some time together.

Grandpa and Grandma Noble were always there for me, even when I didn't know I needed them. They kept the kind of relationship with their grandkids that made us think they lived just around the corner, even though they were close to two hours away. And Dad learned well from them. Although Dad acts a lot like his father, he has never really looked like him too much, especially when he was younger, before his red hair gave way to the gray. Dad stands tall at six feet three inches and in his younger days had the build of a lean high school tight end. He had a Robert Redford look about him, one that only Mom could see. To this day, when she looks back at old pictures, she sees the resemblance. Everyone she mentions it to eases out a slow "I guess so" as they stare at the picture with a tilt of their heads.

I really don't know who Mom looked liked, but she was also tall and thin. A five-foot-seven-inch track star in high school, she held a few records for several years. She had dark hair, like mine, and usually wore a smile. As a hairdresser she kept her hair in the "in" style and always wore clothes that fit with the latest trends, even as a new mother in mid-1976.

The first few months of my life were as normal as could be for any two young parents. Sue and Doug thought they had everything they'd ever hoped for—a nice job, a respectable house, a beautiful son, and a dog named Bugger. Life was grand. Even the lack of sleep didn't seem to be too much of a problem. After all, this is what Sue had wanted. After years of hoping, praying, and taking more than her fair share of fertility drugs, she finally had her baby. Little did she know that the smooth sailing was about to come to an end.

It started at my two-month checkup with the pediatrician. After listening to my heart, he informed Mom that I had a heart murmur. But so did a lot of other babies that he saw. "I wouldn't worry too much about it," he told her. "These things usually just go away with time." That was good enough for her, and the thought of it quickly left her mind.

As the summer of '76 started and the country's bicentennial celebration was looming, the future looked bright, for my parents anyway. Dad was enjoying his summer off work, and Mom was looking forward to my growing up a bit. After all, those sleepless nights were starting to wear on her more and more as time passed. It seemed she could never get me to sleep much at all.

My dad loves to tell the story of coming home one day to a completely frazzled wife. She had been rocking me for hours, as I slept comfortably. The minute she would try to lay me down I would start crying . . . and not stop until I was being rocked to sleep again. "Well," Dad said, "he knows you will pick him back up. This kid has got you trained. Let me have him." I cried for a minute or two when he first took me but was quickly quieted by some wandering around the kitchen. Dad then went up the stairs, laid me down, and let me start my two-hour nap . . . quiet as can be. He loved the fact that he could get me to sleep when Mom couldn't, and still does today. He was always content to let my mom spoil me silly, as he was the firm, yet loving one.

Mom and Dad continued on with this normal little life until my four-month checkup. Mom was curious about whether that little murmur had resolved itself, but not worried. The doctor did his best to change that. He was concerned with my breathing, which seemed to take too much effort, and wanted to run some tests. After the tests, and an "I'll be in touch," a worried mom and I were on our way home.

Mom walked into the house to a ringing phone. It was the doctor. He quickly explained that he believed I was in "heart failure," whatever that was, and told her that she and Dad should get me down to C. S. Mott Children's Hospital in Ann Arbor, Michigan, as soon as possible. He had already contacted the pediatric cardiologists there, and they were expecting my arrival within a few hours.

They got in the car and started the drive toward Mott Hospital, part of the University of Michigan Health Care System, about an hour's drive due south. I've never really bothered to ask my parents what was going through their minds during that car ride or whether they were scared. I guess some things you just don't have to ask.

My parents spent the next week with me in the hospital. One nice thing about pediatric hospitals is that visiting hours never really end. Next to every hospital bed (or crib, in this case) is a bed for the parents. It is actually a firm plastic couch built into the wall that converts into a bed. But when your child is sick, you will take what you can get. My parents would come to know these little "parent spots" all too well over the next several years. Mom would usually be the one to stay, as Dad was about three inches too long for the "bed." Mom fit nicely though, although comfort was usually the last thing on her mind. What was wrong with me was all either one of them could think about. *Was everything going to be okay?*

My parents learned, over the course of that week, that my murmur wasn't going to just "go away." It was caused by a hole in my heart. The technical name for the hole was a double outlet right ventricle. But who really cares about that. It was the fact that I would need open-heart surgery that really mattered to anyone who had ever held me close. The doctors informed my parents that my heart was "very abnormal," saying that they had never seen a heart quite like mine. As I grew, my heart would not be able to handle the additional workload that would be put on it, and it would simply give out. Putting a patch over the hole, however, would solve the problem.

Back then, the protocol with children was to put off surgery for as long as possible. The trick was to wait as long as they could, as the chances of survival went up with each year that I aged, without waiting so long that my heart would start to give out. That one surgery was the key. My parents were informed that if I could get through that one open-heart surgery, my life should be "pretty normal" from then on. With that I was discharged, now on a medication to help my heart pump a little more efficiently.

During the car ride home, for the next several weeks, and to some extent for the following years, they both asked, "Why, God? Why our son?" Was it the fertility drugs, was it the one (okay, two) time that Mom decided to "light up" while she was pregnant? Did they bring this on themselves? Was God punishing them for their sins?

Looking back, it seems funny to me that they would ask God for the answer. Although both were brought up around (not necessarily in) the church, neither one of them was religious by any stretch of the imagination. Yet for some reason they found themselves asking God for the answers. But I guess that's how most of us work; we turn to God as a last resort, when we see no way of fixing a problem ourselves.

They spent the next several months wondering how they would handle the new life they had just been handed. Wondering if the medicine I was now on would work was only the first of many questions that would plague them on a daily basis for those first few months. Would my heart be able to make it until I was old enough for surgery? (At the time, this was generally thought to be at around four or five years old.) Would my heart even make it through today? Would it give out tomorrow? If I survived to undergo the surgery, would I make it through the procedure? After all, the doctors had "never seen a heart like mine." If I did survive, would I be as normal as they wanted their son to be? This was as close to the end of the world as my two young parents had ever experienced. Yet nothing compared to what the future held.

The future would come rolling in a month at a time, as it always did, and things actually seemed awfully normal considering what they'd learned at the hospital. Slipping medicine into the baby food once a day was really the only technical departure. Except, of course, for the weight of not knowing what the future held for their little son. As time went by, neither one of them could let go of the question "Why?" My mom would try to find the answer.

She started searching for the answer from God. To her this problem was so big, and the doctors had so many "wait and see" answers for her, that God was the only one big enough to know the answers and to fix the problems. So one day while folding laundry and flipping channels, she searched out Pat Robertson and the *The 700 Club*.

Robertson spoke of healings and other miracles that were "possible with God," and for the first time, Mom found that maybe she could see God as being of some use in her life.

But what was she supposed to do? She really didn't hang out with anyone who went to church. Was she just supposed to randomly walk in the doors of a church? Her insecurities wouldn't let that happen. She continued watching *The 700 Club* and trying to find a way to connect with God, until one day her pot-smoking companion and friend from high school brought up the subject. Apparently, Mary Jane (okay, that's not her real name, but, come on, what better pseudonym for Mom's pot-smoking friend) had befriended a pastor's wife at work, who invited her to come to church with her. She was also questioning the whole "God thing" as she saw her friend struggle with the fears that my life had brought. So they decided to check it out together.

Over the next few years, my dad found himself married to a complete and total "Jesus-freak." She was going around telling anyone and everyone who would listen that God was going to heal her son. She would read her Bible, hour upon hour, meditating on every Scripture she could find about healing, health, or prosperity. God and the Scriptures are what she came to depend on. God is what eased her fears. Well, God and marijuana. After all, as Mary Jane would tell her, "Why be down when you can be up?" and "God wouldn't want you to be sad and depressed." So she continued her closet relationship with her drug of choice, all the while preaching at everyone who would listen.

She started to get that feeling after smoking, at first only occasionally, that told her this wasn't the way to go. How would getting high really help her deal with her problems? But quitting really didn't seem like an option. She needed that escape from worrying about what the future would hold for her son. So she would keep going to church but just not tell anyone about her smoking.

One church service she attended when I was three years old gave her great hope. She was sitting in a pew with some friends when the visiting preacher said, "Someone here is praying for someone with a heart problem; I believe it's their child." At that, my mom rushed up to the front to claim her miracle. She prayed with the pastor and left knowing that her child had just been healed. As a matter of fact, she came home that night to lay her head on my little chest. She couldn't hear the murmur; I must have been healed. It's not exactly science, but she didn't care. She knew deep down that things would be okay. Her son was healed. What else could it be? In her mind, the only way that things could be okay was if her son were healthy, if he were healed.

As she shared this news with her husband that night, he replied "Oh, really," with a tone of doubt that anyone could have picked up on. Even though he hoped deep down that somehow she was right, it couldn't be. That stuff just doesn't happen. But there was no telling her that.

It was in the middle of this craziness that my little sister, Stacy, was born. It was June of 1979, and, I must say, I wasn't too happy about it. I had always been the complete and total center of attention. I had quickly learned

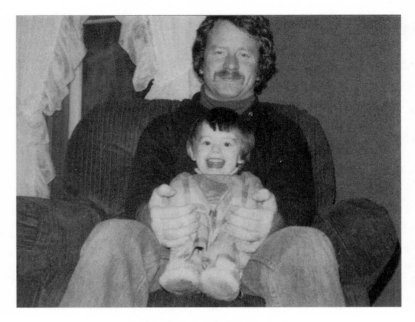

Dad and me at home in 1978

how to use my "heart problem" to my advantage and
would have my mom running for cookies because I was
"just too tired to get up myself." I do, however, remember that, for me anyway, the bright spot of Mom's pregnancy was that I was able to sit on her belly before she
gave birth. I don't know why I remember that, but I do.
Maybe I just saw a picture of it and now I think I remember it. It's funny how the mind works.

To be honest, Stacy didn't really interfere with my
comfort all that much. She was a good fit to the family.
Mom would sit the little, chubby, healthy-looking thing
on a blanket in the middle of the room with a toy and
some food, and she was content for hours. This worked

nicely for me, as I needed, or actually just wanted, the most attention.

And so it continued. I would cry until Mom rocked me; Stacy would sit and eat. Mom would go to church and take me to see faith healers; Dad would watch football and shake his head. Maybe she was doing something right, though, with all this church stuff. I was almost five now and doing pretty good. Was Mom's faith the reason? We would go down to Ann Arbor every six months or so for checkups, each time getting a good report. The surgery didn't have to come . . . at least not yet.

I vaguely remember some of these checkups. They were fun for me. They never hurt, and I got to be the total center of attention for the day (as if that wasn't always the case). I liked my doctors too. My cardiologist was a young guy by the name of Macdonald Dick II, M.D. Yep, that's right. Mac Dick was his name, and he was the best.

A few months after I turned five, Mom came home from a women's church retreat and informed Dad, with absolute conviction, that I was going to have to have the surgery. *What?* he thought. *Where was this coming from? Was this a lack of faith creeping in or what?*

He couldn't remember the last time he heard her talk about anything other than a healing from God. Now she was talking about surgery. When he questioned her, she simply told him, "The lady at the camp said someone is going to have to go through some hard times pretty soon, but not to worry. God will be with them."

"That's all?" he quickly replied.

"Yes," she said. "As soon as I heard it, I just knew . . . I just knew."

A few weeks later I had a six-month checkup with Dr. Dick, and Mom was right. It was time. The doctors decided that I needed the surgery and suggested I get it before I started school. So Mom and Dad took me home and waited for June to come.

Chapter Two

Nineteen Eighty-One

If you're going through hell, keep going.

—Winston Churchill

It was a Sunday in June of 1981, and although my parents were stressed to the max, my sister and I were clueless. In fact, when Mom and Dad told me that afternoon that we would be going to the hospital, I was excited. "What, we are going to get to spend the night there?" I asked with the excitement that only a five-year-old could bring. This was going to be great! Mom and Dad tried to explain what I was in for, but a five-year-old doesn't really understand the concept of surgery.

That afternoon we were on our way to Ann Arbor, dropping Stacy off on the way. No one seems to remember where we left her for the next ten days, but I am sure it was somewhere safe. Looking back on the events of the next few months, where my sister stayed isn't the part of the story you tend to remember. Being pushed aside while more urgent matters were dealt with was a part of life Stacy would be forced to learn to cope with.

We arrived at the hospital and had a great night, from my point of view anyway. I spent most of the evening riding around on a Big Wheel. I did lap after lap around the hospital floor, oblivious to the pain and death that surrounded me and stopping only to say hi to Dr. Dick. The nurses managed to get me off of my vehicle long enough to show me a video about what surgery was and how I would recover and all that. We then went over to the intensive care unit (ICU) and got to see where I would be staying on Monday and Tuesday night. It all seemed pretty exciting to me.

They woke me up early Monday morning (Mom and Dad didn't need a wake-up call) to tell me it was time to go to surgery. I was fine with that until I saw the three

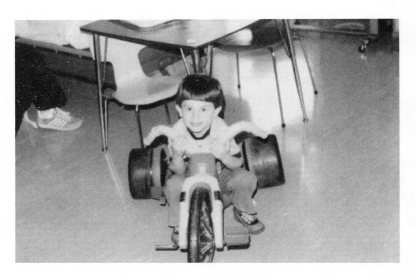

At the hospital the night before my surgery

nurses approach, each of them with a large needle and syringe in their hands containing a sedative, which they simultaneously jammed into my thighs. That hurt. By the time Mom and Dad calmed me down, the sedatives started to take effect, and I slipped off to sleep.

They put me on a stretcher and wheeled me down the hallway. My parents walked alongside the stretcher with a crew of nurses and doctors. Mom simply describes that experience as "horrible." The word isn't what really conveys the emotion when you ask her about it though; it's the tone in her voice and the look in her eyes that she still carries to this day that make you really understand.

As they wheeled me into the operating room, Mom and Dad were confined to the surgery waiting room. They would spend the next eight hours watching the clock there. Between glances at the clock, Dad would pace and Mom would pray. She held on to the last promise that God had given her. Even though this was a miserable and fearful time, she had to have faith that everything would be okay. Somewhere deep down inside she had something to trust, something that was telling her that things would work out for the best. She remembered all the Scriptures she had read about knowing a "peace that passes all understanding" and finding comfort in the "shadow of the Almighty." God was giving her the strength he had promised; she knew things would be fine. That is why she was so surprised when the surgeon finally appeared with news she never expected, only feared.

"Things did not go very well," the young surgeon told them. "We got the patch in place over the hole, but he has lost a lot of blood, and if he makes it through the night, we don't know what to expect." *What?* they thought. *Did he just say "if he makes it?" What did he mean by "don't know what to expect"? Brain damage?* This wasn't happening. They looked to Dr. Dick, who had accompanied the surgeon to talk to my parents, to get the answers. He confirmed all of their fears.

My parents were allowed to come in and see me, and for the first time in my mom's life, she couldn't look at her own son. It looked like tubes were growing out of my little chest, emerging from underneath blood-covered bandages, and my entire body seemed to be swollen. As Mom quickly buried her head into Dad's chest, the nurse showed them the way to the ICU waiting room, where they would spend the night. They would have given anything to get back to that feeling of "horrible" that they had experienced as I was wheeled into surgery. With a little perspective, what once was considered horrific now didn't seem so bad.

After a few hours of letting her mind run wild, Mom reached back for her Bible. She read and prayed all night. Every few seconds or so, as a negative thought would creep into her mind, she would pound it out with a word of hope from God. Reading the Bible got her through the night.

I survived the night with no brain damage. My high school algebra teacher might disagree with that, but for the most part, I came through just fine. I recovered from the surgery quickly, as most kids do, and was able to leave the hospital just a week after leaving the ICU. I was actually back riding the Big Wheel around the halls by the first weekend, just five days after surgery. It was all relatively easy for me, although Dad seemed to have a few more gray hairs by the time we left for home.

Mom's faith was now stronger than ever. She had just lived through the hardest few days of her life, more than what she ever thought she could. She felt much stronger, ready for anything that could possibly come her way, now that this thing my parents had feared for the past five years was over. Now they knew the outcome; I had made it through. The future was bright and "normal" for their son for the first time since that initial week in the hospital four and a half years earlier.

The weeks that followed were enjoyable, and soon it was the end of August, and we were all enjoying the summer. I rode my new bike (a "feel sorry for you" gift) and played outside. Mom and Dad enjoyed life with a little less stress, and Stacy loved having a little control over me for the first time in her young life. She quickly learned, as a two-and-a-half-year-old, how to get her way with me. All it took was a solid punch to the chest. I would run off crying, and she would be left alone feeling satisfied. Dad would simply tell me, "Hit her back . . . then she will leave you alone." I just couldn't do it. This was my little sister. But one day I had had it. I hauled off and hit her back. Dad was right. She stopped hitting me. Mom and Dad were always careful not to baby me too much. It would have been easy to yell at Stacy for hurting me, but I was already the favorite in my sister's mind. Why make it worse?

On one of those August days I was out playing as Mom worked in her beauty shop. She had a one-chair operation that was attached to our house, behind the garage. It was her mom's shop before hers, and one of the few beauty shops in town. It was comforting to always have her there as I was growing up. I used to come in and visit with all of the old ladies to see my mom, usually getting at least a piece of gum or some candy. On this particular day I came in to see Mom more for the air-conditioning that could only be found in the shop than for the company. I sat down for a minute to cool off. As I reached up to the counter for a Kleenex, Mom watched my little body go limp and fall to the floor at the feet of her client, a nurse; a nurse with half-cut hair.

Mom reacted, as you would expect, by freaking out and praying, as the nurse started CPR. Back then, in 1981, there was no such thing as 9-1-1, at least not in Montrose. So one of my mom's other clients, the one under the hair dryer, headed uptown. She drove the mile to the one light, in this one-light town, to get the only doctor for miles. He yelled to his staff to call for an ambulance from Flint as he ran out to the car and rode back to the shop with her; he knew exactly whom he was going to see. He got to the shop just as the nurse started to get a faint pulse. I was still unconscious. He informed Mom that my heart was beating but that I was in a sort of coma, still unconscious; there was no telling how much brain damage I would have if I ever woke up.

In the back of the ambulance on the way to the hospital, Mom sat with her head in her hands. For the duration of that fifteen-minute, eighty-mile-per-hour drive, her mind raced. She once again felt the weight of not knowing what the future would hold for her son; this time it was heavier than ever, as she wondered whether I would ever even open my eyes again.

She could hear me moaning and groaning as the medical supplies clamored about in the midst of the screaming sirens. She felt the need to vomit as she kept getting tossed to and fro with each corner we turned or car we passed. The motion sickness seemed to pile on top of the stress that rested in the pit of her stomach. She was, however, unable to focus on herself, as her ears were tuned into my every noise. As she looked up at me lying there motionless, she felt some relief when I moaned. As long as I was making noise I was alive, although a part of her wondered whether my moaning was a bad sign. All sorts of frightening thoughts raced through her mind. *Why wasn't he awake? Would he ever wake up? How long do comas last? What caused this?*

As her mind continued to want answers that not even the doctors held, she just kept saying, "It'll be okay, Matt. Everything is fine," talking more to herself than her now semiconscious son. As we neared the hospital, she kept her head down while holding my hand and listening to my unconscious groaning, until it stopped. She couldn't look up at me, as her heart fell, exploded. She knew I had died. After what seemed like a few minutes, but in reality was probably only seconds, I said, "I want my mom. Where is Mom?"

"I'm here Matt. Don't worry. Everything is okay."

By the time we got settled into the emergency room at the local hospital, I was fully conscious again. I was back to being what seemed like a very normal, but scared, five-year-old. The doctors in the ER didn't have a clue about what to do with me and prescribed an additional forty-five-minute ambulance drive down to Ann Arbor. After arriving in Ann Arbor, I spent the night hooked up to a heart monitor. I slept as Mom and Dad listened to beep, beep, beep, pause, beep, pause, beep . . . all night long. Each time the monitor paused, so did their breathing, and it paused frequently because I was experiencing what's called an arrhythmia, an irregular heartbeat. As the doctors did tests, they realized that the patch covering the hole in my heart had torn loose. It was flopping around with each heartbeat, causing the arrhythmia. The solution: another surgery.

Just days later it was again the three nurses with needles, the long walk alongside the gurney to the operating room, and eight hours of waiting. Dad was clinging to anything he could find, looking for strength within. Mom was fixed on God, holding to his promise. She remembered the words "Someone is going to have to go through some hard times pretty soon, but not to worry. God will be with them." And so she held on to her faith. That was really her only choice.

She leaned on the wisdom of several biblical verses. She'd read a verse, hear one on the radio, or be given one by a friend and feel like they were written just for her. They didn't necessarily relate to anything special at the time she came across them, but she'd write them down, and, at some point, they'd be exactly what she seemed to need. One of those verses was Psalm 91.

When I was in the ICU following this second surgery, which the doctors said went "much better than the first,"

Mom was again in the waiting room. She recalls that she was there with only one other young man in the room. They both heard the alarms and saw the medical personnel running about. They had each come to know this protocol all too well. Someone was having serious problems; someone's child was dying. As their eyes met, they both wondered who it was. All Mom could do was run through the Ninety-first Psalm in her head over and over for the next twenty or thirty minutes.

> He who dwells in the shelter of the Most High will rest in the shadow of the Almighty. I will say of the Lord, "he is my refuge and my fortress, my God, in whom I trust." Surely he will save you from the fowler's snare and from the deadly pestilence. He will cover you with his feathers, and under his wings you will find refuge; his faithfulness will be your shield and rampart. You will not fear the terror of night, nor the arrow that flies by day, nor the pestilence that stalks in the darkness, nor the plague that destroys at midday. A thousand may fall at your side, ten thousand at your right hand, but it will not come near you. (Psalm 91:1–7)

As the third-shift physicians appeared in the doorway, all Mom could do was pray. Even if they called her name, she knew everything would be okay. Her faith ran that deep. Yet her faith wasn't deep enough to keep out the fear. As she looked up and waited for her name, they looked to that nice young man in the same room with Mom that night. He got up with tears filling his eyes and walked out with the doctors. As Mom watched them leave, she couldn't even feel thankful that it wasn't me having the problems that night. Emotionally she was depleted and all she could wonder about were the next few minutes. After all, at any second the doctors and nurses could start scurrying about again.

That nice young man must have lost his daughter that night, because he never came back to the waiting room. In fact, Mom never saw him again. Mom didn't know why his daughter had those problems while I was okay. For all she knew, he could have been praying harder than she was. But she couldn't think about whether he'd been praying or not because if he was, and it "didn't work," well, Mom couldn't think about that.

For me, the recovery process was going well, and by all accounts it was finally over. Was this the healing miracle that Mom thought she was promised? Did my healing come in the form of a patch that was finally sewn in place correctly? To her it did. She remembered the preacher who knew that "someone was praying for a child with a heart problem," and she remembered the feeling that she had during that prayer with him. She remembered how she knew everything would be okay. That was the promise of healing that she held on to.

During all of the chaos, Dad found himself in the midst of a career change. Not the best time for it, but how was he to predict the problems my surgeries would bring? He always used to tell his students to "make sure you like what you do. Life is too short to get up every day not wanting to go to work." Earlier in that summer of '81, he decided to take his own advice, and he quit his life as a teacher. He started classes and pursued a career as a salesman for State Farm Insurance. One of his final tests was on a day when I was still in the hospital recovering from this second surgery.

That afternoon, after Dad had finished his test, Mom was at the hospital chapel talking with a pastor. She had to interrupt the pastor and dismiss herself; she just felt like she needed to get back to see how I was doing. She knew something was wrong. As she walked onto the floor, unusually nervous, one of the nurses grabbed her and said, "Matt is having problems. You can't go down there." She quickly shoved Mom into a little waiting room. Mom cried as she called out to God, praying as she heard people yelling and running around. With each passing minute she knew my chances of survival went down drastically. She sat in that room alone for a long time.

Dr. Dick finally emerged in the doorway, his shirt and tie covered in blood. With a huge sigh and look of pity in his eyes, he said, "Well, he is alive . . . but that is about all. While doing CPR, his chest split wide open. We split his ribs, and I was able to do cardiac massage until his heart finally started beating. He was down for an extremely long time, and if he makes it through the night, he will have some brain damage; the question is just how much. Also, infection is probable, as things were not sterile in there. We did everything we could." Mom responded with a huge "Thank you, God" and then proceeded to tell Dr. Dick that I was going to be fine. He responded, nonverbally, with a look of compassion that said "He is probably not going to make it." He then proceeded to give her the "Now Sue, we have to be

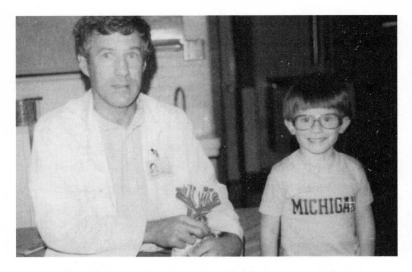

Dr. Dick and me at Mott Children's Hospital

realistic here . . ." trying to bring her down gently. Mom wasn't having it. She wasn't going to let him crush her faith. That was all she had left.

Well, again, my algebra teacher may disagree, but I came out on the other side with no brain damage and no infection. The reason for the cardiac arrest was that the patch had once again torn free. This was uncommon, as the patch was supposed to be put in place once and stay there for life, but this was not the case for me. It was again causing arrhythmias that put me down for the count.

Now the surgeon was ticked. He wanted another shot at it. He knew he could get it this time; his ego wouldn't let him admit that maybe he was missing something. He wanted another attempt at fixing it but would never get it.

About this time Mom was getting advice from her pastor and his wife that my parents just needed to take me from the hospital. "Trust God," they would tell her, "for that healing that was promised in the Bible." She prayed and Dad thought, getting advice from his ever-present parents. Mom approached Dad with the idea of getting out of there and just "trusting God." She didn't know if it was the right thing to do, but it didn't seem that the doctors really had the answers either. Dad responded with "Sue, I'm simply not there yet. You have got this faith, and that's great, but I am not there. I can't do it." She wisely responded with "Well, I do know that as husband and wife, we need to be together in our decision, so let's just pray some more, maybe give the doctors another shot." That was the plan. Wait and see.

Shortly thereafter, Dr. Dick approached them with an idea. He was simply honest: "This surgeon has had two chances at it. If this were my son, I would take him some-where else. This guy is great, one of the best, but maybe there is just something that he is missing." That was all they needed. Dr. Dick set it all up and came back to inform my parents that he would have a plane there soon to take Mom and me to Mayo Clinic up in Rochester, Minnesota. Dad would have to drive up after spending the night with Stacy, who was being shuffled from one family member to the next. Everyone was satisfied with the decision except Stacy and me.

Stacy wanted her parents, and I wanted Dr. Dick. For the first time during this ordeal, my mom tells me I lost it. As they tried to wheel me out, I held on to the curtains crying and yelling, "Dr. Dick is my doctor. I don't want to go!" The nurses had always been amazed with me. It was as if I'd accepted my lot in life and knew, deep down, that the pain, discomfort, and fear were all for a reason. I rarely complained, rarely cried, and was always willing to do "what I had to." I didn't like getting blood drawn and all that kind of stuff, but if Dad told me I had to do it, I did. I remember him simply saying, "Matt, it will hurt, but you have to do it." He would also tell me, "There are some things you just have to do, even when you don't want to," using words a five-year-old could understand. I trusted Dad. If it had to be done, it had to be done. But this time I was not going to listen, not even to Dad. I guess everyone has a breaking point.

We flew to the Mayo Clinic in Minnesota via a medical transport plane and headed into surgery the next day. Again I found myself with the three nurses with needles, and with a long, this time unfamiliar, walk to the operating room. My parents had the usual long wait while I was in surgery, only in Minnesota, the surgery lasted ten hours. Exhausted and frazzled from the trip and the stress, they held on as best they could.

Telling this story, it seems odd that this could have really happened. *Did I go through all this? Did Mom and Dad really do this?* It doesn't seem real. It's like something you hear about on *The Oprah Winfrey Show,* not something that happens to you and your parents. But it did happen, with more to come.

While talking with the doctors after the surgery, after being told that things would be fine over and over again and never seeing that result, my parents weren't sure whether they should believe what the doctors said, but they listened anyway. "Things went well. We think we fixed it." As Mom and Dad walked away and started to make phone calls to relatives, they heard a page overhead to return to surgery. They had been around the hospital long enough to know that this was not good, not in any way. They rushed back to surgery, both fairly sure I was dead or dying. In that moment, Mom lost her promise and the thought of God being with her.

When my parents got back to the surgery department, the doctors explained that during a routine postoperative test, they saw that the patch had torn free yet again. This time it didn't even stay in place for a day. They were taking me back into surgery to try again. Mom and Dad would have to wait some more, after calling the relatives to take back the good news they had given them earlier.

The doctors emerged from the operating room a few hours later with big smiles and sighs of relief. "We figured it out. Matt's heart is very unusual on the inside. There is a bunch of abnormal muscle bundles in there; that is what we, and the other surgeons in Michigan, were trying to tie the patch to. After the heart would beat for a while, the patch would tear loose. We sewed it to a more sturdy structure this time. It is fixed. However, Matt did have a long surgery, so let's see what the next few days hold."

Mom and Dad spent the next few days as they had done two times before, helping me get through the pain and fear, and hoping this was the end of my medical struggles. At one point during those few days of my recovery, Mom and Dad found themselves in the hospital chapel. Although the routine tests in the days following the surgery were all looking good, who knew if we were in the clear? Mom had realized long before that she couldn't get through this on her own. In Minnesota, Dad finally realized that he couldn't do it anymore either. They made a decision to try to find a church that they both liked when they got home, hopefully with their son.

One of Mom's friends organized a prayer team for me at her church. They had a sign-up sheet to fill every hour of the day with someone who was responsible for praying for me. They didn't even know me, but for weeks, every hour of the day, someone was praying for me. Mom and Dad would soon find their way to that church, where they would learn how to depend on God for the rough times to come.

After I got out of the hospital, with everything "okay," Mom and Dad fulfilled their promise to each other and started attending that church (that meant Stacy and I did too), as they tried to learn how to live a life without fear. Mom was now going to church with her family, not with Mary Jane anymore. Mom would still see her friend, however; after all, why would Mom "want to be down, when she could be up?" One day, Mom smoked half a joint with Mary Jane and then just walked away from it. Not because of guilt or because she felt that she needed to in order to be a "good Christian," but because she could. Smoking just wasn't the same anymore; she didn't need it. Her strength now came from something much bigger, much stronger, and something that would never let her down.

She now looks back at her questions to God, wondering if my troubles were because of her sin, with a laugh. How could she have ever really thought that? None of us lives the perfect life. To one, it's marijuana and to another it's exaggerating stories a little too much. We all do things in life that depart from the choices that God would want us to make, but he still loves us. He still wants the best for us. Sure there are consequences to every choice we make, some good and some bad, but it's not about a God bent on hurting us. Nor is it about a God that won't accept us because of our sins. Even though my mom was sinning in the worst way (in her own mind), God still helped her. He kept his promises. She got through those hard times—God didn't leave her and things did turn out okay. She and my dad had learned a lot about themselves and about God over those few months in and out of the hospital. It was a good thing too. They would soon come to find out they would need him again.

The next seven years wouldn't bring the hard times they had known over the past few months but a new set of trials. Home from the hospital, and bent on living a normal life, they were learning how to cope with the daily fears that living with a child with a heart condition can bring. The easy part was over. Like the saying goes, we climb the mountains but stumble over the rocks.

The past few months were hard, but they had no choice but to plow through them. They kept on going as life brought them everything that they never could have imagined. Now, sent home with assurances of health, which they had heard more than once, they had to choose how to live. They could live with an everyday fear or an everyday faith. The choice was that simple.

Chapter Three

Problem Solved

When I look back on all these worries, I remember the story of the old man who said on his deathbed that he had had a lot of trouble in his life, most of which had never happened.

—Winston Churchill

Dad had passed his insurance exam back when I was in the hospital in Ann Arbor; he passed with flying colors. So when we returned from Minnesota, he started his new career selling State Farm insurance. It would be a slow start, but eventually he would look back on that decision to change careers as a great one. With Dad off working the nine to five, Mom back in the beauty shop three days a week, and Stacy part of the family once again, we were ready to live a normal life. I would spend the next seven years living like any other kid.

It was a childhood filled with Little League, middle school girls, and the best Christmases anyone could imagine. Mom loved Christmas and made it perfect for everyone. Christmas was a process that started in early

November when she would begin to redecorate the entire house. Mom has always had a good sense of interior design and would redo the house in good taste and to subtly match the season. Every year it would come, that day in December. Outside it would be snowing, and I would be excited, waiting for Grandma and Grandpa Noble to arrive, bringing my cousin Andy with them. I would sit and wait, peering out the windows at the new snow. Some of my best childhood memories are of enjoying time with my family in a house filled with the smells and sounds of the season, as Mom would brew a pot of potpourri on the stove and turn Christmas music on the radio.

Christmas is what always comes to mind first whenever I talk about my childhood, but as I sit here now I find it hard to encapsulate all the feelings into words. I guess we all have those memories from childhood that we hold on to. Those things that are kept in our minds and over time made better than they actually were.

As I think back on my childhood during these several years, I realize I have far more than just Christmas memories. In fact, I have so many great memories I always find it hard to pick which ones to tell. Which memories tell the story best? Should I tell you about enjoying football with Dad in the fall or of sitting with him every day after work while we watched *M.A.S.H.* on TV? He would always pour himself a big glass of milk and flip through the paper as I watched from his lap. Maybe I should include the countless stories of spending time with Mom and Stacy in our backyard pool, day after day in the summer. We only came inside to make ourselves a pizza

and call Dad at the office. How can I leave out the stories of camping and fishing every summer or the family
vacation to Florida every March?

I really don't have to tell any of them; the fact that I
have so many to choose from reveals the kind of childhood I had. Just like all my friends, I have an array of
pleasant memories to choose from, and not all of them
involve the hospital.

Looking back now I realize how lucky I am, but as a
kid, it never really hit me that my childhood almost
never was. For my parents, however, a lot of those
camping trips and close family moments were a little
extra special, as they were so thankful to still have two
kids. Yet worry was never far off for them. It would
creep up almost daily, and there was always a valid reason for it. A cold, a headache, heartburn, or watching
me bend over trying to catch my breath after running
around—all completely normal experiences for a kid
but heart-wrenching for my parents. Every one of these
activities would have worry and fear trying to take hold
of them. Not for me though. I didn't have much fear at
all when it came to my heart condition. I was just a kid.

My only reminder of the summer of '81 was a scar
that ran the full length of my chest and several "bullet-
hole" wounds where chest tubes once drained blood
from my body. I would also be reminded of my heart
condition about every six months when I would get to
make a trip down to Ann Arbor for a checkup, each time
sent away with a "looks good" and promises of continued hope. It was still fun for me to go down there; they
all loved to see me. I was the miracle kid. Working

among sick and dying kids every day, they always enjoyed seeing those of us who had gone through a lot and came out on the other side alive *and* happy.

These little trips down to Ann Arbor weren't always so great for Mom and Dad. Life was not quite so simple and easy for them. Nor was it as normal. They both had a happiness and a sense of normalcy that went far beyond what it should have, considering what they had been through, but each trip to Ann Arbor would be a reminder of the past and a look into their fears for the future. I was blissfully clueless, while they made an effort not to spend their lives waiting for that other shoe to drop.

At times the stress would be hard on their marriage. On some days my medical struggles brought them closer together, but more often than not my heart just brought more stress. They had made the choice a while back to trust their marriage to God as well. So with each one of them always willing to give more than they got from the other, and a commitment to never quit, their marriage grew stronger over the years.

In spite of their fears, Mom and Dad made a conscious decision not to treat me any differently than necessary. They didn't want their fears to become mine. The doctors had warned my parents about me becoming a "cardiac cripple." The natural tendency is to treat a son or daughter with a heart condition as handicapped, not letting him or her run, swim, or live like a normal kid. Parents become paralyzed with fear, waiting for another cardiac arrest, waiting for their child to drop dead yet again. My parents, especially my dad, were determined not to let that happen with me.

Maybe it was the fact that Dad wasn't actually there for any of my cardiac arrests (Mom was both times) that made it a little easier for him to hold this resolution. Maybe it was just a strength he developed over those first few years out of the hospital, or maybe it was just because that was who he was. My parents' healthy mind-set made all the difference in my childhood; it allowed me to live life just like all my friends.

Just like every kid in America, I wanted to belong, to fit in, and I did. I wasn't the kid with the heart problem who couldn't do anything; I was just another kid playing with friends. I didn't walk around feeling sorry for myself all of the time, because there was no need. I had some tough times, like when I was told I couldn't play football, but I always kept those moments of self-pity between my parents and me. I hated using my heart problem as an excuse. I always wanted to run just as fast and do just as much as everyone else. My condition just made me try that much harder at everything. I think my parents, especially Dad, understood.

My parents weren't endangering my health. They didn't allow me to do anything contrary to medical advice. I was not allowed to play in any school sports, except Little League baseball, but everything else was just fine. Dad stuck to the rule of letting me do just about anything. Mom did too; it was just a little harder for her. She used to sit poolside with me on those summer days with a biblical verse in hand, repeating it over and over in her mind to ease her fears and to reassure her that I was indeed healed. It was the only way that she could let me swim, play football in the yard with my friends, or run around the neighborhood without constantly knowing my whereabouts.

As time went by and I did more and more, letting me go and have fun slowly became easier for my parents. Baseball was hard for Mom at first, as it was the only organized sport I was playing. The doctors debated whether they should let me play. They kept me away from all other school sports because they thought it would be too competitive. Not that I couldn't compete, but that I would try too hard. They let me play baseball because it was the least physical of the sports offered in Montrose.

I remember Little League baseball very well. I loved it. I still love the game. I will never forget one particularly important game. We were playing Joe's team. Joe was my best friend at the time. Actually, he was my "first friend," as in I called him first every Thursday night to see what we were going to do for the weekend. If he was busy, I would move on down the list. He was and still is the kind of friend that is hard to find.

This particular afternoon, Joe came over to my house after school to hang out, before going up to the game with Dad (my coach) and me. Needless to say, Joe and I spent all afternoon talking trash. Frankly, I knew I was outmatched, but we had a lot of fun goofing around while waiting for game time to come. After getting all geared up and posing for some pictures for Mom, Dad finally got home. We made our way up to the ball fields and quickly got into the game. I was as excited as could be.

To be honest, I really don't remember the beginning of the game, but the end of the game I will never forget.

We were in one of the last few innings when Joe was brought in to pitch. He was having trouble finding his rhythm (I know, most fifth and sixth graders don't have a pitching rhythm yet, but this is my story). He walked a few batters, some of our poorer hitters at the bottom of the order, when Dad called all the players on our bench together. "Okay," he told us, "just hang in there. This pitcher has a temper, and when he gets mad, he throws a lot of balls. I can see he is getting frustrated, so make sure it's a good pitch before you swing." He was right. Joe was getting frustrated, and I was on deck, nervous, but making sure not to relay that to Joe.

The next thing I knew it was my turn at the dish. I had to grab hold of my wandering thoughts as I stepped in and took one in tight. It got my heart going a little. Joe could throw fast. In the back of my mind, I was wishing we were in the backyard with a Wiffle ball. I felt much more comfortable there.

I stepped back in and after running the count up a bit, took a fastball right down the middle. I stepped into it with the form and grace of a major league hitter and racked one. I hit a home run. Well, actually, it was a double to the gap with two throwing errors, but in Little League, if you make it all the way around, that's a home run. I was usually in the top of the order, not known for my power, but on this particular sunny afternoon that was not the case. I had hit my one and only home run, and it was off of Joe. As I came across home plate, smelling the freshly cut grass and hearing the cheering of the crowd (seven parents), I was happy. As I looked back at Joe, I'd like to say that he was happy for me too, but he wasn't. He was mad, just as I would have been if

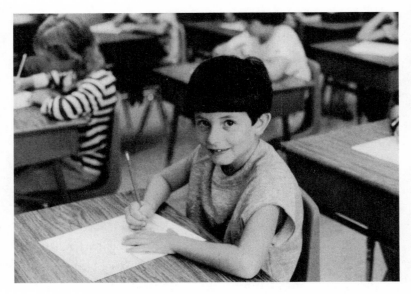

Me at school sometime during the "Red Cross years"

the tables were turned. I'll tell you, life doesn't get much sweeter.

I am sorry to say that I don't remember the score of that game or even whether my home run took us to a victory or a loss. Nowadays, I hate watching Sportscenter only to see some athlete celebrate a personal accomplishment as his team takes a loss.

All in all my life was pretty sweet back then. It was as simple as could be too—fights with Stacy, pond hockey, baseball, backyard football with Joe, and family vacations all filled those first few years out of the hospital. It was all pretty normal. Actually, it was better than normal. I had it made and was living the dream. Yet, it would go on to get even better.

I would get to meet Sparky Anderson, Chet Lemon, Allan Trammell, and a host of other Detroit Tigers from that 1984 World Championship team. A few years earlier, when I was about seven, the Red Cross had approached me to be their "poster child." Apparently I was just what they were looking for. As you can imagine, back in '81, I had more than one pint of Red Cross blood in my body; plus I was cute enough to get the job done. I signed on, a little reluctant at first, until I found out that I would get to be in a TV commercial. I had Joe over, and we played football while they taped us.

So there we were, the family plus Joe, in a commercial. They also stuck me in some parades. I would sit on the back of a convertible, like a beauty queen, and wave to the people. Yeah, I got my fifteen minutes at a pretty young age. The highlight came shortly after that day that I humiliated Joe on the baseball field. (Sorry Joe, but I'm not going to tell about all the times you struck me out. After all, this is my book.) That high point was the making of the actual posters. That was when I got to meet part of the 1984 Tigers team. We made a poster with Sparky Anderson, the team's manager. That was very cool. About fifteen years after I did the poster with Sparky Anderson, my uncle Don saw the Red Cross putting up that very same poster to help advertise a blood drive in the shop where he worked. I guess I was just that cute. Or, maybe their budget was shot. One of the two.

As the next few years went by, playing Little League and starting middle school, I started to become convinced that my life wasn't all that great, or even normal. Although I was lucky to be alive, or at least not drooling all over myself, I was approaching middle school, and just being alive wasn't good enough. I was starting to want to do some things I couldn't do. Most important, I wanted to play football, a must for every boy in Montrose.

I remember sitting on the kitchen counter, going around and around with my mom and dad. I wanted to play football. "Why couldn't I? It wasn't fair. Why did this have to happen to me?" They tried to give me the answers but to no avail. I was finally starting to ask the "why" questions that my parents had asked years before, back when I was just four months old. I guess I would have to start the journey to find those answers, the same journey that my parents had been on for years.

I had by no means found the answers as sixth grade started. While all my friends were off playing football, which in Montrose started in fourth grade, I would sit around and pout, feeling sorry for myself. Dad would try to change this.

A new varsity football coach came to town at the start of my sixth-grade year, a guy by the name of Tony Annese (pronounced uh-NEECE). Being a school board member in a small town, Dad knew everyone at the school, and he arranged for me to work with Mr. Annese. I still remember when Dad told me that Mr. Annese wanted me to help him out with the varsity football team. Basically, I would be the water boy. It was a job coveted by almost all sixth-grade boys in Montrose, a town with an incredible football history. I took on the job, nervous but excited.

Mr. Annese was a young guy who loved the teachings of Vince Lombardi and Lou Holtz, all the great coaches who realized the mental aspect of the game. Life and energy just exploded out of his small frame. I remember him running circles around the players while he played the "scout team" quarterback. "First and ten do it again!" he would yell out after humiliating his defensive players. Mr. Annese was a true student of the game, one who really understood what it takes to win. He was a psychology teacher in the high school as well, and I would eventually be in one of his classes. But I learned as much as I'd ever needed to know about psychology and motivation by watching him with his players on the field, in the weight room, and while goofing off in the gym.

As I think back on it, my dad must have been a little nuts, letting me spend three hours every afternoon with this extreme coach and a bunch of high school guys. During those practices I learned all the profanity I'd ever need to know. I mean all of it. I wouldn't even see my first R-rated movie until *Die Hard* in 1988 or '89. Now I was around a young, hot-tempered football coach and a bunch of high school guys. This wasn't the type of environment my dad, now a pillar of his church, envisioned for his son. Yet he let me go every day. He understood how important football was to me and knew that my being involved in the sport would be for the best. It was one more way to keep me from becoming a cardiac cripple. I know now that it was because he trusted me, himself in what he had taught me, and God.

When it came time to start hanging out with the team again the following year, I was there without question. As my seventh-grade year came around, I was still having fun, and Mom and Dad were getting pretty good at letting me live my life. We all believed that my heart troubles were in the past.

Chapter Four

The Fourth of July

There are only two ways to live your life. One is as if nothing is a miracle. The other is as though everything is a miracle.

—Albert Einstein

It was late June of 1988, and seven years had passed since my last surgery. The anniversary of that first surgery of mine came and went without a word. I didn't think about it one bit. I wonder about Mom and Dad, though; did they still hold a place on the calendar for that day? It sure didn't seem like it to me. We were up north camping at Higgins Lake State Park with about four or five other families, including Joe's, and having a great time.

When we went camping as a family, Stacy and I would have fun together. I was always making up games for us to play. I would usually make the game difficult for a girl who was four years younger than me. Either that or I would simply change the rules midway through. Yeah, I liked to win and usually did. Stacy didn't care though. She was just happy to be playing with her big brother, or should I say, just happy to have something to do. On this trip, however, I had Joe to have fun with, and that left Stacy with nothing to do but tattle on us.

It was a pretty standard camping trip for the family, other than the tattling. We stayed in our pop-up camper, sat by the campfire every night, made hobo dinners, cooked apple pies in the pie irons, and went fishing. I am sure we even made a s'more or two. We had a fun week.

We returned home on the Fourth of July. I am not sure why we didn't stay up there for the fireworks. It could have been the fact that Stacy and I really didn't like fireworks. Ever since we were little, neither one of us liked the loud noises, which were a little scary when we were younger. But now, the noise was just annoying. Most likely, the reason for our early return was to beat the traffic. Dad never liked to end his vacation with a stressful car ride. So this Monday morning we packed up camp and headed home.

I can't say that it was all bad going home on this hot and sticky summer day. At home, we had a pool, which I liked a lot better than some big ole lake. Joe had a pond, so he was used to the constant rubbing of seaweed up against his leg as he tried to relax in the water. Me, I was a city boy (a city of about seventeen hundred) who was used to the clean feel of chlorinated pool water.

Stacy and I hit the pool as soon as possible. Of course we couldn't hit the water until we finished unpacking and cleaning the camper, dragging our feet and muttering under our breaths the entire time.

"I didn't say nothin'." I had learned by now that this was a better response than starting an argument with Dad after he heard our muttering. Stacy hadn't learned this lesson yet. In fact, she wouldn't really get it through her head until well after she started college. Dad never lost an argument with his kids, mostly because he would never let one get started. His favorite response to a whiny "Why?" was simply, "Because I said so." He loved saying that. Stacy hated it. I learned to play the game. Stacy eventually joined me in the pool after serving her sentence.

Later that afternoon, Mary Jane came over with her daughter to hang out with Mom. I am not sure why; she and Mom really weren't that close anymore. Going to separate churches, and with a little less in common now, they just didn't spend a lot of time together. Mom was glad to see her again though. After all, Mary Jane was responsible for getting Mom started with her faith and had been a strong source of encouragement to her back when I was younger. So they spent the afternoon catching up. Mary Jane always cared a lot about me and logged more hours of prayer for me than for most other folks. For that I was and am thankful. Although back then, she kind of bugged me. She felt like an aunt who cares too much and gives sloppy kisses.

As Mary Jane and Mom sat on the deck down by the diving board at the deep end of the pool, Mary Jane's daughter, Stacy, and I were all racing. Yes, I had the idea of racing, a game I was confident I could win. It was a freestyle match, simply going from one end of the pool to the other, thirty-two feet. We were already getting tired after spending hours in the pool, but I sucked it up and gave it everything I had.

I pulled out to an early lead and never looked back, proud to be winning a race with my sister, almost four years my junior, and a girl my age who wasn't the most athletic. As I got to the end of the pool where Mom was, my heart was racing as expected. It was going a little too fast, though, and I just didn't feel right. I looked up and said, "Mom, I feel funny" in a worried tone. She must have seen the look in my eyes because she immediately jumped up to grab onto my arms as I went completely limp. She pulled me out of the water, and as I flopped onto the deck, time slowed and panic set in. Mom screamed, and Mary Jane lost it. Dad was in the house when he heard the commotion and came running out to meet Mom as she knelt over my lifeless, blue body.

Mom had sent Mary Jane off to call the rescue squad, who were headquartered in the fire station just about a mile down the road. When Mary Jane got to the phone, she was in such a panic that she couldn't get it to work. She had dialed the numbers so quickly that not one of them registered, and she was left with a rapid busy signal. She dropped the receiver and ran out into the street in a total panic.

Meanwhile, Mom and Dad were "working" on me. They were doing the CPR that they had learned seven years prior. What part of the CPR technique that time hadn't erased, panic did. They ended up doing very little, besides praying.

As Mary Jane got a few steps out of the door and was heading into the street, she saw a woman. This woman had heard the screaming and was trying to find a way into the backyard, which was protected by a six-foot high wooden privacy fence. The woman spotted her as well and attempted to slow her panic. "Calm down ma'am. What is wrong?" Mary Jane couldn't really talk, so she just took her through the door to the backyard.

As Mom and Dad looked up, they saw this woman coming at them. She was toting a little medical bag, the kind that old-time doctors used to carry. It was almost as if for about half a second they forgot about me as they tried to process: *Who is this woman, and how did she get here?* "Don't worry," she told them, as they snapped back into reality, "I am an emergency medical . . ." something or other. Not surprisingly, Mom and Dad didn't get the details. She proceeded to open up her little bag and get something to clean out my airway. I had vomited as my brain was shutting down and my windpipe was blocked by my lunch from earlier that day. She then rolled me flat and started CPR.

Someone eventually got ahold of the emergency crews; we still don't know who called them, but there were more than enough people around by now. It's amazing how quickly that many people come around during a crisis. I woke up a few minutes later to about thirty people staring at me, with my head in my own puke, just as the ambulance was arriving.

Dad scooped up Stacy, one freaked-out nine-year-old. She was only two when I was going in and out of the hospital. All she ever really knew was a normal big brother. Dad and Stacy, still in slight panic mode, changed, got in the car, and sped off to the hospital, just a few minutes behind the ambulance.

As everyone milled about in disbelief, chattering about what had happened, the emergency medical "something or other" headed back to her car. All we know about her is that she was driving through town that day when her car overheated. We also know that she pulled to the side of the road, just about ten paces from our house. As she sat there, back in the days before cell phones, she probably wondered what she was going to do. She must have stepped out of her car to either look under the hood or approach a friendly looking house to ask to use the phone. Right about then, she heard the screams of terror coming from my mom and Mary Jane. As the woman was trying to find her way back to the pool, Mary Jane appeared and escorted her to the backyard. The woman came back, revived me, and then in the commotion of the ambulance arrival made her way back to her car. She got in and drove off. Apparently her car started up just fine.

A lot of people ask me whether I think she was an angel, just appearing and disappearing like she did. That must be what people think angels do, because whenever I tell anybody the disappearing part, they always let me know "it must have been an angel." I don't know if she was or not. All I can say is that only once in our (mine, Mom's, Dad's, Stacy's, and Mary Jane's) lives, has one of us walked out the front door to find an overheated car, let alone one with an emergency medical something or other in it. It just happened to be at the exact time I was having a cardiac arrest. Coincidence? I doubt it.

I never really thought of her as an angel, though. I always wondered why God would send an angel to Earth to save me, when he has an emergency medical something or other driving around town whom he could utilize. Years later, upon hearing this story, a lady who was working with my mom told us that she took a CPR class with an instructor who recounted a story of reviving a boy by his pool after her car had overheated, saying, "You never know when you might use this stuff." I don't know if that boy was me or not, but I imagine so. Angel or not, I think God's hand was in there somewhere.

Apparently, the ER is a busy place on the Fourth of July. The hospital in Flint was filled with fireworks accidents, drug overdoses, gunshot wounds, and everything else you can imagine. The doctors and nurses were stressed to the max, although totally relaxed compared to Mom. I lay there for hours with Mom and Dad at my side. We don't seem to remember where Stacy was.

We finally got to see a doctor, whose first words to us were, "Does his EKG always look like this?" Not a good question to ask a worried mother and father. They didn't have to answer verbally; after seeing their reaction, he started speaking in his best doctor tone. "Well, everything looks fine now. His blood work is totally normal; everything is great. There are no signs that this had anything to do with his heart. Maybe it was low blood sugar or something. So, I am going to go ahead and discharge you." At that, my dad simply pointed to my mom and replied, "Look at her. You are keeping either Matt or her. I am not taking both of them home with me." He got the point, and, realizing that something slightly more traumatic may have happened, he decided to admit me. The hospital staff simply watched me overnight, as everything looked normal.

I had a strange feeling lying in the hospital bed that night. All I remembered from the evening was telling my mom I didn't feel well and then waking up to a bunch of people staring down at me. Mom and Dad had this look of complete fear in their eyes, mixed with a little bit of joy once I started talking. It was a strange mix, one I would come to know all too well. My chest hurt badly, my ribs too, and I felt totally spent. Every ounce of energy had been drained from my body. I could feel the adrenaline rushing through me, and my mind was piqued. My body, however, was too weak to react to the adrenaline. It's a strange feeling when the body doesn't respond to its own chemistry.

As I lay there in bed that night, with puke caked in my hair, a benefit of being admitted on one of the busiest nights of the year, all kinds of questions went through my head. *Had my heart failed me again?* I didn't remember much of my childhood days in hospitals, but I did realize that I didn't get to be a Red Cross poster child simply because of my good looks. *What would this mean? Would I be in the hospital long? Were Mom and Dad okay?* I didn't remember ever seeing them like this before.

Lying there in the dark, it was my turn to listen to the beeping monitors. It didn't take me long to learn how to hold my breath with each pause, just as Mom and Dad had done seven years before and were doing now as they tried to relax in the room with me. I don't remember for sure, but I think I prayed that night. As I lay there with my questions, Mom had hers too. *Was God letting her down? What was going on?* I was supposed to be healed. Once again, she and Dad found themselves asking "Why?"

The next morning the local hospital quickly shipped us off to Ann Arbor, where we tried to get a few answers. Dr. Dick greeted us as we arrived at the hospital. I still remember lying in my hospital bed as Dr. Dick talked with my parents and me. He sat there, with his legs crossed, not saying anything, just chewing on his reading glasses. You could see the wheels turning, though. Looking back, I am not really sure why I liked Dr. Dick so much when I was younger. Don't get me wrong. He was a very nice guy, but he wasn't the stereotypical pediatrician. He didn't make funny noises or say goofy stuff. That's not to say he wasn't funny. He was more of the absentminded professor variety. He was frequently coming to work with little pieces of toilet paper stuck on his face, from where he cut himself that morning shaving. I would later learn it was because his mind was usually so focused on his patients. By now his hair was almost all gray, as Dad's was. I am quite certain that I caused more than a few of those gray hairs.

As we sat there with him, he began to describe to us what had most likely happened. It was the same thing that had caused me to pass out in the beauty shop and in the hospital when I was five. I'd most likely had a cardiac arrest. Apparently cardiac arrests were not all that uncommon, from a cardiologist's perspective anyway.

Dr. Dick went on to describe what a cardiac arrest was. At its simplest, it is the heart in a bad rhythm, a rhythm in which it is not able to pump blood efficiently. It isn't that the heart is stopping; in fact, usually it is going extremely fast. The heart is going so fast that it is almost quivering instead of actually pumping, or beating. When the heart is quivering, it is not pushing blood to the brain or body. Therefore the body does not have a pulse, which is not, as you can imagine, a good thing.

The reason the heart all of a sudden starts beating in this erratic fashion is quite complicated, but it has to do with scar tissue in the heart. In my case, I was left with scar tissue because my heart was cut open three times in an effort to fix the hole. (My parents were well aware that sudden cardiac arrest was a possible complication to my open-heart surgeries.) Some people have an episode of sudden cardiac arrest after a heart attack leaves scar tissue in the heart. Either way, it's the same problem. Dying from this erratic pumping, or quivering, of the heart is called sudden cardiac death.

Today, doctors know a lot more about sudden cardiac death than they did in the eighties. In the United States, sudden cardiac death kills more people than breast cancer, lung cancer, and AIDS combined. For those people unfortunate enough to have a cardiac arrest, the vast majority die before ever reaching a hospital. Of the remaining few who do reach a hospital, some die there, some survive with brain damage, and a very small percentage walk away normal. By the age of twelve, I had already walked away from three cardiac arrests.

I started to realize that the perplexed look on Dr. Dick's face was caused as much by trying to figure out how to treat me as it was by wondering how I was still alive, and normal. The plan of action would be to start me on some antiarrhythmic medications. (Any electrical disturbance of the heart, as this was, is known as an arrhythmia. Antiarrhythmic drugs try to prevent arrhythmias.) The only problem with these drugs is that you never know whom they will work on. For one patient, one particular drug may work well. Unfortunately that same drug in a different patient could actually cause sudden cardiac death. Therefore, I had to take these medicines while I stayed in the hospital for a few weeks to see how I would respond.

It wasn't long before the doctors found a medicine that seemed to work really well, and after a few weeks in the hospital they sent me on my way. They told us that it may be another seven years before I experience another cardiac arrest, or I may never again have one. We hoped that the medicine would completely fix the problem.

The day after I got out of the hospital, loaded up on my new medicine, I was ready to have some fun. I called Joe and a few other friends and we played football in the field across from my house, underneath the water tower. What was I thinking, you ask? Well, even though the doctors had just told me that, basically, I could fall over dead at any minute, I wasn't too concerned. I was twelve; I wasn't the least bit afraid of dying. I can't quite say the same about Mom and Dad though. I had more than one conversation with my parents about my attitude. It's not that I wanted to die. I just didn't fear it.

I used to tell my parents, "When I die, I'll go to heaven, right?" My parents are the ones who taught me that that's what happens to everyone who dies who knows Jesus. They go to heaven. From what I had heard, this heaven was a great place. So what's the problem? If I'm out playing football and start to feel funny, one of two things will happen. Either I'll wake up in the back of an ambulance, or I'll wake up in heaven. Either way, I would be fine. Mom used to get a little mad and say, "Well, won't you miss me?" To which I would respond, "There is no sadness in heaven, right? So I'll be happy. What's the problem?" I simply believed everything they had ever taught me. I guess that's what you call "the faith of a child."

Mom and Dad weren't quite so at peace with the possibility of me dying, even though they were several years ahead of me at dealing with all of these issues. They, however, decided to remain firm in their decision to let me live a normal life. So with a faith that I still can't wrap my head around, they let me live. Even on the day after I got home from the hospital. They let me live. Mom once again believed this would be the last time I would see any troubles. God was going to take care of me, as he had done time and time again.

Chapter Five

Where's the Limo?

*Read the best books first, or you may not
have a chance to read them at all.*

—Henry David Thoreau

About eight or nine months after I got out of the hospital, I went to seventh-grade baseball tryouts. This was the first time I would be playing an organized sport through school. Up until then it was all Little League.

Tryouts lasted a few weeks, and going into the last few days, I knew exactly where I stood. I knew I would have to do something special to guarantee myself a spot on the team. Back during Little League, I was a pretty good player, but now, as everything got a step faster, I found myself struggling a bit. I still had a little fear of the ball that I couldn't shake, although I never told anyone that. As the final day approached, I knew it was going to be narrowed down to me and this kid named David. He was a friend of mine, although we had been much closer in years prior. David was hanging around the coach and chatting with him all the time while I was trying to prove

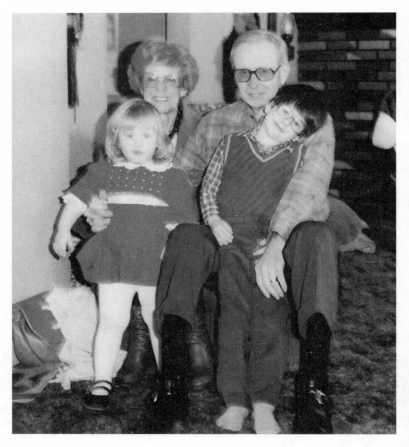

**Stacy and me with Grandma and Grandpa Noble before Grandpa
ever started dialysis**

something. Turns out I should have tried a more social
approach. I got cut.

Devastated doesn't quite do my feelings on that day
justice. Baseball was all I had. Not anymore. I remember
going home that afternoon and sitting on my mom's lap
as we rocked in the rocking chair—too old for this at thir-

teen but that never crossed my mind. I cried and cried. All I remember saying over and over again is "Why?"

I would work harder and really get it done. Lift weights and practice year-round. I would make it next year. The problem is that I knew my parents and my doctor wouldn't let me. My time in school sports was coming to an end, and I knew it. I think that is part of what made my loss so hard. The doctors had already told me this would probably be the last year that they would let me play. Deep down I knew this was my last chance.

That night after being cut, Dad asked me if I wanted to ride down to Jackson, Michigan, with him. Grandpa Noble was in the hospital there, and I wanted to go visit him. My reasons for wanting to see Grandpa were somewhat selfish. I wasn't going so much to cheer him up but to cheer me up. Plus, I don't think there was ever a time that I was in the hospital that my grandparents didn't come and see me.

Grandpa had a condition called autosomal dominant polycystic kidney disease. He was born with it, but it never bothered him until he was in his sixties. In polycystic kidney disease, as you get older, your kidneys start to develop cysts. Eventually, there are more cysts than kidney, and the kidneys don't work at all.

For the past several years, Grandpa had been on dialysis. I never really thought much about him having to go through the hassle of home dialysis; it had just become a part of his life. He never let his grandson see the pain, fatigue, and sickness that he dealt with on a daily basis. All I ever saw was the little thirty-minute procedure three times a day that drained fluids through a tube that came out of his stomach. He was just Grandpa.

We sat in the waiting room for hours that night. It was horrible. I couldn't remember ever being that bored or that scared. Turns out that Grandpa had gotten sicker, quite a bit faster than expected. Tonight he was not doing well at all. I sat there with my dad, now with so much more empathy for him and Mom. I decided it was easier to be the one in the hospital bed, despite the pain.

When you are the patient, you know what you are feeling, and even though in reality you don't have any control, it can feel like you do. I felt helpless just sitting in that waiting room. Time passed slowly, and I didn't know what was going on. *How was he feeling? Were things getting better or worse? Was he in pain?* I thought of all the questions I'd never needed to ask as a patient. All we could do was sit there and wait.

The night was longer for my dad than for me. As we ate some cafeteria food in the waiting room, I had a good time with Dad. I liked the fact that I was the one here for him, in my mind anyway. As it turns out, he, once again, did more for me. He told me that night how sick Grandpa really was and that "there are worse things than death." Grandpa didn't want to suffer, and he was at peace with dying. Death didn't have to be a bad thing for anyone.

I couldn't believe it. *Was he talking about Grandpa dying? That wasn't possible.* We had just come here to visit him, but I never got to go in and see Grandpa that night. Dad said he was too sick. I know now that he didn't want that to be my last memory of him. My cousin

Andy and his mom, my Aunt Barb, came and picked me up, and I slept at their house for the night.

Andy and I spent the night talking, like thirteen- and fourteen-year-olds do, about everything. Tonight though, we mostly talked about Grandpa, every possible good memory we could recall. We talked ourselves to sleep.

Aunt Barb woke us up that next morning, Saturday, April 15, 1989, and told us that Grandpa had died in the middle of the night. I don't remember my immediate reaction or what the next few hours held. I do remember that baseball didn't seem so important anymore. I never felt bad about not making that team again, never shed another tear over it, never even got jealous when Joe and the others talked about the season in class that year. I still missed the game, but I got some perspective that day.

After Grandpa's funeral, I returned to a pretty standard seventh-grade life. I was a little different from most seventh graders in that I knew I could die at any time, whereas most of my classmates never gave their mortality a second thought. Yet those thoughts didn't consume my mind. It was mostly the girls in our class who held my attention.

Back in seventh and eighth grade, I hung out with the "in" crowd. In Montrose, that meant the jocks. I wasn't really a jock anymore but wasn't really close to any of the band kids, so I stayed friends with Joe and all the others through middle school.

In the eighth grade, I got invited to a make-out party, confirming my "popularity." Our parents still called them boy-girl parties, but we were much more mature than that, in our own minds anyway. Although I hung out with the popular girls, and was very social, I never really had much luck with the girls back then. I was too scared and didn't have any "moves." I could feel comfortable in any social situation, not considered shy by any means, but when it came to girls—yikes. I was just flat-out nervous. It wasn't the day-to-day conversations that made me edgy but the "fun stuff." I don't know why I was so nervous— maybe just a fear of rejection. I do know that I had all the normal concerns of a seventh grader, wondering whether I was a good kisser, but I also think I was a little afraid of what else could happen. I mean, how embarrassing would it be to drop over dead while making out with some girl?

I guess those fears kept me out of some trouble but did lead to some serious frustrations. I never quit trying though. I would flirt like a madman. I got pretty good at it too. But without the moves to close the deal, I usually got relegated to the friends' zone. I, however, was always in denial about the friends' zone. I used to think that if I got to be really good friends with them, at some point they would take a deeper interest in me. I'd heard that women like that kind of stuff. I learned that during those after school talk shows and in movies. They all used to say that a great relationship starts with a great friendship, so I thought I was right on track. As it turned out, intimacy works a lot better for career women than it does for eighth-grade girls.

On the last day of eighth grade, Joe and I had a great plan. We had been talking with a few of the popular girls, and it turned out they were renting a limousine for the last day of school. A chauffeur would pick them up, and they would drive around, celebrating the end of middle school. Joe and I had asked them what they planned to do after the first ten minutes of driving around. Apparently they hadn't thought that far in advance. We convinced them to stop by my house where Joe and I would be hanging out. We would cruise around with them and show them a good time.

They agreed! Holy crap! They were going to come and pick us up! Joe and I were pumped. These were the best looking and most popular girls in school, hands down. Everyone knew it. Joe had a thing for the red-head, Kristi, and so he was pretty excited. I had my eye on one of them too—one that was way, way, way out of my league.

After surviving three cardiac arrests, I had heard things like "You are so special" and "God must be keeping you around for a reason" all the time. After hearing such sentiments on almost a daily basis, you start to believe it. I guess that's why I never had much of a problem with low self-esteem. If anything, I had a high self-esteem issue, especially as a cocky eighth grader.

So the girls were coming over, and the plan was to hang out with them for a while in the limo to make some inroads for the make-out party that night. It sounded like as good a plan as any. Actually, Joe and I were convinced it was going to be a great afternoon and night.

We headed back to my house after school and waited. We waited some more, and then after that . . . we waited. Hope started to dwindle as time passed. We tried to occupy the time with Nintendo, but that didn't work too well. We would keep going back out to the road. "They know where you live, right?"

"Yes, everyone knows where I live." Then we'd breathe a collective sigh of disappointment.

With the patience of fourteen-year-olds, we didn't wait much longer. The plan was too good to be true anyway. So we decided to go swimming. We quickly changed and headed out to the pool, trying to come up with a new plan for the party that night. We quickly forgot about things, though, as we were having fun in the pool. We had set up an inner tube in the middle of the water and were jumping off of the diving board trying to slam-dunk a ball. Yeah, we had forgotten about them already. At least we were acting like we had.

I made another spectacular dunk and was just climbing out of the water as Joe set up his approach on the diving board. I stood up and held on to the railing, as things didn't seem right. I bent over with my hands on my knees and looked over to Joe. "Just a minute," I said as I held up my left arm and index finger. I immediately dropped, hitting my head on the edge of the pool as I tumbled in, sinking to the bottom.

Joe dove in and pulled me into his arms. As he got his head above water, he screamed for help, the kind of scream that the neighbors had heard before. Mom looked out into the backyard to see Joe, as if in a movie scene, holding my limp body in his arms. He lifted me out of the water and laid me on the deck.

This time there was no overheated car, no emergency medical something or other. We only had the medicine that I had started taking a few years earlier that was in my system, which obviously wasn't working. Mom wasn't doing a nurse's hair either. This time she had a gym teacher in her chair. It was good timing though, as this gym teacher had just finished her required CPR class a few weeks earlier. She knew exactly what to do. As Mom and Nancy, the gym teacher, tore through the doors to the backyard, once again someone under the dryer called for help.

We never can seem to figure out how long I am out for. The consensus this time was somewhere between five minutes and nine hours. I don't know how long I was unconscious, but I do know that I woke up to hear the ambulance. Hearing sirens, knowing they are coming for you, is quite a feeling. An ever-changing mixture of embarrassment, fear, pain, and anxiety overcame me as my eyes were fixed on the clouds floating by. Again I felt the adrenaline rush, without the physical response, as my ribs, chest, and head ached and as I lay there trying to piece together what had happened. *How long was I out for? Where is Joe?* Apparently he had gotten pushed aside to watch his best friend, turning blue and bleeding from the head, get CPR from afar.

I was miserable again, this time worse than ever. When I fell into the pool, I got a pretty good cut on the back of my head, and so this time I was lying in a pool of blood instead of puke. The rescue squad quickly took over upon arriving. They put me on a backboard, because of possible neck injury, and during the entire ambulance ride, my head was bouncing up and down on this wooden board, right on the cut. That didn't seem healthy to me, but I was not in control here. So my head hurt, but my chest hurt too. "Who did CPR on me this time?" I asked my mom. She responded as the guy in the back of the ambulance chuckled a "this time?" I would have laughed too, but my head was hurting more and more with each bump in the road.

Dad once again found someone to take Stacy and joined us at the hospital. They stitched my head up after getting X rays to make sure I didn't have a broken neck. Once again, they got me out of there as fast as possible. There was talk of taking a helicopter down to Ann Arbor. I was excited about that, but Dad put the kibosh on it. The hospital needed to save it for someone who actually needed it, not for someone the ER doc was freaked out over. We ran into that a lot—most ER doctors wanted me out of there as soon as possible. After hearing my history, they knew there was nothing that they could do for me in the emergency room. This time was no different.

So even though I wanted to take the helicopter down to Ann Arbor, I knew Dad was right. He had learned by now that after I was revived from a cardiac arrest, I would be fine for another few years, at least that was the pattern we'd fallen into. Still he was nervous and scared, as any father would be, wondering if this time would be different—in a bad way.

For that hour-long ride, I got to talk to the guy in the back of the ambulance with me. He listened to all my stories in disbelief—more from my nonchalant attitude after what had just happened than from the actual events, as amazing as they were. I was fairly relaxed about the whole situation. Mom and I pretty much had it down by now and Dad fell into his routine and went to take care of Stacy. The bad part was over, and we just had to spend about two or three weeks in the hospital as they tried to find a new medicine for me. I was really more upset about the fact that I was going to miss the party later that night than I was about the fact that I'd almost died.

Joe went to the party that night, still pretty shook up about what had happened earlier in the day. I can only imagine. As I had learned with Grandpa, I had it easier that day than Joe did. I talked to him a few days later on the phone and learned that things worked out as planned for Joe that night. He got to play the sorrowful hero as he recounted the story to everyone at the party. I was happy for him. I told him, "At least some good could come of this mess," as we both laughed.

And the girls in the limo? Apparently after driving around for a while, they got bored, just as we had predicted. They remembered our invite and decided to head over to my house. They missed the ambulance by about five minutes. I just couldn't catch a break.

Chapter Six

Popcorn on the Floor

Believe it is possible to solve your problem.
Tremendous things happen to the believer. So
believe the answer will come. It will.

—Norman Vincent Peale

I spent the next few weeks in the hospital trying new drugs, just as Mom and I had thought. It wasn't that the drug I had been taking all of a sudden stopped working; it was working more than 99 percent of the time, which is common for this type of drug. Ninety-nine percent was pretty good, but when you are trying to prevent sudden cardiac death, it's not good enough. For those few weeks in the hospital, we would continue to try to find a medication that worked 100 percent of the time.

Joe and three other friends came to visit me. It was a relief having my friends around, as I was getting frustrated about missing out on my "normal" life, and it was cool to just forget about that for a few hours. I got to hang out with my friends in the courtyard of the hospital and pretend not to be the least bit scared.

The truth was that things were starting to get harder for me. No longer was I this carefree kid who lived only for the moment. I was starting to think about the future, what I wanted to do, and who I wanted to be. All of a sudden, I started to see that this condition might never go away. I had never really thought of the permanence of it all before. I had always seen the hole in my heart as a temporary problem, as Mom did. I guess I wasn't that little kid who could easily take things a day at a time anymore.

One night I convinced Mom and Dad to leave the hospital for the night, assuring them I was old enough to stay alone. They didn't really want to leave, and I really didn't want them to go, but I was growing up and needed to learn how to handle some of this on my own. After all, they would be back before I woke up in the morning. On this particular night, I was exceptionally frustrated. Convinced that the reason I couldn't find a girlfriend was because of this heart thing and wondering whether my life would ever be normal, I prayed to God.

I don't remember exactly what I said to God, or for how long I prayed, but I do remember the overwhelming sense of frustration and helplessness. Tears ran down my face as I continued my lament to God. My eyes were fixed on the empty corner of the room, where the wall meets the ceiling, asking God if these medical struggles would ever end. *Would I be okay?* All of a sudden a happiness came over me from within. The next thing I knew I was chuckling instead of crying. I was trying to hold back the grin, given that I was still pissed at

God. He still hadn't given me an explanation for all of this, and I wanted him to know I was mad.

When I was a kid I prayed every night. I couldn't go to sleep without saying my prayers. I would pray and ask God for everything, but that's the first time I felt he'd answered me. I didn't really think about why I had gotten an answer this time, but looking back I've wondered. I don't think it is because I prayed any harder, or because my feelings were more intense, or because of what I was asking for. I think it was simply because that's exactly what I needed—not only to get me through that night but many others to come.

It was a great feeling. I went from knowing that things would be okay to being convinced God would heal my heart. I don't know how I made that leap, or why, but in my mind, God had told me that night that he would heal me. I didn't know when, but I would be healed. Until now, I have never told anyone that story. After all, was that really God speaking to me? Is that how God worked? I didn't know for sure and, even though it felt right, I didn't tell anyone. I really didn't need to. For once in my life, I didn't need to talk about something or process it to understand it. It was between God and me with a clarity and confidence I'd never known.

I would come to depend on the memory of that joyous feeling many times over the next few years, even the next few weeks. Each day that passed, I became more confident that it was really God telling me something that night. For years I had heard my mom and dad saying things like "God told me" or "God gave me a Scripture," and I never really got it. I mean, I had never heard God

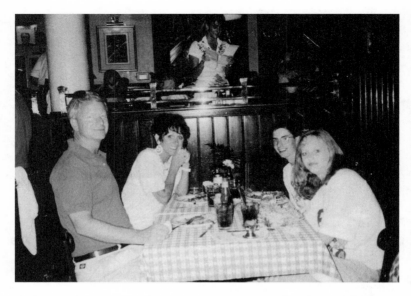

Dad, Mom, Stacy, and me on vacation in Florida just before I started high school

talk and frankly had no reason to believe that he even existed, except for the fact that my parents had told me that's how it was. But that night I came to realize that God talking to Mom or giving Dad a Scripture wasn't nearly as weird as it sounded. God is much simpler than that. God wasn't in the earthquake, or the thunder, or a loud booming voice. God didn't even really talk, at least not to me. God was in the silence. It was as simple as feeling a happiness and relaxation from within, when every-thing, including my own mind, told me that shouldn't be.

I was released from the hospital after a few weeks and ran straight for high school. That August, when foot-ball started up, my friends were at practice with me for the first time. I had been the little kid on the field with the high schoolers; now, I was another one of the high school kids. As much as I like having my friends around me, the situation posed a small problem. It's cool for a middle school kid to be water boy while hanging with the big boys, but not so cool for a ninth grader. I was in serious jeopardy of being taken as the geek who picked up the sweaty socks of his peers, but I had a plan.

For as long as I can remember, I had wanted to be a doctor (gee, I wonder why), so I started studying sports medicine. In the summer when all the other kids went to football and basketball camp, I went to a camp to learn how to be an athletic trainer. As a student trainer, I would tape ankles, tend to injuries, and be the one to go to for medical help. Montrose, being a small school, couldn't afford a real athletic trainer, so I was the man.

The work elevated me above water boy, and I would still get to hang out with my friends. I remember being at these camps wondering why these kids weren't playing football. Even if they were little, or didn't have much talent, that didn't have to stop them. They could adopt a Rudy mentality. Rudy was a guy who went to school at Notre Dame and made the football team through a walk-on tryout. This was extremely rare, as most of the spots on the roster were reserved for scholarship players. Rudy had little talent but a lot of heart. So what if you are small or don't have all the talent in the world. Go play, man! I couldn't understand why anyone who could play wouldn't want to.

Upgraded from water boy to trainer, I headed into high school. It was still pretty dorky, but I managed to pull it off. In fact, going into high school I never got picked on as a freshman; I had the entire football team looking out for me. In Montrose, that was everything. In a school of about 500 students in grades nine through twelve, the 40 or so football players ran the place.

By now, Mr. Annese was in his fourth year at Montrose and hadn't lost a regular-season game since his first year as coach. The students loved him, partly because he taught us what it means to win but mostly because of who he was. Everyone respected him. Players wanted to please him, on and off the field. Mr. Annese was convinced that his players shouldn't be drinking, in or out of football season. His players looked up to him so much that they started to believe that too. Montrose may have been the only high school where it wasn't cool to drink, but because of Coach Annese and the football players, that is exactly what happened. Mr. Annese transformed that school; he made it a place unlike any other.

That's not to say that I had a perfect run at high school. Around my sophomore year I hit a few bumps. I was a pretty easy target. I was a five-foot-eight-inch, 115-pound trainer (skinny more because of genetics than my heart problem), hanging out in the locker room trying to be cool. Trying to be like everyone else. Two kids in particular made fun of me. The hardest part for me wasn't that they would give me a hard time; it was that one of them and I had been close friends just a few years earlier.

In true teenage style, when one would point the finger, everyone else would laugh. That was tough for me. I remember going home on several nights after basketball games feeling totally rejected. Alone.

One morning I woke up to see that our mailbox had been smashed and our new house egged, in a fairly malicious manner. I knew it was because of me. My parents' new house had been damaged. I quickly learned that a good friend was involved. I don't know to what extent, but someone had told me he was there, although I am sure he probably just stood by and watched. I never brought it up with him. I knew he only wanted the same thing all of us at that age wanted—acceptance. I never held it against him in the least. I guess I knew, had the tables been turned, I probably wouldn't have passed up a chance to hang out with that crowd either.

I seemed to be able to keep a perspective uncommon for a fifteen-year-old. I saw the kid leading the charge against me for what he was. He was simply insecure. Realizing his athleticism wasn't going to take him much farther than the junior varsity basketball team, he turned to humor to get acceptance. In high school, actually in life, the easiest humor is always at someone else's expense. He took that path. I was hurt, but I was secure enough to accept the pain for what it was and to brush it off in due time. I was so secure in who I was that not even one of the coolest kids making fun of me could truly bring me down. After all, somewhere down deep I believed that God was keeping me alive—and for a reason.

It wouldn't be long before that part of my life was behind me. I guess my time to get picked on had passed. I'd like to think it was because of the way I handled it. I would always just laugh it off and move on, never holding a grudge. I understood.

As my sophomore year moved on and life was good again, I started hanging out with "the boys" more and more. There was Joe, Zac, Chris, Jason, Dan, and me. "The boys," as we called ourselves, would eventually become the starting five on the basketball team, plus the trainer. We had a lot of fun together.

Whenever we were looking to get into trouble, or just be free from parental supervision, we would go to Jason's mom's house. She lived in a not-so-great part of Flint, about twenty minutes away. We did all kinds of stuff when we were bored, but basically, it was just fun having a town, a car, and no curfew. We usually found trouble, but I was always careful to stay on the edge of it. I was the more conservative one of the group.

When I was in high school, Dad, the insurance agent, used to make me read newspaper clippings about local kids. "One bad choice can change your entire life," he used to tell me, as I read these snippets. They were about kids getting killed while drinking and driving or getting jail time because they were in the car when their friend robbed a store. "One bad choice can change your entire life." I never forgot that line from Dad. It kept me out of a lot of trouble.

Whenever we wanted to just relax and have some good old-fashioned fun, we went to my house. Mom would always entertain the group by chatting with us. Everyone loved Mom. She would recount her stories of smoking pot and how she quit but tell us not to do it or we'd end up as ditzy as her. Dad would talk to each of my friends about whichever sport was in season. It always just seemed like the all-American family at the

Nobles. Mom and Dad got along great, and I think my friends enjoyed the environment at our house—a safe yet fun place to be.

My junior and senior years at Montrose would be two of the best years of my educational career. During my junior year I spent a lot of time hanging out with the boys, and it seemed like before I knew it football was over and we were well into the basketball season.

Atherton was our rival. Every year we would pound them in football and so their only chance to get even was on the basketball court. With our entire school focusing on football, our basketball team wasn't the greatest. On this particular snowy February night, we were in for a battle.

I was sitting in my usual spot down near the end of the bench, but I don't remember actually sitting for much of the game. It was a close, intense, and very physical game. Because of the bad blood, there were a lot of fouls. I don't remember who won, or even how close it really was, but I do remember it coming down to the wire. As the buzzer sounded to end the game, there was still a lot of pushing and shoving on the court as frustrations ran high. It escalated pretty quickly into an all-out bench-clearing fight. I got right in the middle of it as my adrenaline got the best of me.

I don't know if anyone actually landed a punch, as the referees and coaches broke it up and got us all into the locker rooms pretty quickly. We were all seriously geared up though. I started to realize how "up" I was and tried to calm myself down a little. By now, at seventeen years old, I was starting to think things through a little more than I did when I was a kid. I knew that almost every cardiac arrest that I had had in the past was associated with activity, and I was starting to correlate a fast heart rate with problems. As I paced back and forth for a few seconds, I didn't need to reach for my neck or wrist to get my pulse; I could feel my heart pounding inside me. It was going fast. I sat down on the edge of the "doctor's table" in the training room that was connected to the locker room. As I sat there trying to relax, I thought, *Oh God, just slow this thing down. I don't want anything to happen here.* I was hoping to avoid trouble more for the fear of embarrassment than for the fear of death.

I felt my heart start skipping some beats, and I knew what was coming. Yet I just kept saying, "Come on, God" as I tried to slow my breathing. I had only been sitting on the edge of the table for a few seconds, but it had felt like a while. I was suddenly aware of every little movement I made as I felt a fear rise up inside of me. I knew what was coming. All of a sudden I felt my heart take off into that abnormal rhythm. Cardiac arrest here I come. The second I felt the irregular heart rhythm, I looked out through the large window separating the training room from the locker room to see someone walking by. I said, "Hey, come here. I don't feel good," as I lost consciousness.

I fell forward with my head hitting his chest. He dropped his popcorn all over the floor as he grabbed me, laid me back onto the table, and yelled for help. It didn't take long for me to start turning a tint of blue, as my heart wasn't pumping out any blood.

Mom was at home when she got a frantic call, one that she secretly waited for every time I went out. She called Dad, who was at a church leader's meeting, and then quickly got in the car for the five-minute trip up to the school. She prayed the entire time.

By now Mom wasn't the "Jesus freak" that she once was. Her faith hadn't diminished one bit, nor did her relationship with God, but the way she carried herself had. She had started to realize that maybe God wasn't going to miraculously heal me like she had always assumed he would. She used to go around telling everyone that I would be healed, later saying that she was trying to convince herself of it just as much as the people she told. By this time, she was starting to learn that God works the way he wants to work, not the way she wants him to. Both my parents in fact were learning more and more about who the real God was as the years passed.

Mom would think back on that time when a preacher called her out of the crowd. She remembers how she just knew everything would be okay. Looking back, she would almost laugh at herself now that she understood more clearly that everything being okay meant something so much different from what she imagined. Back then, the only way things could be okay was if I were healed. Now she was starting to see that maybe God had another plan—a plan she didn't know about and couldn't figure out but one that would turn out better than hers in the end. I guess that's the only way she could let me start driving when I turned sixteen and going out on my own. Amazingly, she did it without asking one more question than any other concerned mother would have.

It must have been a tough time for her and Dad, always waiting for that call as I started to go out on my own. I would have never known it though. Even though they knew that call might come one day, they also knew that God really did have a plan for me. And they understood that that plan was for the best.

So when that call finally did come, from one of my classmates pleading, "Sue, get up to the school now. Something happened to Matt, and they are working on him now," she was able to pray with a silent strength during that car ride. Her car ride wasn't quite as panicked as one might think.

Mr. Kinter, the high school principal, ran down to meet Mom at the doors to tell her, "They just got him breathing." She relaxed a bit, yet she still didn't know anything. Wondering who "they" were and how long I had been out, she started to worry again. As she was escorted into the training room, now packed with people, she saw the paramedics putting me onto the stretcher. I saw her and sighed, "I'm fine, Mom," knowing she was probably a wreck. She looked around the room to notice two women she knew standing on either side of the table next to me. They were the mother and sister of one of the basketball players, both ER nurses. Apparently they were waiting just outside the door of the locker room when they heard my classmates yell for help. I didn't know who they were. The only thing I knew was that after passing out, I woke up to these two women standing next to me. My heart still didn't feel right; it was pounding way too hard. I was only awake for a few seconds when I felt my heart take off again. I knew I was on my way out again when in a panicked whimper I told the only two people around who looked confident to "make it stop. It's doing it again." Without the support they were used to in the ER, all they could do was wait for me to pass out again and then start CPR. I passed out to their encouraging words. I came to about a minute or two later, and my heart started to slow just before Mom came in the door.

The paramedics got me on the stretcher and wheeled me out through the gym. It looked as if no one had left. Apparently word spread fast that something was going on. On the way out I had an oxygen mask on so I couldn't say anything, even though I am sure everyone in the entire gym would have heard me. It was so quiet I could hear the wheels of the gurney squeak as they wheeled me out. I figured the least I could do is let all my friends know I wasn't dead, so I gave them a little thumbs-up. Everyone started clapping, and I felt like an idiot.

Dad got there just as we were getting into the ambulance. It was the same ole thing. We were in for a long night, as they would take me to the local hospital and then on to Ann Arbor as usual.

Chapter Seven

A Deck of Cards

Be careful about reading health books. You may die of a misprint.

—Mark Twain

We talked to Dr. Dick the next day, after a long night of waiting to see this man with the answers, and once again he had a look that showed how perplexed and amazed he was to see us. This time he had big ideas. He told us about a new device that we needed to consider. He went on to explain the automatic implantable cardioverter defibrillator, or AICD.

Apparently this new device, which they had started implanting in adults a few years earlier and still hadn't implanted in anyone nearly as young as me, was very similar to the external defibrillators that you see on television shows like *ER*. The external defibrillator is the big machine with paddles that are put onto a patient's chest to shock the heart back into a normal rhythm. The AICD worked in the same way, except it was implanted inside the body so it was available 24/7, and it acted automatically, within seconds.

"When going into cardiac arrest, the heart is in an abnormal and fast rhythm. During this rhythm it cannot pump blood out to the body; thus we end up with sudden cardiac arrest," Dr. Dick explained. He went on to tell us that the "defibrillator would work by shocking the heart back into a normal rhythm. Shocking the heart like this is usually the only way to get it back into a normal rhythm." (I know now that he only used the word "usually" because of what I had been through.) We also learned that the reason that almost everyone who has a cardiac arrest doesn't ever even reach the hospital alive is because they don't have a defibrillator nearby. By the time an ambulance arrives with one, it is usually too late. That is why nowadays, with improved technology, we see automatic *external* defibrillators (AED's) popping up all over the place, in places like airports, casinos, and hotels. They are now even available for home use.

Today, more and more people are getting AICDs, as doctors are realizing how many lives they can save and as new clinical trials repeatedly show the device's effectiveness. Even Vice President Dick Cheney has an AICD. In February of 1993, however, automatic implantable defibrillators were not that common. Back then, to get an AICD (also called an ICD) you had to have a documented episode of this abnormal rhythm or have survived an episode of sudden cardiac arrest. Because I had had both, I was in.

Because the ICD was fairly new technology back in 1993, it was used mostly in older people who had been left with this rhythm problem after a heart attack. Dr.

Dick told us that day that it was so uncommon that I would be the first person in Michigan to get one who was under the age of fifty. He stopped and said, "Well, one other girl got one a few months ago but she . . ."

He paused so I filled in the gap. "Died?" He nodded.

Mom replied with a fearful "What!" as I chuckled and thought *whatever.*

"Oh, but she had a lot of other problems," he quickly explained to ease Mom's fears.

So the plan was to get an ICD, even though we didn't know what that really meant. All we knew was that after getting this device, should I have another episode of sudden cardiac arrest, no one would need to do CPR, and I wouldn't turn blue and start the march toward death. In fact, I might not even pass out; if I did, it would only be for a few seconds. After having this device implanted, I would go from having about a 98 percent chance of dying before I reached a hospital to having a better than 99 percent chance of surviving the event. With those kinds of numbers, we didn't really need to think about it.

Dr. Dick's nurse introduced me to this new device, telling me it was the size of a deck of cards. It would be implanted just under the skin on the left side of my abdomen. At the time, the implant technique was to put patches on the heart that would work just like the paddles you see Dr. Carter from *ER* rub together, just before he gives patients a jolt that bounces them off the table. And yes—it would give the same kind of jolt internally should it ever have to work.

She also told me about a new investigational implant technique that would allow them to put the device in place without splitting my chest wide open. This technique, which was still being studied in 1993, would soon become the way almost all ICDs would be implanted. They'd make just two incisions, one just below my left collarbone and the other over where the device would be inserted on the left side of my abdomen. The incision below the left collarbone would provide them access to a large vein that runs directly to the heart. They could then thread a wire that would remain inside my heart and attach to the ICD. This wire would deliver the shock to my heart should it ever need it. It sounded good to me, not having to have my chest split open, so my parents and I signed the papers and we were set for surgery the next day.

I don't remember getting ready for surgery, but I do remember how I felt afterward. How could two little incisions (one was two inches and the other was five) make a person so miserable? As a side effect from the anesthesia, I had a mega-hangover and was throwing up, which didn't exactly add to my comfort. When they told me that the investigational part didn't work (apparently the wire wouldn't stay in place) and that they would have to take me to surgery again the next day, this time splitting my chest open, I didn't care one bit. Although my parents were seriously concerned, as any surgery this serious posed a large risk, I was too concerned with how miserable I felt at the time to be thinking about any pain or risk that was to come.

I did manage to make it through the day and night and woke up feeling much better. I was no longer hung over from the drugs, and the pain really wasn't too bad, especially with the help of Mr. Morphine. However, I only got to enjoy myself (relatively speaking, of course) for a few minutes that morning before I was wheeled off to surgery again. Because the wire they had threaded into my heart would not stay in position during the first surgery, I would indeed need the patches sewed directly to my heart to deliver a shock. In order to put these patches in place, they would have to make a lengthy incision that extended about eight inches, going from under my armpit to the center of my chest, about two inches below my left nipple. The cut was right between two ribs so that they could split the ribs apart, exposing my heart. This would allow them to attach the large patches directly to the surface of my heart.

Now that hurt. The next day I was still pretty drugged up so the pain was bearable, although I was again feeling extremely nauseated. Time went by slowly. But the worst day is always two days after surgery. You don't remember the day of surgery much at all, and the next day you are still fairly beat down and content to just lie there and sleep a lot. This surgery was no exception. By day three, the doctors lowered the amount of pain medication I was on, and I ached all over. I wanted to get up and move around, even just wiggle in my bed, but with every little movement my entire side would hurt like I'd never remembered hurting.

Slowly but surely, though, I got around, starting with just a trip to the bathroom and then a walk down the hall. Before I could even do a lap around the floor, they were discharging me. Things were looking great. I had my new ICD implanted just under the skin in my left abdomen and was ready to start feeling better.

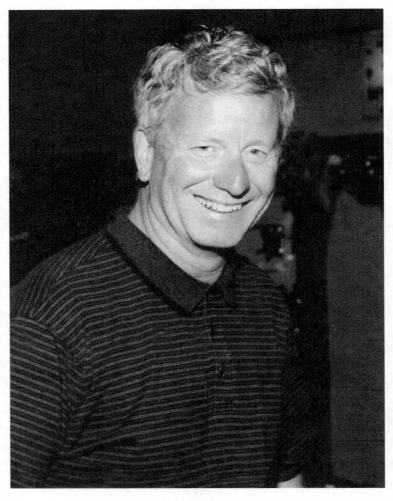

This is how you'll find my dad on most days . . . golf shirt and all

I don't remember the first time I got a look at what my belly looked like. In those first few days, I really could have cared less. When I finally did get to take a look at the incisions, I just laughed and thought, *What kind of huge freakin' cards do these people play with?* The device was about the size of a pint of whiskey, without the neck, and was implanted just below the skin. Because I was now about five feet eleven inches and still 115 pounds, it wasn't hidden at all. It bulged out from underneath my skin. I didn't spend much time worrying about how it looked. I don't know why. Looking back I probably should have as a seventeen-year-old, but I didn't. By that point, I was used to doing what I had to do. So I chose to have fun with it.

I remember one really beautiful day in school toward the end of that year. All the guys were walking around the hallways with their shirts unbuttoned and trying to show off their muscles. I remember Jay, who was a solid six feet eight inches, trying to look buff as he strolled down the hall. I walked right behind him with my shirt undone, imitating his "muscle walk" as everyone walked by. That got a lot of laughs. I would always try to have fun and make the best of it. I guess if you were a therapist, you could say that I used humor as a defense mechanism; after all, if I made fun of myself first, then it wasn't funny if other people did it.

When I first came home from the hospital with my new ICD, though, I wasn't making too many jokes. I was trying to keep up with school, but it was hard to sit and concentrate in that kind of pain. Getting my strength back was a slow process. At first I could only sit at the table and do homework for five or ten minutes at a time before I would have to lie back down and even take a nap.

After several weeks, I could sit at the table for quite a while and do homework. I was not yet good at standing up straight or walking around. I would just shuffle from one room to the other, with my body hunched forward and to the left. When I stood up straight, I stretched the skin that had been cut into. One night, Dad decided I needed to get some exercise. Walking around the house just wasn't cutting it. How would I get better and back to school if I never pushed myself?

We went up to the school that night, with me complaining the entire way, mostly in a nonverbal way. I knew I had to push myself too, just as Dad was telling me, but it was hard. We got up to the school, and I thought we were just going to walk around the halls a few times. Nope. We went for the track. It must have taken us eight hours to walk one lap; at least it felt like it. I was sore and tired, but I wanted to get back to school and Dad was right. This was the only way to do it. So I pushed myself. I walked, and Dad kept saying, "Stand up straight."

Once we had a lap under our belts, the exercise started to feel good. It was a nice night too, especially for March, with a gentle breeze. It was warm enough for just a sweatshirt. I breathed in the air as we walked around. It felt so good to be outside for a while just enjoying Dad and the weather, until Dad said "stand up straight" again, as he did about every thirty or forty steps. As I walked around and enjoyed the spring air, I was glad, for just a minute anyway, that he'd made me come outside.

After being out there for a while, I started to pick up the pace a little and felt my heart rate start to rise. That scared me. I didn't let Dad see that, though. I just slowed my pace back down and complained that my chest was sore from standing up too straight.

I remembered that feeling of a racing heart in my chest that I'd experienced so many times by now; the memories from the night of the basketball game and during the other cardiac arrests stayed with me vividly. I had grown to hate that feeling of a racing heart. I wondered how I was ever going to get back to school and forget about my heart. I might get carried away again and forget to keep my heart rate down. Although I had the ICD, the doctors told me that they programmed the device so it would shock me when my heart reached 200 beats per minute. "What if my normal heart rate gets above 200?" I remember asking. They told me I would get shocked for that too. The device couldn't tell the good 200 from the bad 200, so when it detected 200 bpm it just shocked. Better safe than sorry I guess.

I thought about that information as we walked, and I felt my heart rate increasing normally with the exercise. I wondered what my heart rate was at. *Was this getting close to 200? What did it really feel like when the ICD went off anyway? Did the shock hurt? I'd better slow down.* I didn't want to find out.

That day I started a whole new fight, a fight that would turn out to be much harder than any one I had fought before, but one that was much more important as well. If I were going to enjoy a normal life of any kind, I would have to win this fight—a fight to control my own mind.

Chapter Eight

Fourth of July, *Again*

Weakness of attitude becomes weakness of character.

—Albert Einstein

Shortly after my walk around the track, I was back at school. Making it through an entire day of classes was hard at first, but I was so glad to be back I didn't care. I had missed the social aspect of school. By the time I got back, basketball season was over and baseball season was well under way, so I just enjoyed the rest of the year by hanging out and having fun.

Everyone at school was glad to see me, but no one treated me differently—except, of course, the teachers. I knew how to play them by now and, to be honest, I had things my way. I couldn't get into trouble if I tried. Not that I ever did anything too bad—I was just always way too social for the classroom—but the teachers cut me a lot of slack.

I never let the ICD affect my social life, but it did take some time to relax and forget about this big thing in my stomach. It always seemed like I was just waiting for it to go off. I almost wanted it to at first, to end the mystery. After a while, though, I learned to forget about it. I quit worrying about when it would go off and what it would feel like.

Dad always used to say, "Don't worry about the things you can't control." This was definitely one of those things. So I decided not to let my thoughts dwell on the negative, which became easier and easier with each day that passed. Every time I made it through another day without a problem, it made it that much easier to expect good things in the upcoming days.

By this time in my life, I had a much better perspective on what I had actually been through. I realized how amazing it was that I was still alive. I was also conscious of the fact that no one, even someone with my condition, knows when their time is up. I might die tomorrow, but I might not die until I am ninety.

I knew I had better plan for my future too. I was never the type to say, "I might, die so I better go skydiving." I am more the type to say, "I just better enjoy every day. Enjoy school. Enjoy the weather. Enjoy my family and friends. Enjoy creating a life for myself." I was driven to do just that. I wanted to succeed in life, and so I balanced having fun with keeping up in school. I didn't want to go to Harvard or Yale; I just wanted to find a good college in Michigan. I knew most required a 3.0 grade point average for admission, so graduating with a 3.0 became my goal.

I finished my junior year pretty strong and didn't fall behind because of my surgery. I didn't miss a beat on the social calendar either. I went to the prom (and, yes, I even had a date) and enjoyed flirting with almost every attractive girl in the school, although I didn't have a serious girlfriend. All and all, I remember my junior year as a great one. I've even come to appreciate the few months of recovery from the surgery, when I was given a chance to see what I was really made of.

As my senior year came around, I was living like a "normal" kid. For the most part, I would just forget about my ICD and have fun. I was still hanging out with the boys a lot, but it was a little different this year. By now my little sister, Stacy, was in high school too. She was a freshman, and for the first time we were sharing a school. My friends spent that year chasing her friends around. It was a little strange for Stacy and me, though. All my friends were like big brothers to her, and all of her friends were like sisters to me. We still had fun though. It was actually kind of nice having my little sister around more.

We also fought more than ever this particular year, mostly about normal high school stuff. Her attitude could have been much worse. It must have been hard for her coming into "my" school as Matt's sister instead of as Stacy. She was used to it by now though. She'd been Matt's little sister her entire life. She didn't have any miraculous stories, was never a poster child, and never got to be on television or even in a parade. I should have cut her some more slack because of that, but back then, she was still just my little sister.

That same year, I got into a little bit of trouble for the first time in my life. Mom and Dad went out of town and, of course, I had a party. It resulted in the most severe grounding of my life, even though it was innocent enough, as drinking still wasn't cool in Montrose. Even if drinking would have been cool, I wouldn't have done it. I lived in a small town where my mom worked in a beauty shop. If something happened, she heard about it. Also, Dad was pretty good friends with Mr. Annese, and he knew *everything* that happened at that school. In fact, he stopped me one Friday later in the year to tell me, "You know, if what you are planning tonight actually happens, your dad *will* find out about it. Just like he found out about that last one." I walked out of Mr. Annese's classroom loudly proclaiming, "The party's off!" I knew that if I went through with it, I would come home from school to find that tan 1984 Buick Century that my parents had bought me up for sale.

Dad's threats of making me pay my own car insurance or selling my car altogether managed to keep me out of serious trouble. I also managed to make it through my *entire* senior year without taking home one single book or piece of homework. I was very proud of that at the time. I only pulled a grade point average in the 2.8 range, but I had well over a 3.0 going into that year. So I could afford it, or so I thought. Turns out I would pay the price later for not studying.

As the year-end approached, Zac and I started making trips around the state to check out some colleges. One day we skipped school to visit Western Michigan University in Kalamazoo and Michigan State University (MSU) in East Lansing, among others. Western was actually our last scheduled stop of the day. We did the whole guided tour and were both impressed. On the drive home, we were both pretty much sold. Our trip home, however, took us straight through East Lansing, by Michigan State. We decided to just drive around campus and check things out.

We didn't go on any tours or hear about the curriculum. We just found a parking spot and walked around. We were walking past the football stadium when we saw the tunnel leading out onto the field with the gate left open. We strolled through the tunnel that the players run through most Saturdays in the fall. It was pretty amazing standing on the field looking up at all the seats. As we left there and walked around a bit, I remembered how much I used to love MSU as a kid. In Michigan, you are brought up either cheering for State or for the University of Michigan. I remembered how I used to be a green and white State fan through and through, a tradition passed on down the line from Grandpa Noble.

Maybe it was my childhood memories or maybe just the size and the tradition of the place, but as we drove off that night I knew I wanted to go to Michigan State. Zac became more convinced on that same walk that Western was the school for him. So we came home that night knowing where we wanted to go. I was going to apply to both schools with my first choice being MSU.

As the year came to an end it was a little sad, thinking about leaving. I would miss football and Mr. Annese. I had been by his side since sixth grade, first as a little water boy and eventually becoming part of his team, even though I never played. Toward the end of the school year I got a letter from Mr. Annese that I will never forget. It was simple—just a heartfelt thank-you for my commitment to the team and for my loyalty to him. I had always thought of loyalty as a great quality to have, and I hoped I had it myself. The fact the he recognized that quality in me meant a lot.

As the year continued to wind down and I thought more about saying good-bye, I also thought about what the future would hold. I was excited about college and thinking about it quite a bit. I knew I would need some money for school, so that spring I found myself a job. It wasn't my first job; Dad had made me get one for the summer after my junior year. However, I was much more excited about this new work—no more McDonald's. I took a position at the local outlet mall in Birch Run selling shoes at the Nike factory outlet store. I used to try to see how many shoes I could sell in a day, even though I didn't work on commission. Most of my coworkers just milled about folding clothes and avoiding customers, but not me. I had loved Nike since I was a kid, and so I wanted to do a good job. I sold my heart out. Looking back, I wish I would have kept track of how well I did.

Only once did I hate having that job. I was scheduled to work an eight-hour shift on a Saturday over Memorial Day weekend. All of the boys were going up north camping for the weekend, and I really wanted to go, but I couldn't find anyone to switch shifts with me. I had to either work or call in sick and go camping. It was just a temporary job selling shoes. I could have just blown it off and called in sick. But I am glad I didn't. After all, anyone can honor their commitments when there is nothing better to do.

I made it through the workday, but Tuesday at school was painful. Over and over again I had to hear how awesome the weekend was. I swear they told stories about that weekend for months and months. I would always have to just sit and listen. Even though I wasn't included in the camping conversations, the boys and I shared plenty of other memories before graduating in June of 1994. I honestly couldn't have asked for a better group of guys to finish my high school run with. Now I had to think about leaving them and many other friends. After all, I was off to Michigan State University in the fall.

I remember the day I found out that I had gotten into State. Dad got the mail that morning and saw I was accepted. Knowing that Mr. Kinter, our principal, was an alumnus, my dad called and asked him to pass the news on to me. During algebra class, Mr. Kinter came in and started singing the Michigan State fight song and then shook my hand and said, "Congrats, you are one of us now" and walked out.

I yelled, "Are you serious?" to his back as he walked down the hallway.

He affirmed, "I just talked to your dad." I sat back in my char with an ear-to-ear grin on my face. It slowly faded into a simple little smirk as I thought, *I knew I'd get in; there was never any doubt.* I couldn't really hide my excitement, though, as a smile stayed on my face for the entire day.

The rest of the school year was a blur, as graduation would come all too soon. Before I knew it, I was a high school graduate and on my way to actually starting my life. I spent the early part of that summer working at Nike and hanging out as much as possible with my friends, as I was starting to realize that I would soon be leaving some of them behind. One of them was Jeff, as he was a year younger than me. He and I had been friends since I was six and he was five. At first we were only friends because we had to be—our parents were close—but it wasn't long before we became really tight.

When we were younger, Jeff and I used to go and rent as many video games as our moms would let us on a winter weekend. We would then sit in the basement of either his house or mine and play all weekend. I can still remember that feeling, like we were reluctantly released from the dungeon. We'd be walking up the steps into the light, with tight muscles and watery eyes after having stared at the TV for eight straight hours.

We stayed friends all the way up through high school, as did our parents, and so on the Fourth of July in that summer following graduation my family visited their house. It was a perfect July afternoon, and I say that only because Jeff's family has a pool. It was way too hot and humid to be spending the day anywhere other than at the pool. We were having a great time with the few families who were there, all friends from church, as we swam and had a cookout. It was a typical Fourth of July for any American. It was also very typical for my family as well.

Once again it was the Fourth, and once again I was swimming. We were playing a game very similar to the one that Joe and I played that day back at the end of eighth grade. Running and jumping off of the diving board, stretching out to catch a football thrown just out of reach. This time, however, I had learned my lesson. I was taking it easy. Mom and Dad were watching me like hawks as they tried to carry on their conversations.

I was being very careful not to let my heart rate get up too high. I mean I would be a total idiot to let myself have *another* cardiac arrest in *another* pool. That's why I was so perplexed as I slowly got out of the water to find my heart racing. I couldn't believe it. I stood on the cement next to this beautiful underground pool more amazed and confused than scared. I tried coughing really hard, as I'd been told that might slow my heart rate down, but of course that didn't work. Dad looked up and saw my face and knew something was wrong, even though I was trying my best to hide it. I didn't even think about my ICD, even though I was looking down at my bare chest and stomach as I made myself cough violently.

Over the next five seconds I started to feel myself losing consciousness. As I was still convinced that this wasn't really happening, all I could think about was not scaring Mom and Dad. I was worried more about them than anything else as I started to pass out. I heard Dad, with urgency in his voice, ask, "Are you okay, Matt?" Apparently that's when I passed out and fell over. Mom had heard Dad ask me that question and jumped up to catch my head just inches before it hit the concrete.

As everyone rushed to me and started praying, Mom and Dad thought about my ICD. Just as they did, it gave me a shock. Within about two seconds I was awake. As I came to, I quickly looked around and tried to piece together what was happening. When you pass out, it is nothing like going to sleep. The brain shuts down, and when you regain consciousness, it is pretty scary until you figure out what is going on. It usually takes a few seconds to piece things together and to remember where you are at and what is going on as the brain seems to be recharging. This time as I awoke I saw everyone around me, most of them still praying. I felt my heart start beating fast again. A few fearful words, "Keep praying. It's still beating fast," is all I had time to say before I passed out again. I had no idea how long I had been out and didn't have time to ask before I was out again. Just after passing out, I got another shock from the ICD and quickly woke up.

As I came to this time, my heart was slowed. Everyone had that look on their faces, the look that I had only seen a few times, always after regaining consciousness from one of my cardiac arrests. It was a strange mixture of fear and joy, worry and nervousness. I asked what happened. As they explained it to me, I couldn't believe I had only been unconscious for a few seconds total. It could have been hours for all I knew. I heard the ambulance off in the distance and told everyone I didn't need it, even though I felt just about the same as when I woke up after all the other times.

I felt like I had just run a marathon and had absolutely no energy left. I could feel the adrenaline pumping through my body, yet everything was calm and still, with the exception of my shaking hands. I found out later that I had received two large shocks. Although I hadn't felt them, since I was unconscious, I could feel the lingering aftereffects in my body. My entire torso was a little tight, like I had just finished a tough workout. However, the soreness was nothing compared with the pain I'd experienced after receiving CPR. This was much easier. For the first time, I actually felt safe after one of my episodes. I was still a little nervous and scared, as it felt like I was flirting with death, but underneath it all was actually a little happy.

Mom was a little nervous and not ready to just take me home, but we turned the ambulance away anyhow. The ICD had worked. It had been my emergency medical something or other. It had saved my life. As Mom let that information sink in and her nerves calm down, she was just as happy as I was to be going home instead of to the hospital.

We called Ann Arbor the next day and went down to get a checkup. They were extremely happy. This time they sent us home feeling confident. I now had a little paramedic's kit in my stomach with me wherever I went. And now I—and the doctors—knew it worked.

Chapter Nine

Carnival

I don't measure a man's success by how high he climbs but how high he bounces when he hits bottom.

—George S. Patton

When we returned from Ann Arbor, I think we were all a little more relaxed than we had been in a while. We had nothing to worry about. The ICD worked. It was a relief. Mom and Dad knew the ICD would, in effect, take their place while I was at college. There really wasn't anything to worry about; I had my ICD now to save me. I was a little more relaxed too. I hadn't felt the shock when the device went off, and I liked that. Passing out was scary, but the fear mostly came from the unknown. Now that I knew I would be conscious within a few seconds, I figured that these episodes would be no problem at all. Even so, I was about ready to vow to never go into a swimming pool again.

Before long I had my freshman orientation at Michigan State. I remember driving down to stay for the night. I was a little nervous but really just excited. I couldn't wait to see the dorm where I would be staying and to get a schedule of my classes. How cool would that be to have classes start at 10:00 A.M. or even 11:00! I just couldn't wait to experience college life.

The weather was perfect the night I stayed in East Lansing. I met a few new friends, and although they seemed to be trying way too hard to impress everyone, they were pretty cool. We walked around the campus checking everything out. Although there weren't many students around at the time, the town still had an energy to it. The large sidewalks and beautiful trees and flowers made you want to walk from place to place, and I couldn't wait to go check out all the cool little college hangouts that seemed to sit at each corner. This was a college town, and it felt like it.

As I walked with my new friends, I didn't tell them about my ICD or my heart condition; they didn't have a clue. I was a little nervous that I would do something to set off my ICD, but my nerves were more about the potential embarrassment than anything else. I thought about it every time we would walk up a hill as we were touring campus but just pushed it out of my mind thinking *What are the odds?*

I got home from that one-night stay at MSU having matured by about three years, in my own mind anyway. I was ready to get to school and had no use for a little sister and parents' rules anymore. I of course loved my family, but I was ready to get on with my own life. I was all set to start my premed classes at school and to work toward my future, which I had all mapped out. My plans were bigger than little ole Montrose, and I wanted to get going.

I managed to make it through the next month or so by spending a lot of time with my friends. None of the boys was coming to State, and even though it was only an hour's drive away from Montrose, I wasn't planning on coming home a whole lot. I also spent quite a bit of time with this new girl I had been seeing.

She had gone to school in Chesaning, a little country town about ten miles from Montrose. She had done well in the local beauty pageant and so she was now one of the Chesaning Showboat girls. Chesaning's showboat is the town's excuse to have a carnival, a parade, and some entertainment come to town for one week every July.

I wasn't too happy about it this year, though, because that meant she was busy all week. I would be left to hang out with my friends. I remember one night during that week, hanging out with some friends of mine who weren't so lucky to be finished with high school, as they were all younger than me. We decided to go check out the showboat, partially because we had nothing better to do, but mostly so they could all check out this girl. I wanted them to see how hot she was. I must say, I was pretty proud of myself at the time.

We headed out basically just looking for trouble and being stupid kids. Everyone wanted to find some Chesaning kids to beat up. I reminded them what happened the last time I was in a fight (the basketball game), and they quickly came up with an alternate plan.

I think they were more scared of my heart problem than I was. None of them really understood the ICD or how it worked. I tried to explain it, but unless you had experienced one of my cardiac arrests, the ICD didn't make a lot of sense.

We went into town and got a chance to say hi to the showboat girls. I got my congratulations from the guys and we were off. After wasting a few hours driving around and looking for something to do, we stumbled upon the carnival and ran into some other friends from school. A few of the guys had graduated the previous year. All I wanted to do was ask them about college and see if it really was as good as I thought it was going to be. They said it was, but I did wonder why the heck they were in Chesaning with us if college life was so great. I guess it was just the summer bringing everyone back home.

A bunch of us decided to go on a ride, mostly just to make fun of how lame it was. To me, anything that wasn't in East Lansing was lame. Most of us were also roller-coaster pros. Every year in school, we would get to go to Cedar Point, an amusement park in Sandusky, Ohio, for a field trip. At the time, Cedar Point had the world's biggest and fastest roller coaster . . . or dang close to it anyway. We had all ridden that, so this little carnival didn't get our hearts racing.

We were on the ride and actually having a good time. We weren't thrilled with the ride as much as we were with messing around with each other. We were goofing off, acting like we were scared, yelling to the operator, "You'd better stop this thing! I am really scared!" with as much sarcasm as we could pile on. He looked up at us like "Gee, that's the first time I've ever heard that one." You could tell it was getting old for him.

I was laughing really hard by now when I felt someone from behind punch me in the middle of the back—hard. As I jerked around to see who did it, I realized that everyone was leaning back and looking elsewhere; they couldn't have done it. Totally perplexed, I stopped laughing and must have looked confused. I was. All of a sudden I felt this hit again. This time it felt as if my insides exploded. I jerked forward as I let out an uncontrollable "ugh." It was almost as if my diaphragm locked up for a second, along with every other muscle in my chest and torso.

It had to be my ICD. I looked at my friend and told him to get the operator to stop the ride. He knew something was terribly wrong; I must have had a look of fear in my eyes because all of a sudden I didn't like the look on his face. It didn't take long before they all started yelling at the carnival guy to stop the ride. Now it was his turn to have fun with us. I had no idea what was going on with me. My heart wasn't racing, or at least I couldn't feel it racing. I wasn't light-headed. I hadn't passed out. I felt fine. *Why was this happening? Why was I being shocked?* I wondered whether it was done or if it would happen again, as I tried to look dead so the carnival guy might actually realize we weren't joking around. He started laughing at us, feeling in control for the first time in a while I imagine. I would get shocked again before he stopped that stupid ride.

As I stepped off of the ride and quickly made my way down that rickety metal ramp and out onto the grass, I was in a mental panic. I didn't know what to do so I just kept walking. My friends followed, never taking an eye off of me and also wondering what to do. As I walked, hunched over, looking at the ground, I don't know what I was thinking. I don't think I really was. I just wanted out of there. It's as if I thought I could walk away from my ICD. Obviously that didn't work too well. I got another shock, this one the first I'd had while standing up. The jolt was so big that it caused me to stumble a little and to almost fall to one knee. I let out a noise that was a pretty good blend of a yell, an ouch, and a whimper. I just wanted this to end. Someone finally made me lie down in the grass, right in the middle of the carnival.

As I lay there I could feel my heart beating fast, but it wasn't like it'd been in the past. My heart had always just felt different when I had an episode. It always beat very fast but also just felt strange, as if it were beating the wrong way, fluttering and pounding. This time it felt fast, but normal, like I had been running around playing basketball or something and then suddenly just stopped to lie down. I didn't like the feeling; it wasn't natural. I hadn't been up running around. I was simply lying there.

Dar was there with me. He was one of the guys who had graduated the year before, and I knew him from the football team. He just knelt at my side as I told everyone, "I'll be alright. Just give me a minute," and then commanded them, "Whatever you do, don't call my parents." I knew the story of what was going on would get convoluted and throw them into a panic. I lay there, waiting for another shock, looking up at the crowd start-

ing to gather around me. It was a strange mix of embarrassment, fear, surrealism, and more fear.

I got shocked again as I lay there and helplessly
looked up at Dar. "I just want it to stop," I think I whim-
pered. I have no idea what he said to me as he knelt
there, but I remember that just having someone there
gave me some comfort. I tried to take some deep
breaths and relax, but my heart was beating so hard I
imagined it was bouncing me off of the ground with
every beat. I continued to breath deep and tried to just
look up at the stars and think about anything else. Over
the next minute or so, my heart slowly started to calm. I
took my pulse and finally my heart rate was normal.
Even though every other physical indicator inside me
told me that things were way out of control, I felt fairly
confident that I would be okay now that my heart rate
had slowed.

Thinking that my heart was back under control, I
started to sit up. My friends weren't so keen on that idea,
but I told them to trust me. None of them trusted me, not
even a little. I was getting ready to stand up when the
paramedics arrived. Shortly thereafter, Chris H. came running up to tell me my parents were on the way. He had
found a phone. I told the paramedics to go away and that
I would be fine. My friends looked at me as if to say, "You
are not coming home with us!"

I quickly signed the papers releasing the paramedics
of their liability, as I was concerned about Mom and
Dad. Chesaning was the middle of nowhere, and so I
couldn't just grab a cell phone and call them to let them

know I was okay. We walked (slowly I might add) to the entrance of the carnival and stood there waiting for my parents. I was just flat-out pissed by this point but tried to maintain a cool appearance as I answered my friends' questions every ten seconds with an "I'm fine, honestly," even though my hands were visibly shaking, as if I'd had way too much caffeine.

At about this time, Mom and Dad were fighting in the car. It was a fifteen- to twenty-minute drive under normal circumstances and Mom was mad that Dad wouldn't speed. "If we get pulled over, it will just take us that much longer to get there, or what if we get in an accident, so just shut up and pray," he told her as he drove at a speed within reason. Apparently it takes a lot to get an insurance man to speed.

After their bickering ended, they prayed until they got to town. As they approached the carnival looking for an ambulance, they saw me standing by the side of the road waving my hands yelling, "I'm fine." I knew they would be a mess.

I got in the car and we headed for home. "Sorry," I told them, as if it were all my fault. I felt bad that they had to go through all this with me. I remember thinking, *I can't wait until I get to school; then it will be easier for them*. I knew it would be that much harder for me, not having their support, but as I saw the look on their faces I just wanted to get away from them. I realized how much pain I was causing. I hated doing that to them.

Through all of this, Stacy had been at Chris H.'s house hanging out with his little sister. His house was always at the center of excitement in downtown Montrose, and tonight was no exception.

Apparently Mom had called Stacy at Chris H.'s house when they were on the way to get me. She said, "Matt had another cardiac arrest. We are on our way to get him, but that's all we know." So Stacy got to sit there and worry. After Mom and Dad picked me up and we got closer to Montrose, Mom called Stacy again and told her I was fine and that we were going to go to Ann Arbor. Stacy wanted to go. She was worried, and I think a little sick of being left behind. Mom told her that we would pick her up in a few minutes.

Of course, Chris H., an excited seventeen-year-old, beat the insurance agent to his house by a good five or ten minutes. When he and my other friends got there, they saw Stacy and wouldn't say anything. They just acted really weird. She told them, "Guys, I know," and they all came unglued at once. Each one of them raced through their version of what had happened, none of them afraid to admit he was still scared out of his mind.

We picked Stacy up and drove down to Ann Arbor. Mom and I sat there just pissed for the entire car ride, as all this was getting really old by now. Dad sat quiet in prayer as he drove, and Stacy looked out the window for the hour-long ride. We finally got there and after a few hours I got a hospital bed. My family quickly got a room at the Med Inn, a hotel attached to the hospital, where they would stay for the night. Once again we would have to wait for the morning to try and find some answers.

Chapter Ten

Simply Surviving

*Character may be manifested in the great
moments, but it is made in the small ones.*

—Winston Churchill

My night at the hospital was a long one. I didn't
know why my ICD had fired, as I didn't think a
little carnival ride could ever get a person's heart rate up
that high under normal conditions, and I didn't know if
it would go off again. In my mind it had shocked me for
no apparent reason, and so I was scared of that happening again. I just lay there, all tense. It was as if I were
home alone and had just heard a strange noise in the
house, only the tenseness lasted all night. Mentally, I
was on the edge of my chair, and I would stay that way
for quite some time. It was a hard thing to deal with. I
had just gone through the scariest moments of my life,
and there was no promise that it wouldn't happen again.
On the contrary, it most likely would.

The next day we talked to Dr. Dick and tried to figure out what had happened. Upon interrogating the ICD with a specialized computer, they discovered that my heart had gone above 200 beats per minute and stayed there, causing the device to fire several times. Because I had not passed out, the thought was that I didn't go into a bad rhythm (ventricular tachycardia) as I had in the past. I agreed; this time felt different. Dr. Dick concluded that I had had an episode of atrial arrhythmia, a nonlethal rhythm problem that comes from the top chambers of the heart.

I still didn't understand why I had gotten so many shocks, though. Dr. Dick explained that the ICD is placed strategically to work best on ventricular arrhythmias, the life-threatening kind that come from the bottom chambers of the heart. Oftentimes, ICDs do nothing to the atrial arrhythmias. Naturally, I asked, "So, if I go into an atrial arrhythmia again, I could just keep getting shocked over and over and over until I get to the hospital?" He told me that usually doesn't happen, but, theoretically, it could. "Gee thanks, Dr. Dick, that should really help me to relax."

He quickly assured me that there were things we could do to prevent this from happening, and although these shocks were inappropriate, my ICD was working perfectly. (These shocks are called "inappropriate" not because the ICD acted inappropriately—in fact it did exactly what it was supposed to do—but because it was an inappropriate reason to shock my heart.)

The plan was to start me on some more medicines, in addition to the ones I'd been taking for years. These new medicines would help keep my heart rate slow and help keep the top chamber of my heart from getting into a bad rhythm and causing an inappropriate shock. It was all very sketchy though. The doctors weren't entirely sure whether an atrial arrhythmia is exactly what I was dealing with. Today's defibrillators actually record an EKG—automatically storing it internally—of the heart whenever it delivers a shock, so doctors can tell exactly why it went off and can try to prevent it from inappropriately discharging again. Most ICDs in 1994 didn't have this, and so everything that the doctors did was based on speculation and what information I could give them about how I felt during the episode—information I wasn't even sure of myself, given that I wasn't exactly taking notes.

Over the next few days I tried to digest all this new information. I wondered whether my heart was getting sicker. *Is that what caused the new problem?* I wondered if this new medicine would help things, and I wondered whether I would ever be able to leave for college. But mostly, I just wondered if I would get shocked again.

As that first week rolled into a second, I started to feel a little safer, but not much. I would try to forget about the "what ifs" and move forward—a task much easier said than done. I had to stay in the hospital for a few weeks as I started this new medicine. This hospital trip was different because, for the first time, they let me leave the floor. Now that I had my ICD, they weren't as concerned about keeping an eye on me every second. If the new medicine happened to make this rhythm problem worse rather than better, well, I would just get a shock and then we would try a new medicine. The doctors weren't quite as worried as they had been in the past. I, however, was more worried than ever, as passing out and getting CPR sounded much better than getting a shock.

One afternoon my parents and I walked outside around the hospital grounds. We went up a big hill just outside of one of the hospital's back doors. The hill actually leads up to the dorm where my cousin Andy had lived the fall before on the University of Michigan campus.

As I walked up the hill with Mom and Dad in tow, I thought about a night a few months before when I had visited Andy at school. I had gone to one of his fraternity parties with him. They put me in charge of working the door, with specific instructions about whom I could let in. I loved it. The entrance seemed to be the social center of the party, and I was having a blast.

Even though that great night had taken place only a few months earlier, and a few hundred yards ahead, it seemed a lifetime away. As I slowly walked up that hill and tried to think about college, thoughts of getting shocked took center stage. I felt my heart beating faster and feared I was going to get a shock. We got to the top, after several rest stops, and I could still feel my heart skipping beats. It seemed as if every other beat was a skipped beat. I didn't get shocked or pass out on that trip, but I didn't like the feeling. I was convinced that things were not right, but when we got back to the fifth floor, the doctors assured me that according to the monitors everything looked perfectly fine. So I tried to forget about it, without any success.

The day eventually came when I could go home. I was a little timid, still fearful of getting shocked unexpectedly, but glad to be out and ready to get on with my life. I hoped that things would be okay so I could get off to college, but I just didn't feel right. I didn't like the new medicine I was on. It made my heart skip a lot of beats, and I associated that with problems. All I could do was try to focus on the future and move forward.

I was just starting to get out on my own a little when I had another little incident. I was at home one afternoon with Stacy and one of her friends while Mom and Dad were out and about. I was trying to convince myself that things were indeed okay, so I started to push the envelope. I was trying to get a little excited and get some exercise, trying to get my heart rate up to convince myself that I was ready to go to school and that I could handle things. I was playing a mental game with myself. I just had to get my heart rate up, even though it scared me, just to see if I would be okay. I would rather have an incident here and now than in a few months when I was alone at school.

I wasn't even really doing all that much when my heart took off. I quickly went into ventricular tachycardia (VT), the life-threatening heart rhythm from the bottom chambers, and I knew it immediately. My heart rate jumped from about 100 to 250 in one beat. I yelled for Stacy in the other room and quickly lay down on my bed, hoping that by some miracle relaxing would get it to stop. I lay there for those first few seconds just waiting—waiting to pass out, waiting to get a shock, waiting for anything. Time actually stopped, I think. I was completely helpless as I just waited. I was wearing a heart monitor at the time that I had been prescribed to wear upon my hospital discharge. The monitor displayed my heart rate and recorded any bad rhythms. It read, 180, 190, 200, 220; it was trying to catch up with my heart, like a speedometer on a car when you take off too fast.

I watched the monitor, fully aware that my ICD was programmed to fire at 200 bpm. As it approached 200, I tensed up waiting for the shock, but it didn't come and I got scared. It wasn't going to work. I yelled for Stacy to call 9-1-1 as she was running into my room. I forgot about the fact that the device had to charge up before it could deliver a shock. So as I lay there, all tense, fearful, and helpless, it finally shocked me. I hadn't passed out. Once again I felt the electricity explode through my body as I jerked and let out that strange combination of a yell and a whimper. I quickly reached for my pulse and found it was normal. I took a deep breath and told Stacy I was okay as she stood there on the phone.

I didn't take my hand off of my chest, as I was afraid the ICD would shock me again. It would. All of a sudden my heart took off again, and again I waited for the shock. The panic built inside me, as I wondered if this cycle of fast heartbeat followed by shock would continue indefinitely. "Ohhhh, Stacy, it's doing it again." Instead of panicking like a little sister should have, she calmly said, "Don't worry, Matt. The ambulance is on the way. You will be okay." Then she gently took my hand and sat on the edge of the bed with me. I got hit with another thirty-one joules of electricity and my heart steadied. Again, I hadn't passed out, and I was not happy about that.

As I lay there things started to calm down, my adrenaline rush slowed, and I thought it was over. I didn't know though, and so I was still tense. I just lay there and waited, waited for something to happen.

At about this time Mom and Dad were on their way home. They were chatting about routine matters of the day as they pulled onto our road. Actually, I'm sure Mom was chatting as Dad let out the occasional "mmm-hmmm." When they got about a mile from home an ambulance quickly approached from behind, with lights flashing and sirens screaming, and they pulled to the side of the road to let it pass. As they always did when seeing an ambulance, they each said a little silent prayer for the person in need of help and reminded themselves that they didn't need to worry. It wasn't me. As they quickly started back down the road, both thinking the same thing, they saw the ambulance slow down. They caught up with it just in time to follow it into our driveway.

The arrival of the ambulance and a scared Mom and Dad didn't help me any. I was still mentally torn up as we continued on with the normal routine—to the hospital in Flint and then on to Ann Arbor.

During the trip, I thought about those shocks I had gotten and hoped I wouldn't get another one—ever. The worst part wasn't even the shock, which is over before I even know it's hitting me. It's just not natural for a heart to beat in this bad rhythm. Your mind hits the panic button and everything inside you tells you to do something to stop it, yet there is absolutely nothing you can do. Waiting for the ICD to go off is tougher than the actual shock and fearing that it won't work. Not getting a shock would be easier, but I didn't want to die. I had already pushed my luck by surviving several cardiac arrests before getting my device. If my device was going to fail, I knew I didn't have much of a chance. I knew that they almost never failed, but, even so, lying there with my heart beating at 250 beats per minute, I wasn't exactly thinking rationally.

When we got down to Ann Arbor, Dr. Dick did what he had done years before when he sent me off to the Mayo Clinic. He asked for some help. I love that about him, the fact that I can trust that he will do his best but also not be afraid to ask for help. He called on the doctors from the adult side of the hospital. They were cardiac electrophysiologists (heart rhythm specialists) just as he was, but they worked with adults instead of kids. They saw the same kind of stuff, with a few twists. Dr. S. Adam Strickberger came over to see me the next day.

Adam was a tall, young doctor who seemed to have his act together. Later I would get to know him as a big fifteen-year-old in a doctor's body. He was the kind of guy who said and did things just to see people's reactions and was a lot of fun to be around. This day, however, he was professional and suggested starting me on two medicines, a little drug cocktail that he often prescribed. The hope was that this would help keep my heart out of that bad rhythm so the ICD wouldn't need to go off. I liked that idea and Dr. Dick took his advice. I started the new medicines right away. I spent the next few days in the hospital, once again wondering whether these new medicines would work.

I tried to act normal around my family, but mentally I was falling apart. I was extremely conscious of every heartbeat, a phenomena doctor's call "cardiac awareness." It is common for heart patients to feel, and in fact concentrate on, each and every heartbeat. You become so aware of your heartbeat that you can feel each and every one, as people with normal hearts can when they lie on their chests.

I would feel a "skipped" heartbeat and hold my breath, waiting for my heart to take off into some sort of an arrhythmia. In that half a second, part of me would wish for the ventricular kind of arrhythmia, knowing that I had a better chance of passing out before I got a shock. However, passing out is also scary. On the other hand, I wasn't in the mood for the four, five, or ten shocks an atrial arrhythmia could possibly bring.

Those "skipped" heartbeats that many people feel after drinking some caffeine were driving me insane. In fact, in those first few days, even getting up to go to the bathroom was hard. I would get out of bed, take a few steps, and feel my heart rate start to rise, as it should. An activity like that would have many people's heart up to 90 or even 100 beats per minute. I was so sensitive to the change that the normal rise in my heart rate frightened me. All of a sudden those 100 beats per minute felt like 300. I would take two steps and stop to try to count my pulse . . . just waiting to get shocked.

My ICD, a gift from God, was a big part of the reason I was alive. It had saved my life a few times already, but I couldn't help but wonder whether it was worth it. *How was I going to live?* I couldn't even get out of bed and walk to the bathroom without being paralyzed by fear.

The doctors and nurses weren't much help in teaching me how to cope with this new problem, mostly because I was too cool to let them know about my mental struggles. Mom once tried to go to an ICD support group to get some help but came away more depressed. Every patient there was at least sixty years old. Their issues were slightly different from mine. Not one of them was worried about starting college in the fall. I felt like I was pretty much on my own.

I would later learn that their issues were actually quite similar to mine. I was worried about getting shocked while in class; they were worried about getting shocked while holding their grandkids. Either way it was fear: fear about change in our lives, fear about pain, and fear of the unknown. I would also find out later that had we looked beyond the surface, we could have learned a lot from this group. Many elderly people deal with their shocks and devices much better than younger recipients do. The elderly seem to be more grateful for the extra life given them, while us youngsters tend to feel we are owed a certain amount of this life. I would learn this lesson in time, to simply and honestly be grateful for each day that God puts before me, but it sure wouldn't come within the following week.

Over the next week in the hospital, I tried to take it minute by minute. I remembered Mr. Annese talking about mental toughness. He always talked about that. He talked about being mentally focused and giving it everything you've got for thirty seconds . . . just make it through that one play and then worry about the next one. It helped some, but this wasn't football. I didn't have to stay strong and hang tough for the duration of one play; I was looking at the rest of my life. I would try not to think about that though. I would just try to get to the bathroom and back without having to stop and take my pulse. I wondered what it would be like to live without this battle. What would it be like to never have to question my own heartbeat, wondering if the next one would come? This mental anguish was hard—and getting old.

All I could do was pray, but it felt like I was praying on a cloudy day, as if my prayers were just hitting the clouds and falling to the ground. I tried to remind myself of the one time that I had prayed and just knew that things would be okay. I held on to the memory of that feeling. I knew this anguish would end, eventually; I just had to make it until then. "God make it come soon," I would pray over and over. "Just get me through and give me strength." I don't know if I ever really stopped praying for a while there, even though it didn't seem to be helping.

At times I worried about whether I should even be going to college, given my condition. Now, I was starting to wonder whether I'd even be given the chance, as it looked like I might not be out of the hospital in time to start the fall semester. A part of me wanted to stay in the hospital forever, but I knew it would get easier when I left. There was nothing else to do in the hospital but think about my heart and listen to the beep of each heartbeat on the monitors. Forgetting about my heart was the plan, even though I knew it wasn't going to work too well.

As the next few days passed it became clear that I wouldn't be out of the hospital in time to go to college. I was upset; I had been excited about going. I became even more sad and angry after talking to friends on the phone as they packed and said good-bye to leave for college. I am sure I would have been even more ticked if I hadn't been so scared. There was a part of me that wasn't too sure how I would have made it anyway. I was nervous just walking around the fifth floor at Mott Children's Hospital, where I was surrounded by some of the world's best medical care. How would I handle a walk on campus at MSU?

For the first time in my life, I left the hospital feeling scared. Mom and Dad were old pros at handling the fear that followed discharge, but it was new to me. I probably should have gone to them for more help than I did, but I didn't want them to know how scared I was. I had put them through enough, so I did my best to act as if I were fine, even though I'm sure I wasn't fooling them nearly as much as I thought I was.

Needless to say, I didn't call my friends to come over and play football when I got home. In fact, I remember sitting in the basement watching television one night and thinking about sleeping down there on the couch, just so I didn't have to walk up the flight of stairs. I didn't let myself do it though. That would have been the easy way out.

If I were going to get back to a normal life, eventually getting out of my hibernation, I would have to keep pushing myself to do what scared me. If I could get over one or two hurdles each day, before long I would be back to the pre-carnival mental state of mind. I had to conquer those basement steps just like I conquered that walk to the bathroom at the hospital. I had to learn how to relax again and eventually to leave the house. Ahead of me was what seemed like an endless set of hurdles. Now was no time to take the easy way out.

I still remember the first time I rode to the grocery store with Dad. I swear he was walking twenty miles per hour up and down those aisles. I strolled behind pretending to be in a happy-go-lucky kind of mood as I did my best to hide my fears. I could have just stayed home, but I knew I had to get back to living in a hurry. It would be only a few weeks before I would need to sign up for classes at a local community college.

I enrolled at that local community college because it was the only school that hadn't already started classes when I got home. Looking back, it was a good thing I started there. Classes weren't too tough, and I didn't seem to be able to focus much on my schoolwork. I still remember starting to worry about the five-minute uphill walk back to my car about halfway through math class each day.

The community college environment didn't feel like college; it felt like Montrose-south campus. It was so easy, and I hated every minute of it. I mostly hated it because it wasn't State. Most of my friends were gone, and I was still living with Mom and Dad. I was anxious to grow up, get out, and do things my way. Those little "to-do lists" of household chores I would get were really starting to make me mad, even though I was living rent-free and Dad was paying for college. I had no choice but to continue on, taking it a day at a time.

I would soon find myself back in the hospital, this time for just one night. Dr. Dick assured me that absolutely nothing had happened, nothing was wrong, that the episode I had had the night before was all mental. I tried to argue, mostly because I was embarrassed that I came to the ER and then talked my way into getting admitted into the hospital when there was nothing wrong. He calmly explained everything to me. Apparently, feeling like my heart was out of control when it was fine was normal. He told me that he understood how hard this mental struggle must be for me but that nothing had happened. I didn't get a shock, I didn't pass out, and nothing had happened to my heart.

Deep down I knew he was right. I knew it was all mental. That morning I sat there on the edge of my hospital bed waiting for Dad to come and get me. Mom and Dad had even returned to Montrose that night, leaving me alone in Ann Arbor for the first time ever. Their farthest departure from my hospital room in the past had only been to a local hotel; this time they drove the hour home, apparently not too worried about me. I guess they knew nothing was wrong too. I sat there staring at the floor in the midst of busy nurses and doctors running about. I was in my own little world as I promised myself I wouldn't let this happen again. This is not how I wanted to live my life. I prayed and asked God for help, because I wasn't sure I could keep the promise I'd just made to myself. Again I got no tangible response, but I didn't let that deter me. Mom and Dad had worked hard not to turn me into a cardiac cripple. I wasn't going to let myself become one either. I wanted to live life, not just survive it.

I went home thinking I would try to do more than just survive, but mostly I just hung out around the house. I

spent much of my time watching television and breaking up fights between my fifteen-year-old sister and my
parents. Stacy hadn't learned how to "play the game"
and just tell Mom and Dad what they wanted to hear.
Like most fifteen-year-old girls, she was struggling at
school, more socially than academically. All those years
of being handed off to neighbors, relatives, and friends
so the focus could be on her big brother was starting to
bear its consequences. High school is full of rejection,
and apparently she had had about all she could take.

Regardless, I was thinking more about myself than
her at this time in my life. I had a deadline for getting
myself ready to go out and face the world. I was going
to go to Michigan State the following semester. One term
at the community college was one more than I had
planned on. I wanted out. For now I would just try to
get out of the house and live life.

A few of my friends were still around, but they were
seniors—in school all day and at practices all afternoon.
Thank God one of the boys, Chris W., stayed home and
went to a local college too. Chris was a good friend, but
it would be a while before I would hang out with him.
I was still working my way up to going out and having
fun. It was hard enough trying to do the simple tasks in
life, activities most people do without even thinking. I
just tried to keep moving forward and to not let this stuff
slow me down too much. I still had Michigan State and
medical school in my future, and I was bound and
determined to get there.

My first night out, Chris and I went to a local pool
hall. Chris had fun—he always has fun playing pool—

but I was miserable. I sat on a stool waiting for my turn, which takes a while when playing with Chris, when I felt my heart start skipping beats. I quickly tried to take my pulse without anyone knowing what I was doing. I was getting pretty good at it by now. It wasn't beating too fast, but it kept skipping. I didn't know what to do. I was just scared. *Don't shock me here,* I thought. *I'd almost rather die. Wait, no, I don't want that! Oh, God, I just want to be normal and enjoy a game of pool.*

Those two hours of pool felt like six. It was as if I were being tested to see if I would keep my promise to myself. Every few seconds I would tell myself to *just pretend you don't feel good, your stomach or something. Just going home wouldn't be breaking your promise.* Had I left, I wouldn't have broken my promise, but I knew that the only way to get around this mountain was to climb straight over it. I couldn't let myself fail. I had done that too many times over the past few months. I had to win one of these battles if I were going to make it over the mountain. I just kept praying, trying to get God to make my way easier. I didn't pray anything too special or too religious. I just kept asking for help and strength. It felt comfortable to have someone in the fight with me, a fight that no one but Dr. Dick knew of, let alone understood.

I made it home that night and went to bed mentally exhausted. Although I didn't have any fun with Chris that night, I had made it over the mountain and was happy about that. I knew hundreds of mountains still lay ahead of me, even though I couldn't see even one of them. I just wondered how tall they would be. *God, I hope they aren't any worse than tonight,* I prayed as I slipped off to sleep, even though I knew they probably would be. They always are.

As the winter of '94 came, Chris and I played more pool and had philosophical discussions about politics, God, women, and life in general. I still wasn't ready to really get out there and throw caution to the wind, and I think Chris understood that. He was a good friend to just hang out with me.

I didn't date much during this time (the showboat girl was long gone by now), partially because I wasn't enamored with any of the Flint junior college girls, but mostly because I had no idea how to bring someone into this world I was living in. Even though I ran into fewer and fewer situations where I would think about my heart, I was by no means back to my old self.

I had to keep fighting the mental battle. It was getting easier as the days passed without problems. Each day I had more and more time without thought of doom. Also, I had gained a new perspective. As I looked back on the carnival a few months prior, it didn't really seem quite as bad. Time dulls wounds and eases the pain. I was starting to realize that if that carnival hell did happen again, I could handle it. It would be hard, but I would get through it. The problem was I didn't want to have to prove that to anyone.

As each day passed I got more and more excited about leaving for school and more confident that I could handle it. I was still a little nervous and annoyed about the idea of living with someone I didn't know. I never liked bringing anyone into my problems, but I knew I would have to. I kind of wished that Chris would be going with me or that I would have chosen a school that a friend from high school was at. I never liked it when people picked their college based on where their friends were going. Even though at this point, a large part of me wished I'd done exactly that. I guess God knew that and decided to step in.

Chapter Eleven

I'm Going Where?

*An optimist is someone who goes after Moby
Dick in a rowboat and takes the tartar sauce
with him.*

—Zig Ziglar

Zac came home from college for Christmas break; I
still remember that day when he walked into our
house for the first time. "What's happening?" he said, as
he nodded his head upward. He looked older and even
sounded different; in Montrose everyone said, "What
sup?" But I liked the new greeting that he had picked up
from Western. We chatted for a while about college life;
man, I was ready to go.

He asked me about my upcoming schedule and
classes at State. "Ya know, I haven't gotten anything in
the mail yet," I told him. He suggested I make a call to
figure out what was going on. I should have heard from
them by now. I didn't know how college worked. I just
thought I would be living in the same dorm and would
have the same classes I was slated for before my hospitalization. Zac explained that it wasn't quite that easy.

137

I quickly jumped up, grabbed the phone, and called State. "Well, Mr. Noble," the woman on the other end of the phone explained, "we have you down as a no-show for last semester."

"No," I quickly snapped back, "I sent in doctor's notes and everything documenting what was going on. You knew I wasn't able to come."

"Well, we don't have it now," she rudely replied.

At this point in the conversation, I figured I would have to do a bunch of paperwork and it would all be straightened out. I was a little frustrated but willing to do what I had to do to get out of Montrose. "Okay," I said, "what do I have to do to reapply? I want to get this straightened out. I am going to be starting in just a few weeks."

She informed me that that wouldn't be the case. "I'm sorry, sir, but you will have to reapply for next fall. Because you were a no-show, we cannot accept you for this next term." I argued a little longer but soon realized there was nothing I could do. I hung up the phone totally frustrated.

As I walked away from the phone, I about lost it. "What the heck am I going to do?" I asked Zac. After giving me the requisite sympathy, he came up with the idea of calling Western Michigan University. He loved it there, and it was my second choice anyway. I was already accepted at Western and had slated the school as my backup.

I sat there wondering if my acceptance was still good when he suggested, "Just go there for the one semester. You'll be out of here and then you can transfer to State next fall." That sounded like the perfect plan. I quickly called Dad to tell him what State had said and asked him whether he cared if I tried Western. He was fine with it; he knew I wanted to get on with my life.

It was a long shot. If State required that much of an admissions process, what made me think Western could have me all set to go within a few weeks? I gave them a call anyway, just hoping someone would answer the phone during winter break. I got someone right away, explained to her what had happened, and sheepishly asked whether they had my acceptance from last semester still on file. She quickly came back with a "Sure do . . . and it's still good, but . . ." Oh crap, here it was . . . "we'll have to see if there is any place for you to live." She transferred me over to the housing department, and I explained my story again and asked about getting a dorm. "Well, you said you had a friend here, right?"

"Yeah, why?"

"Well, where does he live?" Zac told me he was in Bigelow Hall, and I relayed the information. "Well, we've got a room on the first floor of Bigelow. Will that do?" *Perfect*, I thought. *Near Zac yet no stairs.*

I was starting to get excited, thinking this plan might just work, when she asked if I had registered for classes yet. She sounded concerned when she transferred me to an academic adviser to try to get me enrolled. My adviser was in her office and quickly picked up the phone. Now, let me just say that I went to college for four years, and not once during those years did I get my adviser sitting in her office, able to take my call. Yet, miraculously on this day, I got her on the phone; plus she was able to schedule me for all of my classes. In one phone call I had everything taken care of.

About three weeks later, in January of '95, Mom, Dad, Stacy, and I made the two-hour trip over to Kalamazoo to move me into the dorm. We unpacked, and I spent the afternoon getting settled. They took off, Mom with tears in her eyes, and all of a sudden I was on my own, as I wouldn't even be assigned a roommate for a few weeks. I remember lying in bed that night thinking, *What have I gotten myself into?* I didn't have a clue how I was going to make it through. I was still gun-shy and timid, afraid that any little thing would set my heart off racing. The only plan I came up with was to just keep acting like I knew what I was doing and hope things would work out.

When the semester first started, I wasn't feeling well at all. Not only was I always worried about my heart; I was just plain sick a lot. Later, we figured out that it was because of a medicine I was on, but at the time most doctors, and I, thought my illnesses were stress related. One morning I got up for a 7:00 A.M. chemistry lab— that's like the middle of the night for most college kids. I went to the cafeteria to eat, just like every other day, hoping some food would make me feel a little stronger.

On this morning, like most mornings during this semester, I was mentally exhausted, physically tired, and feeling sick. It seemed to be an everyday thing, but this was the hand that I was dealt, so I played it. In my mind that was my only choice. But on this day I would get a dose of embarrassment added to my pain. I took a bite of food and all of sudden it just came back up. I was throwing up into my bowl of cereal. I wasn't heaving it up; it was just as if my stomach said, "Not today," and politely sent it back up. I looked up to see the one other person in the cafeteria get up and leave, too disgusted to finish his meal.

I got up and threw my food onto the dirty tray conveyer belt, mad more than anything else. I schlepped across campus like every other day, this time in the blowing snow. This is what my life had become; this is what I had waited so long for. *Gee, this is great,* I thought.

At times, when I wasn't feeling too sick and when I wasn't waiting for my heart to go out of rhythm, I was able to enjoy myself. It was freeing to be away and to just hang out. I loved that part of college life. Just go to classes for a few hours a day and then do whatever you wanted. It was my kind of fun. Zac and I spent a lot of our free time together, and I got the impression that the friends he had made during the first semester were all of a sudden getting blown off for me. I guess I didn't really gel into the clique he had formed up there on the third floor. I was too timid to go out and do a whole lot. Heck, at first I didn't even like climbing the three flights of stairs to go up to his room. Zac was great though; he would just hang back with me. I appreciated that, although I never actually told him so. I think we had the kind of friendship where I didn't need to tell him. He knew.

Zac and I hung out a lot with Kacie too. She was a Montrose grad as well, only one year ahead of us. I knew Kacie back in high school. We were partners in a speech my junior year. When I started that semester, neither Zac nor I knew she was at Western. On my first day of chemistry class I remember sitting in the lecture hall of about two hundred students and seeing a girl who

looked a lot like Kacie. Sure enough, it turned out to be
her. Having another friendly face around, someone else
who already knew me and my story, seemed to make
the college experience a little easier and brought some
much needed comfort.

Like most college students, Kacie had roommate
issues and liked to get out of her apartment. She spent a
lot of time with Zac and me because of it. At times we
would get sick of the dorms, so it was nice to have Kacie's
apartment to get away to as well. The three of us ended
up living in our own little world that semester. I worried
less about the "what ifs" when I hung out with them.
*What if my ICD goes off? What if I go into that bad atrial
arrhythmia and get a bunch of shocks? What if I pass out?*
It was just easier because I knew they would understand.

As the semester wore on, I was having more and more
fun and feeling better and better. I still had difficult
moments though. I remember going to a hockey game
with Zac and a bunch of other guys from the dorm. We
were having fun; plus it was Western vs. Michigan State,
and this was a sport that we could dominate in. I was
happy to put it on State too, after they had blown me off.
We were making a lot of noise, just being stupid college
kids and getting rowdy. I was feeling fine when all of a
sudden I remembered getting rowdy at the basketball
game a few years earlier. I quickly found myself sitting
down taking my pulse while my friends pounded on the
glass. With a normal pulse, physically I was fine; however, I had the hardest time convincing my mind of that.

I sat there and tried to calm down. I was too excited.
Or at least I thought so. Just when I was starting to feel

better and get some confidence, this moment brought me to my knees mentally. I started to pray and remembered how long it had been since I last talked to God. I used to pray every day, but it had been a while. I wasn't going to church while I was away at college; I guess that was a part of me doing things my way. I went a few times, but didn't feel like I fit in. Not having my parents there to make me go, I stayed home almost every Sunday morning. Plus, the time had come for me to decide for myself what my thoughts on God really were. Was I going to adopt my parents' religion and make it my own or go my own way? Those answers would come in time, but, for now, I would pray. It's what I knew, and it helped. Once again, prayer gave me someone who understood and who could help me through, even in the midst of a wild hockey game.

I was much quieter the rest of the night; I suspect Zac figured out what was going on. None of the other guys did. Again I went home frustrated, just wanting to know what it would be like to live without these worries.

It wouldn't be long before we finished up the term and headed home for the summer. Zac and I already had plans to get out of the dorms for the upcoming fall semester. We were going to get an apartment in the complex that Kacie had been in the year before, while she upgraded to a house. I never even thought about transferring over to State, as I had initially intended. In fact, that thought left my mind about two weeks into my first semester at Western. Despite the hard time I was having physically, I was enjoying Kalamazoo. I felt like I belonged.

Early that summer, Zac and I met Dad for lunch near his office. We were working for him on breaks from school, doing basic home inspections around Flint. As we sat there for lunch, the natural topic of conversation was our report cards. Zac got a 3.3 or 3.5 or something like that. I pulled a solid 1.45. It wasn't exactly the strong start that medical schools were looking for, but it was what it was. I think my poor performance had a little to do with how I was feeling mentally and physically. I mostly attributed my grades to my senior year at Montrose. Although I had done a great job of getting by that year with as little work as possible, I wasn't exactly prepared to study in college, and, frankly, I didn't really know how. I had never really studied before. Dad had warned me over and over about that very thing during my senior year. I didn't listen. This day at lunch he wasn't mad a bit. He just made sure, in his own comical way, that Zac and I knew that he had been right. He knew I would figure it out and so he just supported me. It was exactly what I needed.

That summer I also got a job at the University of Michigan hospital where I had spent so many nights. I had a few connections, needless to say, and got hired as a tech in pediatric cardiology. I would be working in the electrocardiogram (EKG) lab. I was making more money than any of my friends, and I was getting experience that would look good on my med school applications. I was captivated by the subject and eager to learn. I just soaked it up. I also befriended two new fellows in the department. (A fellow in pediatric cardiology is someone who has finished medical school, finished his or her residency, and is working on a pediatric cardiology unit before becoming a full-fledged pediatric cardiologist.) Pete and Ian both took me under their wing.

I took call with Ian a few nights, just to see what it was like. I also did it because I enjoyed the hospital at night. When I was confined to the hospital, as a child I slept most of the day and stayed up all night. I would watch prime-time television, then the *Late Show with David Letterman*. Mom and Dad would usually leave for the Med Inn at about the time I perked up and when the third-shift nurses started duty. The nurses at night usually had time to sit around and talk with me. I was always sociable and enjoyed these conversations. The first-shift nurses used to get so mad that the other nurses let me stay up late. The third-shifters weren't quite so uptight. I liked that.

Although I did enjoy the peace and quiet only the darkness brought to the hospital, I quickly learned that I didn't like taking call all that much. I mean I loved the people at the hospital at night, and it was fun to be hanging out and learning from Ian, but I also loved to sleep. The doctors would tell me that they got used to sleeping less, when taking call as interns, so I didn't let my love of sleep deter me from pursuing medical school.

That summer at the hospital went by extremely fast, and it wouldn't be long before Zac and I were back at Western. After hitting the garage sales looking for top-notch furnishings, we were ready for that apartment just off campus. We decorated it perfectly. The highlight of the décor was the tape outline of a dead body placed in the middle of the living room floor. We were fully equipped with a black light, a lava lamp, and a basketball hoop. We had the college apartment look down pat.

Kacie was again having roommate issues, so despite our less than inviting environment, she was still around quite a bit. Our quasi-Seinfeld cast became complete when we met Quan, our neighbor from across the hall. Quan was a tall and skinny guy from Detroit. He was always good for barging in and helping us eat our food. Just like Kramer, he was occasionally annoying but always fun and always welcome.

Zac and I would spend a lot of time with Quan and his roommate Brian. Brian was premed also, whereas Quan seemed to be in college just for the lifestyle. We spent hour upon hour playing video games with those guys. They were a lot of fun, often in an unpredictable kind of way. One night Quan busted in at about 3:00 A.M. He woke us up to quickly say, "Guys, if you hear gunshots, just get down on the floor, below the windows. I know you country boys don't know that kind of stuff." Then he was gone, out the door. We both laughed, "He must have smoked more than he sold again."

I was having a great time and would think about my heart less and less, although it never seemed to be out of my mind completely. It had been a year since I had any problems at all. I was trying as best I could not to let those past issues affect my college "experience." I wanted to live life, not just survive it. I wanted to enjoy college, not just make it through. The definition of enjoyable is different for different people. Even though I was trying to get the college fill, I never smoked with

Quan and his boys. If it hadn't been for my heart, though, I probably would have.

I was still trying to figure out the whole God thing, and even though I never stopped talking to him, I didn't really know if those church "rules" were right for me. I think the real reason that I never tried pot had little to do with my mom's past struggles and the lessons she passed on to me or with my church upbringing. I was just too scared to try it. I knew that if I did, I would end up getting shocked; I didn't need that stress. So I would just pass it along to the next guy and say, "It's all you, man." Having my health as an excuse really did make it much easier to "just say no."

Zac grew up going to church like I did. We both did a decent job of following the rules of the church, partly because it made our parents happy. We had, however, gotten to the point where we needed to discover God and religion on our own. Western didn't necessarily give me a better education than State, but being there did give me Zac's company. He and I helped each other out in many ways during our time at Western. I know he helped me anyway, especially on this journey to discover who God really is, the journey that has turned out to be the most important of my life.

Although Zac started going to church in Kalamazoo before I did, I think we both came to the conclusion at about the same time that we needed to figure this God thing out. I had always just assumed that God was real—that's how I was raised. In addition, how could I ever doubt God after what I had been through? How could I question him after finding comfort in prayer time and

time again? Yet I needed to figure it out for myself and
not just believe it because my parents did, and even
though I had found comfort in prayer, my doubts still
loomed. Maybe the doubts were a product of the environment I was in; maybe they were there because I let
them stay, wanting to try it my own way for a while.
Whatever the case, I would spend the next several
months of my life searching for the truth.

It didn't happen overnight, but slowly Zac and I came
to believe what our parents had been telling us, most of
it anyway. The following year, Chris W. and Dan transferred to Western and moved in with Zac and me. Chris
and I would have some more late night discussions
about God and politics, like we used to do back in the
community college days; now Zac was there to join us.
A lot of the beliefs that I still carry today were formed in
those late night discussions, and I wouldn't trade those
memories for anything.

As I was loving college and enjoying life more than
ever, I started to see the rules of the church in a different way. I started to see the rules as simply the best way
to live. We've heard it before—if God made me, then he
would know how I could live this life to the fullest. He
would know how I would get the most out of this life.
That's all those rules are—God telling us the best way to
live.

As I thought about becoming a better person and living this life to the best of my ability, I saw that the way
was with God. Sometimes we all act like little stubborn
two-year-olds and want to do it our own way. We want
to figure it out for ourselves. Even though someone

points us in the right direction, we insist on going our own way. We've got to do it the hard way. I think that's what those few tough years had been for me.

As I sat there in college, having had some great times both from a social and physical standpoint, I looked back over the hardest year of my life. There I was going through hell as I finished high school and started college, and for the most part, I tried to do it on my own. I had come to the same point my Dad was at back in 1981 when he said, "I can't do this on my own anymore." I don't know the day, or even the month, but my epiphany was sometime during these "good years." I realized that if I had to go through the hell I'd been through before, I wanted to do it with God and not without him. It was as simple as that.

I've never had anyone call me a wimp, laugh at me, or even look down on me for being too religious or for turning to God when I was dealing with my life-and-death issues. As I would wonder if my heart would beat its next beat or as I lived in fear of another shock, I don't think anyone ever said, "You can do it without God. What do you need him for?" I began to wonder why in our culture it's okay to turn to God for the big stuff, for life-and-death issues, but not necessary to try to trust him on the little things.

Through these good years, I was starting to lean on God with each day, occasionally finding a Scripture, as my mom had been doing for years, that I knew was written just for me. One of the Scriptures I somehow memorized on the first read was Romans 8:28: "And we know that in all things God works for the good of those who

love him, who have been called according to his purpose."

It was true too. As I graduated college in June of
1998, four years after I had started, I thought about all
the tough times I had been through. I looked over my
life with gratitude for the hand that I had been dealt. I
stood there on graduation day thinking about how I got
there and who I was. I knew I would be a different person, much weaker and with much less character if things
had been different. I saw how God used some problems
with the admissions department at State to put me here
with Zac and Chris W., and I was thankful. I also saw
how each and every long night in the hospital helped
me grow as a person. As I stood there in my cap and
gown, I felt ready to go out and tackle the real world,
trusting that God would help me through every step of
the way.

It is easy to say you believe something; it's a whole
different thing to put it into practice when the time
comes. The time would soon come for me to prove
whether I really believed what I thought I believed.

Chapter Twelve

Preparation

*People become really quite remarkable when
they start thinking that they can do things.
When they believe in themselves they have
the first secret of success.*

—Norman Vincent Peale

As I was finishing college, I was still gung ho for medical school but decided to take a year off before starting. I didn't want to graduate in June and have only two months off before diving into medical school. I decided to use that year to relax a little and to bolster my med school applications with some "real-world" experience. I got a job at the University of Michigan yet again, this time working in the electrophysiology (EP) lab on the adult side. Adam, the doctor from the adult side that I had seen when Dr. Dick called on him for some help a few years earlier, was still working in that department, along with a lot of other well-respected cardiologists.

I moved in with John and Sandy Barber, friends of Mom's from high school. They used to live in Montrose, and their son John and I were friends before they moved to Ann Arbor. They let me live with them every summer during college and now again after I had finished school. I never did thank them as much as I should have, even though I wouldn't have been able to take those jobs in Ann Arbor if it hadn't been for them.

I worked as a tech in the lab, where physicians implanted pacemakers and ICDs and performed other procedures dealing with the electrical part of the heart. I was working twelve-hour shifts and only had to work three days a week. I was exhausted at the end of each workday, but the six-day weekends made it worthwhile. I spent some of those six days doing research with Adam and a few of the other doctors and did some substitute teaching in Montrose, as I split my time living with Mom and Dad and the Barbers.

I enjoyed all the work but viewed it simply as a stepping stone. With everything I did, I thought about how it would affect my med school applications. I had finished Western with a GPA in the 3.4 range and had scored just slightly above average on the Medical College Admission Test (MCAT), so my academic record wasn't exactly stellar. I needed whatever help I could get. My experience working in the hospital proved to be valuable. After that first summer in college working in the EKG lab, I was moved up to the electrophysiology lab and also got to spend time doing research with Pete and Ian over the next few summers. Our research led to an abstract being published in a small medical journal, and the research that I did while working on the adult side after college got me published in the *Journal of the American College of Cardiology.*

Medical school admissions officers used to tell us, back in 1998, that the average med school applicant applied three times before actually getting into med school. I knew I had my work cut out for me, especially when I got my first round of rejection letters, without even getting an interview. The application process is multilayered. First you fill out primary applications, then secondary applications, and then if they still like you, they interview you and then possibly accept you. Not getting an interview was a sign that I was a little ways off, but I still had one more try to beat the average, so I wasn't deterred in the least.

Dad had always told me to have a backup plan, just in case. He would even go so far as to try to get me to take business classes while in college. He'd say, "You can do a lot with a business degree." I would always just tell him that I was going to get in no matter what, even if it took ten tries. He wasn't satisfied with that, so he forced me to look into a backup plan a little more. Medical sales became the forced backup plan, just as much to make him happy as anything else. Don't tell him this, but I still wish I had taken a few business classes while in college. Yeah, that's the kind of dad I have; he is always right.

That first year out of college, working in Ann Arbor and living between Ann Arbor and Montrose, made everything that was to come possible. It was a time of preparation. The life of a tech wasn't what I wanted to settle into. I wanted more, and I was going for it.

Although it was inconvenient living in two different places, and a little boring with most of my friends still away at college, I kept looking forward with a positive attitude.

As I was preparing for what was to come in my career, I was also inadvertently preparing for the next bout of personal troubles that was to come my way. That preparation came in the form of some spiritual discoveries. For the first time in my life, I had a real hunger to find out what was in the Bible. It started simply with the influence of a good friend, but I would later look back on the help that my hunger would uncover with such gratitude that I could only contribute it to divine intervention. I was starting to see that this is what religious people mean when they say that God gave them something or did something for them. This spiritual growth would become of such value that it could only have been from God, even though it was nothing more than the influence of a good friend. I would later thank God for the "coincidence."

Because I was at home on most weekends, I had started going to church with Mom and Dad again, only now it was because I wanted to go. I started working with and hanging out with the youth pastor who was now at our church. Tim was only about five or six years older than me but married and with a mind set on having a large family. He quickly became a great friend and a mentor of sorts. I guess you could say that about any great friend though. A great friend becomes a mentor because just being with him or her makes you a better person. Tim did that.

We were a lot alike too. We both loved the fun of competition, especially in sports, and were both driven people. Tim's wife, Amy, would often find herself shaking her head saying, "You two are so much alike," as I started to hang out with them more and more.

In some ways, we weren't all that similar though. Those five years that he had on me had shaped him in a way that I was a little jealous of. When you spend any amount of time with Tim, you get the impression that he could handle anything that comes his way, although outwardly it looked as if he never really had any serious struggles. He wasn't the type to go around spouting off Bible verses either, even though he probably knew more than many scholars. In fact, he was the least religious pastor I knew. He simply lived what he said he believed. Why tell someone when you can show them?

Watching Tim live this life inspired me to want to learn more about living like a Christian and to stop just claiming to be one. I started by reading the New Testament, with the book of Acts. I read about this guy named Paul. Turns out he wrote about half of the New Testament and really went through a lot in his life, mentally and physically. This was a dude I could relate to. I started soaking it all up. I knew there was a better way to live, and I wanted to find it. I read about Paul, how he went through so much suffering, yet was able to look back on it with gratitude and joy. Needless to say, I looked at my own life and realized I could learn something from this guy.

For the first time in my life, I was reading the Bible because I really wanted to. I would sit in my room at

John and Sandy's house and read, a first in my life, as I've never enjoyed reading. I underlined passages that jumped out at me. I still use that same Bible today, and 90 percent of what is underlined was done during this period of my life.

Every time I started to seek answers, whether out of compulsion or desire, good things came. This time was no exception. I read things that I had heard over and over in Sunday school and even used in debates with Zac and Chris W., but this time they really hit home. As I read about Paul and his life, I started to put my own into perspective.

I came to realize that we all go through struggles, mine just happened to be of the physical variety. Paul was no different. He had been shipwrecked, blinded, beaten, and stoned. Yet through it all he remained positive, upbeat, and showed a genuine love for life. Although I already had some of those qualities, I wanted more. I wanted to live my life like he did. Looking back on the hard times in my life, the roughest being the year after the carnival, I realized I never wanted to live like that again, and I could choose not to.

In the year following the carnival, I would consistently choose to do what came naturally. The problem was that what came naturally were all bad things, things like fear and worry. I would have to choose to ignore what felt natural and right and do what God wanted instead. I would have to do it the way Paul did—God's way. That choice, I would soon find, was not an easy one by any stretch of the imagination. It would, at times, be a constant mental battle, but one that I was ready for.

I once heard someone say that God will prepare you for hard times in your life. As the summer of 1999 approached, that thought occurred to me while I was reading through the underlined passages in my Bible. Nearly every one was about overcoming, persevering, and suffering. I remember thinking, *I hope this isn't God preparing me.*

Just a few weeks later, I sat in front of Dr. Dick as he told me that I would need another open-heart surgery. I couldn't contain a crooked smile as I shook my head and thought, *Whatever . . . I'm ready.* Dr. Dick looked at me a little funny; I guess a little smile wasn't quite the reaction he was expecting.

I had finally begun to put on some pounds and, as it turned out, the weight gain wasn't natural. For the first time in my life, I was more than 140 pounds, even though I stood six feet tall. Most people had been joking with me about putting on a small little "beer belly" and getting "pudgy." It was about time for that, as I had just finished college, but the extra weight was all water that my body had started to retain, a symptom of heart failure.

After years of being beat up, the right side of my heart was starting to fail. I had gone into mild heart failure, which is characterized by an enlarging of the heart. Unlike other muscles, for the heart, getting bigger isn't better. When the heart is enlarged, it is usually "baggier" and tends to slosh the blood around more than pump it out. Blood hadn't been circulating through my body efficiently, causing a fluid buildup. Another side effect of my enlarged heart was severe damage to the valve that separates the top and bottom chambers on the right side of the heart. As the heart enlarged it stretched this valve to the point where it wasn't working much at all anymore. The solution to these two problems would be to start me on some medications to help the heart pump blood more efficiently and to replace the damaged valve.

I remember the hour drive home that afternoon. It was a beautiful day, the kind that makes you happy to be alive, no matter what is going on in your life. I enjoyed that drive home as I thought about Paul saying that he had learned how to be content no matter what was going on in his life.[1] When I first read that verse, I wondered how that was possible. As I drove home, enjoying the beautiful Michigan summer, his words made a little more sense to me.

I had come to liken this life to running a race. As I drove home, I thought about this new obstacle that I had found on my racecourse. I thought about how I'd been running my race for the past few years on what felt like a flat surface with a little wind at my back and that it was time I had a mountain to climb. The ground only stays flat and straight for so long. I thought about searching for the easy way around this mountain that I was looking at but quickly realized there was none. If I could have taken the easy way around, I probably would have, even though it would mean getting to the other side a much weaker person. That's one simple gift God gave me—an obstacle with no easy way around. I would get home that night and tell Mom and Dad what was going on. I relayed

---

1. Phil 4:11.

Dr. Dick's message to them in layman terms, translating the "doctor speak" as I went. They both handled the news quite well, as I had done earlier that day. With a "Well, we gotta do what we gotta do" type of attitude, they simply asked, "When?" My surgery was scheduled for a month down the line, so we had time to prepare. It was refreshing to have a few weeks notice. Ironically, for the first time I didn't need the notice. I had been preparing, unwittingly, for a few months.

The day of the surgery came fast. I found myself once again riding down to Ann Arbor with Mom and Dad early in the morning. I got checked in and was ready to go. We sat in this little waiting room and did just that, waited. I wasn't the least bit nervous. Honest, I wasn't nervous at all. I kept thinking that I should be, but I wasn't. We sat there and made a little chitchat as we waited, but, really, what do you talk about? Finally they came out to get me, and I gave Mom and Dad a hug and a "See you later," very intentionally avoiding "good-bye," and was off into the operating room (OR).

It felt strange walking into the OR without a mask on, so much so that I even commented to the anesthesiologist about it. Not that I had anything better to talk about. I noticed that there were a lot more instruments around than there is for a pacemaker or ICD implant. Even though I knew what instruments to expect in the room, it still caught my eye. I saw the rib spreaders that in just an hour or so would be exposing my heart. I climbed up on the table and tried to get comfortable. As soon as I stopped squirming and said, "Okay, I'm comfortable," I got nervous.

I don't know what I was nervous about. I wasn't afraid of dying. Maybe I had just seen one too many late night news shows about patients waking up in the middle of surgery. I took a deep breath and said, "I'm all yours" to God in my mind. I smiled as I started to relax. The anesthesiologist leaned over me to place a mask on my mouth. I looked up at her and said, "Thanks," knowing exactly what it was that she was giving me, as I'd seen this done from both sides of the table more than once. I jokingly took in a giant breath, acting as if I were trying to suck all of the nitrous out of the tank. She laughed.

The next thing I knew it was post-op day three, the bad day. Dad was reading the paper and rocking in the chair next to me. The surgeon came in to see how I was doing. I quickly told him how miserable I felt, to which he simply said, "Yeah." After he left, I commented on his lack of compassion. Dad laughed as he said, "He was probably thinking, well, duh, I just cut your chest open." I didn't think it was so funny. I just hit the little button that would deliver morphine on command, but it didn't seem to do anything. That day lasted forever. I don't remember exactly, but I don't think I'd describe myself as being content that day.

Over the next few days I seemed to be recovering well. I don't really remember much about those days in the hospital, just that I believe I enjoyed them a little more than most people would have. In fact, the doctors and nurses were starting to look at me a little funny, in a good sort of way. Almost daily I would get comments about how great my attitude was. I would just say, "Hey, I have to do it, so I might as well enjoy it as much as possible."

I felt like I was skillfully climbing over this mountain. I was proud of myself. I got home and enjoyed the recovery period. I relaxed outside on the deck in the sun, as thankful as could be. Maybe this was the time that I had been waiting for. I felt so good, considering what I had been through, I wondered whether this could be the fulfillment of that promise I knew God had made me years ago. I remembered that night in the hospital when God was telling me things would be okay. I took that as a promise of healing; after all, how else could everything be okay? So as the days went by, I convinced myself that this really could be the healing I thought I was promised. I guess that's why what happened next surprised me so much.

Just a few weeks after my surgery, I was still moving slowly, yet well enough to be left home alone. Mom and Dad were at work, and Stacy was out and about. I was sitting on the toilet. The next thing I knew I was lying on the bathroom floor with my pants around my ankles. My forehead hurt too. Apparently, I had just done a faceplant onto the floor. I got up unsure of what had just happened. I hadn't felt my heart beating abnormally, but what else could it be? I quickly called Mom at her beauty shop uptown and she rushed home. I also called 9-1-1, because I realized that I didn't even know how long I had been out for; I could have been lying on the bathroom floor for hours.

My heart was pounding hard and fast now, but that didn't tell me much. I was nervous and a little scared about what had just happened. I lay down on the couch and tried to relax as Mom arrived. I assured her I was okay but couldn't explain what had happened. Shortly thereafter the ambulance arrived. While the paramedics were taking my blood pressure, I felt my heart take off into a bad ventricular rhythm. In a panic, I told them what was going on, hoping they could fix the problem before the ICD shocked me, even though I knew they couldn't. I got blasted with a shock and never passed out. It scared the hell out of the ambulance guys. In a bit of a role reversal, I assured them that my heart was back in a normal rhythm. They were happy to hear that as they continued to hook up the heart monitor.

In the ambulance on the ride to the hospital, I was once again without any faith. I was nervous and scared. Again I was feeling every heartbeat, hoping the next would be normal as well. How quickly I went from knowing things were going to be fine to being completely frightened of what the next minute would hold. In a matter of minutes a faith that had been building, a faith I thought was strong, had tumbled away. That hard-won faith seemed to be lost too easily. Looking back, I see that it wasn't as strong of a faith as I thought. My faith at the time was based on ever-changing circumstances, strong only when things looked good. An uneasiness started to rise up in me as I thought about how quickly the fear had rushed back in. As I waited in the local ER to be relayed down to Ann Arbor, I thought, *I am not ready for all this.* I wanted out. I wanted the easy way out, but there wasn't one.

By the time we got down to Ann Arbor, I had collected my thoughts and remembered that I was in a mental fight. I knew it wouldn't be easy, and it wasn't.

Every time my mind would try to focus on what could possibly happen, all the bad stuff, I would grab hold of my thoughts and bring them back. I would try to remember some of the things Paul wrote about in a letter to some of his friends and followers. He wrote about keeping your mind on good things. Focusing on what is admirable, noble, pure, holy, or praiseworthy, telling them to simply "think about such things."[2] I remembered the fact that he wrote this letter from a prison cell, going through hard times of his own as he encouraged them to not lose heart in their struggles.

In the emptiness of a hospital room, it was easy to feel alone, even though Mom and Dad sat at my bedside waiting with me. Somehow it was a comfort thinking about Paul, a regular guy, just like myself, who had been through so much. A regular guy, chained in prison, waiting to see if he would be beaten yet again, who made it through in an extraordinary way. I thought about how he had every reason to worry as much as I did, probably more, when he wrote those words of encouragement to his friends. Instead of worrying, however, he was helping his friends, telling them to not be anxious about anything, as God is always near. He told them instead to thankfully take it to God, and a peace would come to guard their hearts and minds.[3]

Every few seconds my mind would want to wander back to the negative, but I couldn't let it. I remembered Paul talking about focusing on eternity, and not the here

2. Phil 4:8.
3. Phil 4:5–7.

and now. Somehow that helped, as I understood what he meant when he told his friends that sometimes it feels like our physical bodies are wasting away, but not to get discouraged, as inwardly God is renewing us day by day. He went on to tell them to stop fixing their eyes on what is seen, as it is only temporary, but instead to focus on what is unseen, as that is what lasts forever.[4]

I hadn't memorized these verses word for word, but I remembered them as best I could. I also tried to think about perspective, knowing that I was going through this hell and torment for a reason, even if I didn't know what that reason was. I tried to keep my mind on better things than the fear and suffering I was dealing with. I was a long ways away from sharing Paul's perspective about his troubles. I wasn't yet rejoicing in my sufferings, but I was in a far better frame of mind than I had been before. I had found a little more of that peace that Paul had spoken of. I also had something to hold onto and to fight with. So that is what I did, hour after hour.

By the next day I was still a little nervous, but had my thoughts and fears under control for the most part. Dr. Dick came in with some great news. My ICD had gone off in the bathroom, and apparently I was only out for a few seconds. Better than that, they gained a little insight into my problem. A few years earlier, they implanted an ICD that recorded my rhythm when I got a shock. I had gotten this newest ICD when the battery on the old one was about dead.

---

4. 2 Cor 4:16–18.

The recorded rhythm showed that my irregular rhythm started with a short pause followed by an extra heartbeat. That was the "trigger," as they called it, for my heart to take off into an abnormal rhythm. They thought that if they could upgrade my ICD to the kind that was able to pace my heart all the time, like a pacemaker, they could prevent the pause. Made sense to me. The best part was that preventing the pause would stop my heart from going into a bad rhythm. It was no guarantee that I would never go into the rhythm again, but it could greatly reduce the number of times my heart would misbehave, thus reducing the number of times I would get shocked.

I quickly signed up for the upgrade. The new ICD would have two wires going into my heart—one for the top chambers of my heart and the other, which was already in place, for the bottom chambers. It turned out to be a painful surgery, partially because I was still recovering from the previous one. The hope that it brought, along with my newfound perspective, helped me though.

As I was recovering in the hospital, Adam came to visit and brought me a pizza. I was surprised that he would take the time from his overwhelming schedule to come over and see me. He stayed for a while chatting with Dad and me while we ate. Adam's visit meant a lot to me. The only side of Adam his coworkers usually get to see is the fifteen-year-old boy part, so it was nice to see this other, more caring, side of him.

Pete and Ian stopped in often too. One day Pete brought me a gift and could hardly contain his smile as he gave it to me. I opened it to find the ugliest tie I had ever seen. It had a giant picture of Elvis on it. I looked at Pete as if to ask, "What's this all about?" He tried to hold back the laughter as he said, "Well, you almost went out like Elvis . . . on the toilet, so . . ." My laughter wouldn't let him finish.

Needless to say, I made the best of the recovery time yet again. I had some good times in the hospital, especially when either Pete or Ian was on night call. If I was feeling even close to up to it, I hung out with them for most of the night. I tried to learn everything I could from them as well, as it was all so interesting to me. Just as I was starting to feel good, Dr. Dick sent me home.

Once again I was sent home with high hopes, and once again I found myself back at the hospital before long. In that short time at home, I was confident that my situation was improving. The doctors had found out how to prevent the bad rhythm, or to make it happen less often at the very least. It couldn't get much better than that. I was happy, and, to be honest, I was giving all the credit to God. I couldn't wait to get back to work and to try to get into medical school again. I couldn't wait to get out there and do all kinds of things again. After all, God had finally come through on his promises to Mom and me.

I don't remember how the next one got started, but soon after I was home I found myself in a bad rhythm again, praying it would stop before I passed out or got a shock. It didn't and again I got two shocks before my heart started to calm down. This incident seemed worse than most of the others. Maybe it was looking in Dad's eyes and seeing his fear and weakness; maybe it was because I thought I wouldn't be experiencing this again at all, let alone just a few weeks after I had gotten the new ICD.

I must have looked like an idiot at the time. It was late at night and I was in Mom and Dad's room. I don't know why my heart went out of rhythm yet again, but I remember going in their room looking for help once it did. I lay there on the bed with Dad sitting next to me, his eyes full of fear. I started yelling at God as I was waiting for the rhythm to stop. "I am not going to quit; whatever you want to do, do it. I am not giving up. I trust you. Thank you, God, for taking care of me 'cause I know you will." I stopped to tell Dad, "The shock is coming." He gave me this big bear hug, as if to try and cushion the blow, even though it was coming from inside. I was drained and scared; I just wanted it to stop. *Why was this happening again?* Once again I was living in pure misery. The hell would only last about five minutes, and, after the second shock, I was left to once again deal with my thoughts and fears, wondering whether a third shock would be coming at any moment.

The ambulance came and we went to Flint but didn't get to Ann Arbor until very early the next morning. I was exhausted mentally and physically. I hadn't slept all night. Everyone who came to see me had a look of pity in their eyes—Sarah, the ICD nurse, then Dr. Dick, and then Ian. He was the worst. I tried to get some sleep but was unable to relax my exhausted body. He stood at the foot of my bed with a look of pity on his face. His head was cocked to the side as he asked me how I was doing. His eyes welled up with tears. I lost it and started to cry. I hated that he felt bad for me; I just wanted to be normal. Even though I appreciated how much he cared, I didn't want to have someone feeling bad for me.

Over the next day or so I don't even know what we did. I am guessing I started a new medicine, or they reprogrammed my ICD or something. I do remember wondering how I was going to get back to life. How was I going to get off to medical school? I just didn't want to live life like I had after the carnival. Shortly thereafter, I remembered I didn't have to. Again I took this mental battle head-on. I managed to get home and get back to living. I remembered that promise I had made myself all those years ago, while sitting on the edge of that hospital bed. I didn't want to just survive life. I wanted to live it. Now I had the tools to be able to do just that.

Even though this mountain had ended up being so much higher and steeper than I had thought it was going to be when summer started, I had made it thus far. I didn't know if I was still going to be climbing up either. For all I knew, I would get out of the hospital and have another problem the very next day, but I didn't let that deter me. I had made it this far without seeing my next step; I could make it through whatever else was to come.

I also started to see that even though my experiences had all been hell, each of them had come to an end. Some lasted seconds, some minutes, some hours, but each time I found myself on the other side knowing I had made it. I was starting to believe that I could get through just about anything, even though I still wasn't ready to be joyful in hard times, as Paul wrote about time and time again.

Luckily for me, I would get some more chances to try.

Chapter Thirteen

A New Direction

*Our greatest glory is not in never falling, but
rising every time we fall.*

—Confucius

I got home from the hospital and continued making
plans for medical school and to get back to work at
the hospital. For the most part I was dealing with things
really well. As I looked toward the approaching winter,
I wasn't quite ready to hit the ski slopes again, a sport I
was introduced to in high school and really enjoyed in
college, but I was back into my day-to-day life without
problems.

It was so much easier dealing with trying circumstances now that I had a reason, now that I had some
biblical wisdom helping me along. For the first time in
my life I had a sense of purpose to drive me through the
hard times that would come each day. I was no longer
striving to find my identity or purpose in a job or anything else that really doesn't matter. I now saw a reason
for what I was dealing with; I started to see the big pic-

ture. My faith wasn't anything temporary either and that was the best part.

My experiences were making me who I was; they were shaping my character. I think Paul said it best in the book of Romans when he wrote, "We rejoice in the hope of the glory of God. Not only so, but we also rejoice in our sufferings, because we know that suffering produces perseverance; perseverance, character; and character, hope. And hope does not disappoint us, because God has poured out his love into our hearts . . ."[5] Those hard times, the suffering, had indeed produced perseverance and character. They had made me who I am.

I was starting to understand how Paul could say that he took joy, or rejoiced in, his sufferings and hard times. He saw who he was becoming through those tough times and liked what he saw. I saw myself as a person of much better character than I would have been without the hard times. I looked at each tough or painful event in my life and saw what I'd learned. I could see where I had grown as a person with each hospitalization or struggle while at home. My perspective shaped the way I responded to my latest batch of problems as well. Other people noticed too.

One day that fall I was talking with Sarah, a nurse working with Dr. Dick in the pacemaker and ICD clinic. She was planning a weekend-long support group meeting for patients with ICDs and asked if I would speak at it. Although I really enjoyed speaking, I hesitated. I never liked the idea of going to one of those meetings.

---

5. Romans 5:1–5.

I guess I didn't really like the idea of people thinking that I was there because I needed help; I had handled things and didn't want to appear weak. Thankfully, Sarah encouraged me to come to help other people. She told me that at the time she was following about twenty ICD patients in their clinic. I was just about the only one who wasn't medicated for depression or seeking help from a mental health professional. This was a tough thing to deal with, and I was doing well. She would later refer to me as a role model for other patients. She really wanted me there, so I told her I would do it, more as a favor to her than anything else.

I started to collect my thoughts over the next few weeks on what I was going to say. How do you tell people how to deal with a problem as complex as this in twenty minutes? Everyone who hadn't been shocked was scared about what it would be like, and those who had were scared that it would happen again. How was I going to address this? I could talk about how it really wasn't that bad and that before you know what it is, it's over. How could something that lasted less than half a second be painful? I could talk about how after all I'd been through I learned that no matter what had happened there was always an end. Or, maybe I should just tell them about how much I love life and how I had learned to enjoy every minute I could, because you never know when it would end. I could talk about being thankful that we have this device to save our lives. I could tell them to have some perspective; after all, wouldn't you be willing to go through five minutes of hell if it meant that you would get to go on living? I guess I knew that they had probably heard all that before. I mean, that is the kind of stuff a psychologist would tell you, or so I thought. I wanted to find something more. I wanted to find the real reason why I could live my life without this heart problem or this device controlling me.

One day the Discovery Channel aired a special about the U.S. Navy Seals. I was half paying attention when this guy, apparently the one in charge, came on to explain the navy's philosophy. He talked about how they beat the crap out of their recruits and made them endure everything imaginable. He went on to say, "In this training they made them suffer, because when they suffer they develop perseverance, and perseverance develops character in their troops; this then gives them a hope, a hope that they can get through just about anything." Now I don't know whether he realized it or not, but he was quoting Paul, almost word for word.

As I sat there watching this, I realized I had found the focus of my speech. I would talk about taking joy in the hard times, looking forward to the good things that will come because of the difficult ones. It seemed radical, but it was simply looking at life through a different set of glasses. I had learned to see the benefits that had come from being forced to climb that mountain. I got up on stage that day and relayed my message to about one hundred patients and family members from around the state. I simply encouraged everyone to keep on pushing through the tough times and to try to keep a good attitude. I was several years ahead of almost everyone else there in this process of dealing with these issues from the ICD. I just let them know that they would someday look back, happy they went through it all.

After I finished I stood in the corner for quite some time talking, one at a time, to what seemed like almost everyone there. I was glad Sarah convinced me to come, not only because I was able to help, but also because I found a little comfort that day too. Although I was the old veteran at dealing with the mental struggles that the ICD brought, there were several people there who had grown and learned a tremendous amount from all of their other medical battles. I was reminded that in the grand scheme of things, I wasn't too bad off.

After telling this large group of people my way of dealing with the mental battle, I was challenged to walk the talk. I already was to some extent, but I was now forced to adopt this new way of thinking in everyday life or be a hypocrite. As I got back to work I did just that. I got back into the swing of things without hesitation. I now had less to be afraid of, as I looked at what the future might hold, because I knew whatever it was, God would "work all these things for the good," as Paul wrote.

I quickly returned to the job of pursuing my goals. I thought and worried about my heart daily, but I pressed on into my future headfirst. As I dove in, a funny thing started to happen. I was working at the hospital and applying to medical school, but my thoughts about the future started to change. It was a slow process, but I started to see that old backup plan as a better and better option every day. I realized I would be pretty good in the world of medical device sales and thought it looked like a better gig than this doctoring stuff.

I had gotten to know the representative from the company that made my ICD pretty well over the years. Keith was a big guy who always carried a smile into the room with him. He would check my device when Sarah wasn't around or when he had something new to teach her. I had always thought he was a technical or a clinical representative, but he was in sales. I got to see this sales side of him as I worked with Adam and the boys all that year in the EP lab.

Late in the fall of '99, I started to spend as much time with Keith as I could while he was at the hospital. He would come in for almost every pacer or ICD implant. I learned a lot from him about pacemakers and defibrillators and even got to hear a little bit about what it would be like to work in medical sales. The more I learned the more I loved it, and I was starting to believe that maybe my backup plan was a better choice than medical school. Most people who work for medical device companies, however, come from strong clinical backgrounds, spending at least five years in an EP lab, like the one I was working in, before a company like the one Keith was working for would hire them. I only had one year of experience, so I kept pursuing medical school as an option. Five years seemed like a long time.

That October I heard of a possible opening at the company Keith worked for, and asked him about it. It couldn't hurt to ask, even though I thought the chances of getting hired were slim. He picked up the phone and made a few calls. About five minutes later he came back and, hand-ing me a piece of paper, told me to call this guy for a phone interview.

Later that night I got on the phone to talk to Mike, a manager for some other area, but I didn't care where he was from. This was a great opportunity, and I wanted to see what would happen. We talked for several minutes and then he asked, "Are you familiar with the Flint and Saginaw area?" *Oh great,* I thought, *back home.* I had gotten out of Montrose and loved life in the bigger cities of Kalamazoo and Ann Arbor. The last place I wanted to end up was back around Flint.

About two weeks later I found myself moving back in with Mom and Dad so I could start my new job as a clinical representative with the company I was first introduced to when I was seventeen years old. My parents' house was smack dab in the middle of this territory they needed help in. Although I wasn't enamored with the location, the opportunity was an incredible one, and I was thrilled.

The night before I was supposed to start my new job turned out to be an eventful one. I was in my room getting ready for the big day that was to follow when my heart started racing. All of a sudden, for no reason, it was going 180 beats per minute. *What the heck was this?* I felt horrible. My adrenaline was rushing as I quickly grabbed for my pulse and braced for a shock. After a few seconds passed and I was able to relax a little, I realized that my heart had probably gone into an atrial arrhythmia, the bad heart rhythm coming from the top chambers of the heart that isn't life threatening. That's when I realized it was beating at about 180 bpm—not quite fast enough to cause my ICD to fire. Although I was a little more relaxed, I didn't feel well. I had only been in this rhythm for about a minute, but I wanted it to stop, and soon. I became a little short of breath and everything inside me was trying to panic. I calmed my mind, hoping my body would follow.

I ended up in the hospital for the night. By the middle of the night, the doctors got my heart back into a normal rhythm but wanted me to stick around for a while so they could try to figure out why this had started and if there was anything they could do to prevent it from happening again. So I spent the day that was supposed to start the opportunity of a lifetime with Pete at the hospital. It eventually just got chalked up to "one of those things," and I was sent off knowing it would probably happen again.

Needless to say, my first few weeks on the job were a little nerve racking. At twenty-three, I was already the youngest person to ever work in the field for this Fortune 500 Company of more than ten thousand employees—and slightly intimidated, as I would be the guy giving clinical and technical advice to physicians. Now I wondered whether I would be in the middle of talking with a doctor, or helping one with a surgery, and have my heart take off racing. I basically tried not to think about it. I just had to go into my job trusting that no matter what happened, God would make sure things would work out for the best, as Paul had written.

Trusting was starting to get easier to do. Here I was a graduate of my second-choice college, working at my second-choice job, living in a town I once wanted to get out of, and absolutely as happy as could be. Looking back over my life, I started to see that even when things didn't go as planned, or maybe even especially when things didn't go as planned, it always worked out better than I had dreamed. This job that I had started was no different.

I'll never forget the first day I met Jeff, the sales rep for the area I would be working in. As a sales rep in the device industry, Jeff couldn't possibly attend every device implant that one of his customers did, so I was there to help him. Whenever one of his customers needed someone to check a patient to make sure his or her device was working properly, to give an in-service for a new product, or to join the physician in the operating room for an implant, I was the guy.

I met Jeff in the lobby of a hospital in Saginaw, Michigan. Jeff was in his late thirties, tall, and in good shape. His suit fit like none I had ever seen, far better than the suit I had been proud of up until that moment. The best part about Jeff, though, was how easy he was to talk to. He was the kind of guy who could carry on a conversation with anyone and be genuinely interested. We chatted for a few minutes before heading off to meet some of his doctors. It didn't take long before I realized that Jeff was very good at what he did. As an aspiring sales rep, I watched every move he made. This was a guy who had other reps calling from around the country asking for his advice, and I got to work with him every day. Over the course of that next year, Jeff started to become a friend as well as a mentor, and I gave him all the effort I had.

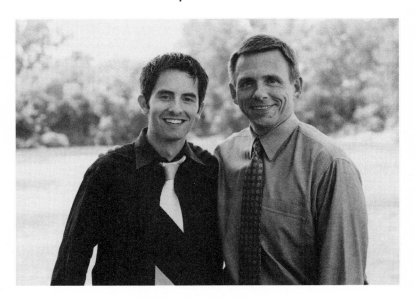

Jeff (right) and me in Saginaw

I worked my butt off that first year. Jeff and I were the only two people covering one of the biggest territories in the country. I was so happy and loved it so much I hardly noticed how much I was working. In fact, after about three months of working with Jeff, I threw out my med school applications, never even filling out the secondary apps that I had received. You could have offered me medical school for free, and I still wouldn't have gone. I felt like I was made to do this job. I had found my niche.

I will never forget our national sales meeting in January of 2001. Here I was, just twenty-three years old and only on the job for thirteen months, when they awarded me with the Field Clinical Representative of the Year award. I had achieved my extremely lofty first-year goal on the job. My next big goal was getting myself promoted from a clinical rep to a sales rep.

Chapter Fourteen

The Longest Night

We should be careful to get out of an experi-
ence only the wisdom that is in it—and stop
there; lest we be like the cat that sits down on
a hot stove-lid. She will never sit down on a
hot stove-lid again—and that is well; but
also she will never sit down on a cold one
anymore.

—Mark Twain

I had moved out of my parents' house a few months before that national sales meeting, after saving up some cash. I bought a condo in the neighboring town of Clio. I loved it because it was right on the golf course but also closer to the highway that I was traveling daily. My original plan was to get promoted up to a sales job and to move to wherever it would take me, hopefully to a bigger city. Now, Clio is no New York or Chicago. In fact it isn't even a Kalamazoo or an Ann Arbor. I had, though, started to enjoy it there.

I was still going to church with Tim and working with him with the youth group. I was also giving baseball a go once again. I had originally gone out to a church slow-pitch softball practice with Tim with the idea of coaching. I soon figured out that the rules of church softball are pretty relaxed and fun, so I could actually play. I would simply get a pinch runner when I got on base so I didn't have to push it too hard. I could have run, but I didn't trust myself. I am not very good at going at 80 percent; it's either all or nothing. If I ran my own bases, I knew I would eventually get myself into trouble trying to stretch a single into a double.

I even recruited Stacy's new boyfriend to play with us. Aaron was a great guy and we all loved him, but I really loved him on our softball team, as he was quite the athlete. Out there on the field it just didn't seem like it could get much better—the sun low in the sky, a nice warm summer breeze, and the sweet smell of the grass.

One game late in the summer made me question whether I should continue playing. I was warming up with Tim and we were joking around when I started to feel funny. The next thing I knew I blacked out and woke up to everyone standing around me. Stacy had been there to cheer on Aaron in his efforts on the field but was the first one I saw when I woke up. "How long was I out for?" I asked her after taking my pulse to discover that it was nice and regular. "Did my ICD go off? Did I get a shock?"

"You just hit the ground and then woke up within seconds," Stacy nervously replied, almost puzzled with the fact that I had lost all sense of time. I sat there for a few minutes before calling my dad to see if he could drive me to Ann Arbor to see what was going on. This didn't seem normal (for me), and I wondered if it was even my heart. After thinking for a moment, I realized that this time I didn't even have to go to Ann Arbor. *I* was the guy who checked ICDs and who helped the physicians figure out what had happened. I grabbed my programmer (the computer that pulls information out of the ICD) and checked out my own ICD. I faxed the strips down to Dr. Dick to figure out what was going on. Once again I had had an episode of ventricular tachycardia and was on my way to brain death when my ICD brought my heart back into a normal rhythm. My device was working. It had saved my life again.

The season was soon over, and so I didn't have to decide whether I should continue to play. I just went to work the next day and didn't let the episode affect me too much. I continued to put everything I had into work and helping Tim out at the church. Although the Clio and Montrose area wasn't exactly a haven for young single people like myself, I was starting to appreciate being around my family more and more. It was pretty obvious that things were getting more serious with Stacy and Aaron, as talk of marriage started to come up. I was sure they would stay in Montrose, as they both enjoyed the small community that they had grown up in.

Mom started decorating her house for Christmas, and I was inspired to trim the condo a little and even got myself a tree. It was fake, but I didn't have time to water and clean up after a real one, even though I missed the smell it brought to the house. I was enjoying the holiday season unaware that my next opportunity for growth would be coming soon.

I went to bed one night after my normal routine. I have always loved getting into a cold bed in the winter, quickly curling up into a ball to try to get warm. It's one of the small things that make life so enjoyable. On this particular night I drifted off to sleep as usual.

The night would not go on as usual though. I woke up in the middle of the night feeling a shock from my ICD. I sat straight up in bed and felt my heart. It was beating fast, but I thought that was just because of the adrenaline rush that a dream had brought. It is common for ICD patients to mistakenly think they got shocked; usually this occurs during sleep or when just drifting off to sleep. The mind is such a powerful thing that a dream of swimming in a pool and getting a shock can seem real. I had that dream more than once and so my first thought was that I had indeed had one of these "phantom shocks," as doctors call them.

I couldn't remember any dream though, and I just didn't feel right. I was a little shaky and my adrenaline was rushing like I had had an episode. I couldn't believe that I had gone into a bad rhythm in the middle of the night; nothing like that had ever happened to me before. Most of my problems, the serious ventricular kind anyway, were usually with exercise. I felt funny enough to get up and check it out though.

I got out my programmer and retrieved the information out of my device. The EKG showed my heart beating normally, then going into that bad rhythm, then the shock came, and then I was back to normal. It wouldn't even hit me until the next day that without a doubt I would have been found dead the following morning had this happened before my ICD was implanted. For the first time, I was totally alone when I had a problem. My ICD was the hero for sure.

I hadn't thought about that fact when I first saw the printout, though. All I could think was *Why?* In medical terms, I mean. I wondered what had caused my heart to misbehave. After coming to the conclusion that I wasn't in any further danger, I tried to go back to sleep, but it wasn't easy. Because I had never had this problem when sleeping before, sleep time had become a bit of a sanctuary for me. No matter what I was going through or how much I felt my heart racing, I always knew that if I could just get to sleep, then things would be okay. Or at least I wouldn't be worrying.

After an hour or so of wrestling with my thoughts, I dozed off. That was a testament as to how well I was doing at dealing with stress at the time. I could have been consumed with thoughts of how and why. I could have been worried sick, waiting with every breath for the next big shock to come. The opportunity for worry was perfect, yet I was able to pass it up.

The next day I called Dr. Dick and let him know what was going on. He was pleased to hear that my ICD was working so well. I also had lunch with Dad that day and told him about it. I didn't want to, because I didn't want to worry him and Mom, but I realized I needed to. They would want to know. They didn't seem to be too worried; after all, I was fine now. Hard information is sometimes easier to accept after the fact.

It took me a while to get into bed the following night. I've always been prone to stay up late, but on this night

I was simply avoiding bed. Again I faced the mental fight. I prayed for quite a while as I paced around the house before I got in bed. I was able to find peace before drifting off to sleep quickly.

I didn't sleep too well that night, but I knew it would take a little time. I had realized that this getting shocked thing was a lot like a mouse with a piece of cheese. If you shock mice when they are getting cheese, they won't go after the cheese anymore. Day after day, I saw ICD patients who got shocked while walking "too quickly," and so they paced their gait from that day forward. Other patients felt a skipped heartbeat before their shock, so every time their heart skipped from then on they would stop in their tracks, paralyzed with fear, waiting for the shock to come. I had done this myself time and time again in the past. This time, however, I knew there was no avoiding it. I could stop swimming or playing softball if I wanted, but I had to sleep.

I worked that next day, still tired after a few nights of rough sleep and anxious to get home and relax. I was confident about getting a good night's sleep, as those days of taking weeks and weeks to get over my troubles were gone. After putting off bedtime for only a few minutes this night and pacing and praying, I got into bed. I even enjoyed settling in and getting comfortable as I usually did. I was off to sleep fairly quickly around midnight but would only get about two hours of good sleep that night.

Again I woke up to what felt like a shock. Sitting up as quickly as was humanly possible and gasping for a big breath of air, I grabbed my chest. I pretty much knew this time that I had been shocked and quickly went to see what had happened. Again I pulled up the EKG strips and again I had been shocked. This one got to me—mentally, I mean. I thought about calling Mom and Dad and the doctors but decided to do neither.

The rule of thumb is that if your device goes off once, and you feel okay afterward, you can wait until morning to call and talk to the doctors. That is exactly where I found myself, and I knew that no one at the hospital at 2:00 A.M. would have any answers as to why this was happening anyway. I tried to figure it out but couldn't. Basically, my mind just raced to anything and everything, the good and the bad.

Again I thought about calling Mom and Dad but realized they couldn't do anything either. When I was younger and I would wake up feeling funny or having extra heartbeats that would unnerve me, one of them would come and sit with me. They would pray for me and talk me back to sleep. It always made things better. I knew if I called them this time, it would just scare them for no reason. Tonight I was on my own.

After about an hour of wrestling with my thoughts as I paced around, I again convinced myself that there was nothing I could do. I couldn't prevent a life-threatening heart rhythm if it was going to happen again, and so I might as well try to go back to sleep. That would be the easiest way to get to the morning. I got in bed and tried to pray myself to sleep. I was drifting off much quicker than I had expected when my body jerked awake. Once again I was wide awake and sitting up.

Most of us have been on the very edge of sleep when our bodies jerk themselves awake for no good reason. Startled, we awaken as if to say, "What's going on?" We then usually relax and roll over within about two seconds and easily fall back to sleep.

Well, imagine that with the thought of a large shock looming in the back of your head. That is what was going on with me. I had this hugely exaggerated instant wake-up, like a ten-foot alarm clock resting next to my head would bring. I realized it pretty quickly as my heart was racing but none of the other signs of a real shock were there. I took a deep breath and fell backward onto my pillow. I would just have to try again.

As time passed, conscious of every heartbeat, I eventually managed to start to relax again and again, and as I was on the verge of sleep, I experienced another phantom shock that sat me up. It was like having a terrible nightmare every time I relaxed, without ever getting the chance to fall asleep. After another hour or so, I was so mentally and physically exhausted that I couldn't take it anymore. At least that's what I told God. Thankfully he would give me the opportunity to prove myself wrong.

I went into the living room to my favorite chair. Maybe that would work. It didn't. After more time passed I found myself lying flat on the floor staring at the television almost in a trance, hoping to trick myself into sleep. I watched television for as long as I could and then fell asleep without knowing it. That didn't work. Just as I was drifting off, my subconscious would jerk me awake. I must have had six or seven phantom shocks by that point, each one feeling as real in my mind as any of the shocks that I had actually gotten. I was tired and sick of fighting my own thoughts. I wondered if I would ever sleep again. I felt like I was at the end of my rope, but I didn't know what to do. There was nothing I could do.

I watched music videos on television as I tried to pass the time and think about anything but what I couldn't get out of my mind. A song by Allison Moorer called "Send Down an Angel" came on. The song is actually about a boyfriend or something, but all I could do was repeat that chorus to God, saying "Send down an angel to get me through." I would go on asking God to "Send someone or something to get me out of this. Give me some peace, relax my mind, help me through."

As I lay there I felt like he was leaving me out on my own for this one. I didn't understand why; I was so frustrated. My mind was a mess. I thought about God and how all he had to do was give me some peace of mind. He could do it. I knew he could. At least that is what everyone had always taught me. That is what I read about in the Bible. Heck, I'd even experienced it myself. I felt like he wasn't, though, as I jerked back awake yet again.

That night turned out to be the longest of my life. I spent the entire night wrestling with my thoughts, trying to get some control over them. I tried to convince myself that I wasn't worried or scared; I tried to tell my subconscious not to worry. I tried to get some sleep, but I couldn't. I experienced five hours of hell like I'd never known. I had dealt with some long nights with some serious physical pain, but nothing like this. I was begging to be in the middle of one of those nights as dawn approached.

I finally decided that I wouldn't be able to sleep so, not having anything else to do and wanting to occupy my mind, I got dressed and went to work. Now, I am not a morning person so I am never up before the sun, but as I got dressed this morning it was still dark. I got in the car and headed out, counting the hours until I could reach Dr. Dick at the hospital.

I got just a few miles down the road when I was stopped at a red light on the overpass to I-75. I had sat at this light hundreds of times looking out over the array of fast-food joints and car dealerships. Looking down the road, I noticed the horizon. Way off in the distance was the beauty of a few trees, as the road seemed to go on forever. As I sat at that light for what seemed like ten minutes, the sun started to come up over the end of that road, up over the trees. The timing was precise as the tip of the sun edged its way above the trees just as I was pulling to a stop. I sat there and watched that sunrise totally amazed, as if I'd never seen a glowing sun with a velvety orange sky behind it. It was the most beautiful thing I'd ever seen.

I sat there and suddenly started to cry. Tears quickly filled my eyes, and I choked back the large lump in my throat. I felt as if God brought the sun up just for me that morning. I had made it through the dark night and God had been with me, even though I felt so alone. I felt so thankful for every little thing and was ashamed that I'd rarely gotten up to see the sunrise. I was so thankful in those few moments as I thought about the long night before. When the light changed colors, I quickly wiped my eyes dry and cleared my throat. I then sped off onto the highway.

I don't remember what I did that day, or even where I went. I don't remember the phone conversation I finally got to have with Dr. Dick, and I definitely don't remember what I wore. I do, however, remember that sunrise as the perfect end to a perfect night. I wouldn't trade the experience for the world. That one night helped shape me more than any other five hours in my life had. That one night gave me a strength I couldn't have imagined having.

I had reached that place that Paul had written about in his letter to his friends in that town of Philippi. Paul wrote about enduring hardships and persevering to the end with joy and thankfulness, all the while chained to a guard in prison. I could hardly wait until my next battle came, just to see if I would remain as thankful.

Chapter Fifteen

Hassles and Rewards of '04

Don't measure yourself by what you have accomplished, but by what you should have accomplished with your ability.

—John Wooden

Within a few days of that long night I found out that one of my medicines was enlarging my thyroid. The enlarged gland was causing an increase in heart rate and abnormal activity, thus the shocks even while sleeping. Within a few days I was off of that medication and on a new one. As I changed medicines, I had to sit in the hospital yet again, this time working from my bed whenever possible. I took calls from customers and played on my laptop, trying to find work to pass the time.

The change in medication went smoothly, and I was soon released, heading home curious and a little worried to see if this medicine would cause problems or prevent them. I was a little nervous but able to move on quickly, as I looked forward to our annual family vacation to Florida.

This year's vacation would be different for me. I had just been taken off of a medicine that I'd taken for more than ten years and that made my skin extremely sensitive to sunlight. During that time, I had to wear large hats and long sleeves no matter how high the temperature got. Since my early teen years, enjoying the sun was something I simply had to give up. I'd get around it, though, usually starting by applying SPF 50 every half hour or so. To play golf, I scheduled tee times at either 7:00 A.M. or 7:00 P.M., and I was always looking for beach chairs in the shade. After a while, you start to forget what you are missing, but this year I would get the chance to remember.

As I went down to Florida with the family and Aaron, now Stacy's fiancé, I had already forgotten how nice the sun was. I remember riding in the car from the airport leaning out of the window trying to get as much sun as I could. "This is how the sun is supposed to feel?" I had honestly forgotten. Not only had my old medicine made me sunburn easily, but the feeling of the sun had changed as well. Whenever I would be in the sun for more than a few minutes, I could feel my skin start to prick as sunburn was setting in. It was incredibly unpleasant.

As we drove out of the rental car garage at the airport and onto the highway in our rental car that day, I was truly amazed at the feeling the sun had brought. The warmth was so perfect it felt like a hug from God. I kept commenting over and over to my family about how amazing it was. They just laughed at me, puzzled that I could have actually forgotten what the sun was supposed to feel like, but I didn't care. I loved it. I spent so much time outside on that vacation, simply lying there and soaking it in, with a little grin on my face all the while.

As time went by, I made sure not to live my life waiting for my next bout of troubles but to appreciate the small things in life. Although I had learned to appreciate what those struggles brought to me, I didn't want to depend on them for my happiness. I remember talking with Dad once when he warned me about people who can only seem to find happiness when they are going through a struggle. If they go long enough without running into a tough time, well, they usually just end up creating one for themselves. It's as if they need the drama in their lives. I wanted to appreciate and make the most of every tough time that I found coming my way, but I didn't want to create unnecessary struggles for myself. That's one reason why I try to appreciate the easy times as well, enjoying simple things like being in the sun and spending time with family.

As the next year or so went by, we found our family growing. Stacy and Aaron got married on June 1, 2002, and bought a little house in Montrose just as predicted, only a few miles from Mom and Dad. I was still in Clio just ten miles away. I was promoted to sales rep later that year, having waited for a position that would allow me to stay close to my family. I guess the big city no longer held all of its appeal when compared to family. I also found the opportunity to continue to work with Jeff in this new position, as he brought me in as a partner, sharing a few of his accounts.

One day I was called to a new account of mine because the patient had requested that I be present for

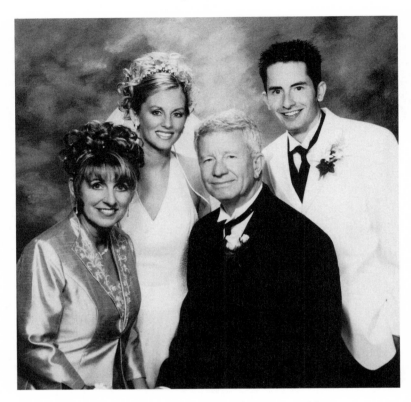

Mom, Stacy, Dad, and me on the day of Stacy's wedding (Photo courtesy of Rick DeLorme www.delormephoto.com)

his ICD implant. He requested me and my company, even though the doctor had planned to use a device from another company. Special requests from the patients, although nice, were rare in the ICD business, but I got there, brought the ICD in, and put on scrubs to join the doctor in the OR. The surgery went well. I didn't know the patient who had requested me, only that he was a friend of my parents. I called Mom and asked her about him that night. As it turns out, he was the husband of the nurse who had saved my life in 1981 in Mom's beauty shop. His wife was the nurse with half-done hair whose feet I passed out at. Here I was, twenty-some years later, now helping to keep her husband alive.

I didn't come across many more patients like that, but all in all things were cruising along great, both at work and at home. I had quit playing softball to coach the team, which was more fun than constantly trying to restrain myself. We had a lot of fun together and won the league championship.

By the time May of 2003 rolled around, the battery on my device needed replacing. Because it is actually easier to replace the entire unit than just the battery, I got a whole new device, one that was much smaller than the first two devices I got years back. This one was actually a little smaller than a deck of cards—a real deck of cards. The surgery went well, and I was home recovering that same night. Mom and Dad came over and spent the next few days with me at the condo to help me get around. I was moving pretty slow for a few days, but I enjoyed the time.

As 2004 approached, the family grew yet again as Stacy and Aaron had a son. Ty Aaron Emmendorfer was born on November 1, 2003, and I must say he is the coolest, cutest, and smartest kid ever, even though he was only half-Noble. I love that I live so close and can watch him grow up and watch Stacy and Aaron as first-time parents who no longer give Rocky the dog all of the attention.

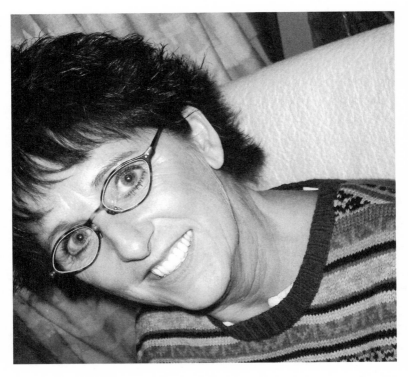

My mom, hair done perfectly, after staying up all night when Ty was born

About this time, I started getting less attention—and was liking it. Ty had become the new day-to-day entertainment for the family. Gone were the days of everyone asking how I was feeling, sometimes more out of boredom than concern. I was, however, having more and more of the atrial arrhythmias, which always bring a little unwanted attention my way. They seemed to pop up at the most perfectly inconvenient of times and were tougher on me mentally than physically. These episodes don't feel good, as my heart starts racing for no reason at all. I would be sitting, walking, or even sleeping when my heart would jump from 60 or 70 bpm to 170 or 180 bpm in one beat. It is not a comfortable feeling by any stretch of the imagination. Each and every time I would have one of these episodes, my mind would start to race. It was as if my mind were filled with thousands of little drawers, each one containing a possible scenario of what could happen now that my heart was racing. I could get a shock, I could get a lot of shocks, I could pass out, it could trigger the bad kind of heart rhythm, or I could die. All these little drawers would pop open in my mind, some realistic and likely, some pretty farfetched.

I had to make the choice to close the drawers. When I would think about a possible negative scenario, I would chase it from my mind. The worst thing I could do was open it up and explore it in more detail . . . *I could get shocked, and that could possibly do this, and then this could happen and then that* . . . If I opened up that thought and explored it, it would always lead to unnecessary worry. The battle would take place when I went into the abnormal rhythm, when I thought I might go into the abnormal rhythm, or simply when I found myself in a situation where I didn't want to go into that rhythm.

In February of '04 I again flew down to Florida to join the family for the annual vacation. We were on separate return flights for different reasons. Aaron flew back one day, Stacy, Ty, and I were out the next, and then Mom and Dad came home later still. As Stacy, Ty, and I got to the airport, I was a little nervous about flying with Ty. He was only four months old, and I was expecting him

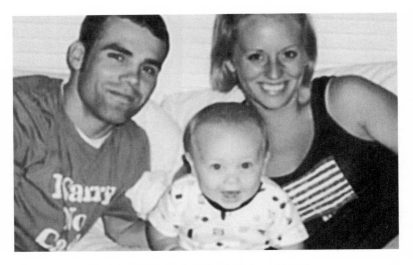

Aaron, Ty, and Stacy in July of 2004

to scream the whole way home. Stacy also didn't feel good, having a bad earache. I had my own issues, but I was trying not to think about them. All day I had been having a lot of extra heartbeats, usually a sign that an abnormal rhythm could start.

As Stacy and I sat there at the gate waiting to board the plane, Ty was as content as could be. I was not. About thirty seconds before we were to start boarding the plane, my heart took off. I was in the atrial arrhythmia going about 170. "Crap," I sighed.

Stacy quickly asked, "What?" I told her and she gave me a look that said, "What do we do?" I took a deep breath and sat down, my mind racing, trying to figure out what to do. I didn't want to get on the plane and be trapped forty thousand feet above the ground for two and a half hours.

Just as I was starting to think of a plan that might be feasible, my heart all of a sudden reverted to its normal rhythm. I assured Stacy that things would be fine. "I'm fine now," I said, as I tried to convince us both. "Really, I am." She agreed and we started to pack up to get on the plane. I didn't want to get on the plane, but Stacy needed some help with Ty. She was feeling sick with her earache and would have a tough time making it through the flight without me.

Although my heart was in a normal rhythm, it kept skipping beats. I would have two normal beats then a skipped beat, as if my heart were teasing me. We got on the plane and had to move seats three times because of some ticketing errors. I was fighting myself mentally, all the while keeping a cool face for Stacy. I fought that battle the entire flight home. My heart skipped and paused and flipped and flopped and flirted with the idea of getting out of rhythm for the entire two and a half hours. None of us enjoyed the flight.

I tried to fill my mind with good things, with the truth. The truth was that no matter what happened, I would look back on it with fondness, even if I were looking back from heaven. What was happening was making me a stronger person, the person I wanted to be. I tried to give up control and let God handle it.

Time seems to go slow when you are fighting a mental battle. The physiology doesn't help. When your heart is beating erratically, your body sends out a signal to your brain that something is wrong, even though there is nothing you can do about it. Even when your thoughts are right where they should be, you still feel "geared up" due to your body's response. That two-and-a-half-hour flight seemed to last forever. But the fun didn't stop there. Three quarters into the flight, Ty puked on me and then leaked diarrhea all over my pants. That didn't help my mental battle either.

I face this mental battle just about every day. Sometimes it is just for one split second as a thought enters; other times its lasts for hours. Either way I have to respond in the same way. I shut those drawers and put my thoughts where they should be. Life is a mental battle for all of us, and I am no different. Some people worry about losing their job and others worry about having enough money to buy food. Worrying if my next heartbeat will be a normal one is just my battle.

The atrial arrhythmias went from happening once every few months to every few days. It even happened once while I was walking down Bourbon Street in New Orleans with Jeff during a conference. That was one of the few times the rhythm corrected itself without any intervention. Thankfully. I couldn't imagine going to the ER in the middle of the night in New Orleans.

As this problem started interfering more and more with my life, my job, and my peace of mind, I decided to have a procedure know as an ablation. An ablation is a lot like a cardiac catheterization, only instead of going in to unclog arteries they go in to ablate, or selectively damage the part of the heart causing the bad rhythm. It usually works well for atrial arrhythmias, and there really isn't a lot of risk. So that was the plan.

Most people would come out on the other side of this with either a cure or a "Sorry, we just couldn't get it."

Well, as you can probably tell by now, I am far from the norm. The ablation worked well, and the bad rhythm was gone, but because my heart was so beat up, I would almost certainly have the rhythm pop up again someday. When that would be, no one knew.

The diagnosis was a little frustrating. I didn't want to have to think about it anymore. I didn't want to have to worry about it while traveling or living my daily life. It would have been great to hear "It's gone; you can quit worrying about that." Again, I wouldn't get the easy way out.

People inevitably reach a point in their lives where they can choose to take the easy way or the hard way. In almost every difficulty, be it marriage, career, or something else, people get to choose how to deal with it. If a couple hits a rocky spot in their marriage, they can avoid the situation by spending more time at the office. Or, they can do the work required to improve the relationship. But I can't take the easy way. I don't have a choice. I've got to deal with it. My only choice is to deal with it in the way that comes naturally, with worry and fear, or deal with it God's way, which at the time always seems to be harder.

If you were able to choose the right way every time, even though you knew it would be harder, think of how strong you'd be. As I ask myself that question, it makes me realize how lucky I am not to have the choice, because I know I would have taken that easier road just about every time. Although initially I was disappointed with the news that I would have a problem again someday, I thought about the good things it would bring. I would be forced to deal with this, again and again.

How do I deal with it? Day by day. Every day I simply have to make the choice to shut those drawers in my mind when they pop open. Have I totally conquered it? No. But I must say that I am a lot better off than I was when I tried to do things my way.

I try not to compare myself with other people when I think about things like this, because frankly I am doing better than most folks in my situation. I could easily become content with where I am at by comparing myself to others. So each day I get up and compare myself to me. I get up every day and try to be better than myself, better than I was in days before. Some days it seems easy, and some days it's hard.

Although the ablation went well, I had a problem with one of the wires that runs from my ICD into my heart. It was a complication from the procedure that I had never seen, only heard about, even after all my years in the world of cardiac electrophysiology.

Chapter Sixteen

Really Living

If one advances confidently in the direction of their dreams, and endeavors to lead a life which they have imagined, they will meet with a success unexpected in common hours.

—Henry David Thoreau

I went to Ann Arbor to see Dr. Dick and Pete to try to figure out what to do about the complication from the ablation. Pete was done with his fellowship and working alongside Dr. Dick at the hospital. I was glad to have him around; I now had a replacement for Dr. Dick when he decided to retire, one I trusted as much as Dr. Dick. It was interesting to have this little meeting with them. I was now playing the role of patient and technical consultant from the company. It was a situation with no clear answer, and because I was so knowledgeable, the decision basically fell to me. I decided to wait and see what would happen; we would do nothing. I wanted to keep things status quo because the procedure to fix this wire in the ICD was not as simple as it would have been for most patients.

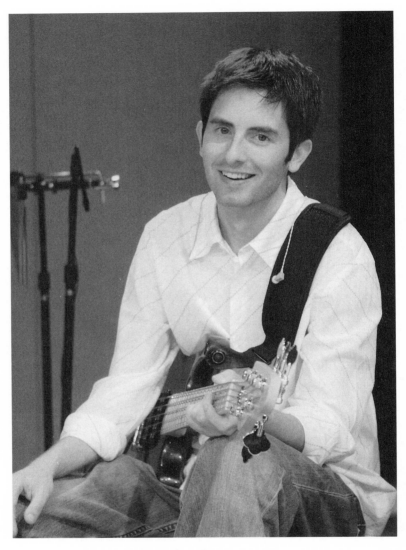

Me with my bass at church (Photo courtesy of Lisa Stone.)

I knew as I left the hospital that day that, by deciding to do nothing, I was at a higher risk of getting a shock. The pacemaker part of the ICD was no longer working, and my heart could have these little pauses (of less than half a second) that could help trigger the life-threatening rhythm. It could happen, but would it?

Yep, just a few days later, but this time it wasn't so bad. After the shock, I just relaxed for fifteen minutes or so. I used that time to look at the rhythm strip. I saw the rhythm that would have ended my life had it not been for my ICD and then simply went on with life. I didn't take a nap, didn't stop everything, didn't go to the hospital. In fact, I even played bass at a church event a few hours later after inhaling a Happy Meal. This time it was much easier to handle, even though nothing was different. It was the same rhythm, the same shock; I even started to pass out just the same as in previous times. The only thing different was me.

I was finally treating my ICD as it should be treated. My ICD is an awesome life-saving device that only causes less than a tenth of a second of discomfort every few years, in the form of a shock. I may have painted the picture here of the big bad ICD, but I've been thankful for it since the day I got it. It didn't come without its fair share of struggles, but none that has stopped me from achieving great things in life. In fact, the ICD has made my life possible.

Once I'd gotten that shock, a medical indicator that the surgery would indeed need to take place, I talked to Pete and scheduled it for the following Tuesday. As I

prepared for the surgery to fix this device that I had
been carrying inside of me for the better part of ten
years, I thought about how great it really was. It had
kept me alive. I couldn't blame the ICD for my mental
battles.

As I went in to get this device fixed, and thought
about the thousands of people who would be getting
one that year and in the years to come, I smiled. They
would also have a chance to live a little longer and enjoy
a little more because of this little device that I was selling. It was just another sign that I had stumbled upon
the right career path.

Coming out of the surgery in the spring of '04, my
recovery time lasted about three weeks, triple the
amount of time it would be for most ICD patients, as my
device wasn't implanted in the usual position just under
the collarbone. My device was still in my abdomen,
where they implanted them in the early '90s before
improving the technology, which complicated things.

I was sore, but the worst of the pain only lasted a day
or so, and I actually enjoyed the next few weeks. I
kicked back in my favorite chair (I know I am not supposed to have a favorite chair until I'm fifty, but I don't
care) and found a comfortable position. Once comfortable, I relaxed and enjoyed the break.

That spring I had been going through a bit of a
"quarter-life crisis." I was twenty-eight years old and already settled into the career of my dreams. What was I
going to do now? Was this it? My success seemed to have
come too soon. I had chased after this thing for so long,
now it was here, and I wanted more. I was also thinking

about finding a wife and making a family for myself. I never expected to be single at twenty-eight—a part of me didn't expect to be alive at twenty-eight—but I always thought if I were around, I'd be married.

As I recovered, I thought about this stuff yet hadn't resolved anything in my mind. I decided to find someone who could help me get some resolution about my "crisis." For the first time in my life I went to see a counselor.

I didn't want to go; I wrestled with the idea for quite a while. The questions, however, didn't go away. As I kept myself from going I soon realized that to me, this life had always been about doing the best I could with what I had been given. I wasn't doing the best I could if I couldn't stop and ask for some help. I could be a better person if I had someone helping me along. Friends go a long way, and I had some great friends who have been there to help me out, but it's amazing how someone trained to ask the right questions can get to the source so much quicker.

With all I've been through, it's funny how what got me to a counselor had nothing to do with my physical heart, but rather with matters of the heart. I saw Nancy, the therapist, only about five or six times, but with a few simple questions she was able to help. I realized that I was indeed doing it right, living I mean. I wasn't put on this earth to find a wife, have a family, or sell pacemakers and ICDs, even though those are all good things. I was put here for so much more. To me, this life is simply a preparation for eternity, and I felt like I was doing that well.

Some may say it's the fact that I dream of living a life without any type of worry that makes me believe in an eternity. It's the thought of being able to swim and run without any threat of a shock or death that makes this dream stick in my head. They say that when faced with the hard realities of this life, I believe in a heaven to give me a hope for the things I'll never know on this earth. That could be. However, we all have at least one thing in this life that we dream of escaping. Why is the dream of escaping to that eternity there? Is it because there is something more?

As I watch my nephew, Ty, approach his first birthday, I see so much frustration as he tries to move about. He gets so mad when he wants something but can't get to it. This frustration makes him unhappy for most of the time, but, without it, he wouldn't have the drive to try to walk. He would never want to take the risk. I can see how scary it is for him. He stands there holding on to his mother's hand, scared to let go. What gets him to let go and move forward? It's that drive that is deep inside him, encouraging him to take that step of faith. It's that desire inside that makes me know there is something more. After all, why would we have the desire for more, if there were no more to be had?

Facing death on a daily basis tends to force you to decide what eternity holds. Maybe it is the beauty of creation, or maybe the miracles in my life, but I have come to the conclusion that there is a God. After that realization, the next logical questions are numerous. Who is he? Can I know him? Will he help me? What does he

want me to do? How do I get close to him? After searching out these answers through all of my battles over the
years, it has started to become clearer to me. In searching, I've come to believe that death is not the end for
me. I've come to believe that this life is simply a preparation for that eternity in which I will live, an eternity in
which I will know true satisfaction and happiness.

So great, I've gotten eternity taken care of, but I have
to be honest. Most days I don't want to feel better later;
I want to feel better now. How does all that God stuff
help me now? I've asked myself that question more than
once. The answer came when I looked not only to Paul,
but to the one he was following. Paul often spoke of the
one who was greater than he, Jesus.

For me the clarity came when reading that Jesus said
that he had come so that we could have life and have it
to the full. Just by following him, as Paul did, we could
have life and have it to the full? That sounds great to me,
but as I look at some of the people around who claim
to be followers of Jesus, I don't see them living life any
differently than anyone else. They don't seem to have
the life Jesus spoke of. Is that because this Jesus is full
of crap, and his ways aren't really any different, or just
because people fail from time to time?

It's easy to judge an entire religion based on a few
people who are trying to live it, but, as humans, we
inevitably fail. No one here on this earth has it perfect,
or entirely right. I've seen Christians whose actions have
scared me away from the church, but thankfully, I've
also seen men like my dad, Chris W., Zac, and Tim, who

have made me want to find out who God really is, simply because I like what I've seen in their lives. I'm just glad I never stopped looking.

When going through a hard time, I tried to learn from friends, but I also learned to go to Jesus and Paul, one of the first ones who tried to live life as Jesus taught. Living by his principles has made my life richer.

Trying to continue on this path, and live this life to the fullest, is what causes me to go out and learn from Paul and everyone else who wrote that book. Living this life to the fullest is what makes me get up every day and try to be better than myself. God didn't make us all alike, so I can't imagine he is expecting the exact same from all of us. Therefore, I try to avoid comparing myself to the people around me. Instead, I simply try to improve daily, striving for the perfection spelled out in the Bible.

With the parents I've been given and the situations I've been put through, it would be impossible for me not to be the person I am today, and I'm thankful. I feel like I am standing on third base, and I know I didn't hit a triple. At the same time, as I get up each morning and face the day, it doesn't always feel like I'm on third base, and it doesn't usually feel like I've got it made. Each and every day I make about a hundred choices that determine how I am going to live. Some of my choices are better than others.

It's easy to say "I want to be a loving father," or "I am going to be a great husband," or "I am going to live my life, not simply survive it," but it's an altogether different thing to actually do those things. To succeed you have to continually do them; they are not onetime actions. A loving father is not just loving when he feels good, a great husband isn't just great on Mondays, and I wouldn't be living my life if I didn't try to tackle those mental battles each and every time they came. I would simply be surviving.

Feeling like I've been given so much, sometimes I wonder whether I'm doing with my life what I should or could be doing. I wonder how I am doing compared to my own potential. If I could look at my life as God does, knowing my genetics, my environment, and all of the circumstances in every situation, how would I stack up against my own potential?

The great thing about potential is you never know how high it goes. Not until you exceed it do you realize that there could be more. I had handled "all I could" dozens of times in my life only to find out a few months or weeks or days later that I could handle more. With each year that passes, my self-expectations rise. What once used to be a daylong mental struggle is now dealt with in seconds.

I'm often asked, "If you could do it all over again, without the heart problem, wouldn't that be great?" Sure it would, as there are times when I do wonder what it would be like never to feel the effects of any medication, as I have taken pills nearly every day of my life. I wonder what it would be like to never have the "what ifs" creep up in my mind, and I wonder what it would feel like to have a normal heart. Would I feel any better than I do right now?

Sure it seems nice at first thought to take that "redo" and live this life without these questions, but as I think about what it would be like to live that "normal" life, I can honestly sit here today and say "no thanks." I wouldn't trade my life for one without the heart problems if offered the chance. I am who I am because of each and every experience that is written on the pages of this book. Each and every struggle has brought me to where I am today, to this place that God wants me to be, and for that, I am thankful.

I've also realized that these questions that come up in my mind are not so special. I ask questions about living without medication, while others ask entirely different questions. What would it be like to feel more loved? What would it be like to love myself? What would it be like to have two parents? What would it be like to have one parent who really loved me?

What keeps me from getting bothered by these questions of mine, besides knowing that we all face our own personal struggles, is knowing that I still may see the answers on this side of eternity and will surely see them all on the other side. As I look at where I have come from, and where I am at today, I can see that I still may conquer the "what ifs" if given enough time. I can't help but wonder how much more I will grow before I no longer have the chance to.

As I look into the future, I try not to think a lot about what it holds. When I do think about growing old and raising kids, I wonder if I'll live that long, as I am sure I still have more struggles with my heart ahead of me, unless of course God decides to intervene. Yet, I wouldn't want that fear to keep me from experiencing something so great. All I can do is take it day by day and trust that

God will take care of my tomorrows, just as he has taken care of me up through today.

So I guess I'm going to enjoy the autumn as it approaches, my favorite time of year in Michigan, and keep my eyes open for a woman who is willing to share this life with me. I'll keep on selling devices and helping patients when I can, until it's time to move on. If I wake up tomorrow, I will try to do a better job at living than I've ever done before, not becoming complacent in my strengths and not giving up on my weaknesses. If I find myself living in the days to follow, I will love those close to me with everything I have. As struggles come my way, I will try to keep trusting them to God, knowing that he is working them for some sort of good, praying that they are not any harder than they have to be, yet knowing that they will be as hard as they need to be.

Yes, I am going to keep on loving this life, for as long as I'm around, enjoying every bit I can.

Epilogue

Today as I sit here putting the finishing touches on a book that I never thought I would pen, I am enjoying this life. Enjoying the simple things. Today I am relaxing in the peacefulness of a Saturday, while yesterday I had fun with the craziness that the end of the quarter usually brings at work, stopping mentally just long enough to enjoy a beautiful car ride, which made the day great. For the hour trip between two small cities in mid-Michigan, I had the window down and enjoyed the cool in the air. I enjoyed every bit of that simple little ride, looking out at the fading summer. I saw the beauty of the color-filled trees, with the perfect music playing on my iPod. I guess that's all it really takes to keep me satisfied anymore—something that simple.

Mom and Dad are enjoying the little things in life too. As I look at my mom and see how far she has come, I'm encouraged. She is now a grandmother like no other, loving her family as I can only hope to. She still enjoys life more than anyone I know, always looking for an opportunity to laugh. She, like I, has also found her peace with God. She looks back on the struggles of her life and ahead on the ones surely to come with thankfulness. For they have shaped her too. She now sits back with her quiet confidence in God, accepting whatever comes next.

She left the questions of "why" behind long ago, finding a peace without an answer. Could it have been the pot or the fertility drugs? She, like I, would tell you it doesn't matter in the least. She takes the life that has come her way with joy, thankful for all of it. Dad would tell you that it is always good to ask why as you look back, just to see if you brought your troubles on yourself. If you realize you have, learn from it and move on. If you haven't, just move on.

I know I haven't talked about Dad as much as Mom in this book, but frankly, to know me is to know a part of him. His fingerprints are on each and every page of this book, even though he hasn't directly helped me type a word.

As I look at him now, his hair covered in gray, I see glimpses of my grandpa Noble. The way he scratches his stomach or the stupid names he makes up for people remind me of his dad, and it makes me smile.

I worry a little about him though. The biggest inspiration of my life, the one I've learned the most from, is getting older. Like his father before him, he sits in his late fifties looking ahead to an inherited kidney disease that is causing problems. He sits now on the verge of being added to the kidney transplant list. I can't help but wonder if we will switch places, me watching from the sidelines while he battles in the game. I wonder if we will get a chance to see our past through each other's eyes as this problem starts to present itself. I try not to think about it, except in prayer, because as Dad has taught me, there really is no point in worrying about what I cannot control.

As I watch both of my parents with Ty, their first grandson, I am reminded of my youth. I can't help but smile as I sit back and watch Mom rocking and singing Ty to sleep with kid songs I haven't heard in over twenty years. I watched Dad tie a long rope from his belt to Ty's walker to keep him moving as he walks around the roads that overlook the golf course in their new neighborhood. It's just like him to think of an easy way to entertain a child for hours. He walked around those streets with Ty until his little legs were about to fall off, even though Ty wanted to keep going.

As I watch Ty, the new center of our family, I can't help but notice my little sister all grown up. Stacy is twenty-five and the best mother I have ever seen, second only to our own. She and Aaron are happy, having a few struggles like any other young married couple, but doing well. As I watch her as a mother and wife, I am truly amazed at the woman she has become. Her entire life she was put in second place yet she was willing to give more than she got. I still find her giving, giving everything she has to her new son and husband.

She's dealt with her own struggles, especially as a teenager, but has grown up well. Never knowing what she wanted to do with her life besides raise a family, she finally started listening to her mother at about age twenty-three. She entered beauty school and was a third-generation natural.

She works two days a week now. Mom works the other three at the beauty shop where they share a chair. When Stacy works, Mom has Ty. Grandma has managed to spoil him completely. At only ten months old, he cries and reaches for his grandma every time she walks in the room. He has already learned that she will give him everything and anything he wants, spending hour upon hour catering to his every whim.

I guess that's what grandmas do though, and Mom has a lot of practice. After all, she has been treating Stacy and me like grandkids ever since day one, spending too much money at Christmastime and always there to listen. She has always given of herself whenever possible.

As I sit here, I find myself feeling both proud and thankful for the family I have been given. Each one of them has made sacrifices for me and because of me. For that, and their love, I am truly thankful.

Matt Noble
October 2004

More about ICDs and Sudden Cardiac Death

Though Matt Noble's medical issues are relatively unusual, sudden death is not. Sudden cardiac death (SCD), also called sudden cardiac arrest (SCA), is the leading cause of death in the United States. The Centers for Disease Control (CDC) estimated that in 1999 as many as 460,000 people succumbed to sudden cardiac death in the United States.[1] More people die from SCD than from any type of cancer, stroke, or AIDS. Yet very few people, even few medical professionals, understand that SCD is a public health problem. Why is this?

Unlike most other disease processes, SCD happens in most patients only once, and then the patient is dead. The acute disease process is remarkably brief. Contrast this with most other types of devastating diseases, which usually evolve over months or years. Media attention

---

[1] MMMR Weekly. February 15, 2002 / 51(06);123–6. http://www.cdc.gov/mmwr/preview/mmwrhtml/mm5106a3.htm

and research efforts tend to be focused on these diseases, while SCD has received minimal attention until very recently.

Sudden death is generally due to a heart rhythm disturbance (ventricular tachycardia or ventricular fibrillation). Usually, this arises in a region of prior heart muscle damage (heart attack, cardiomyopathy, or other less common processes). In most cases, patients will have established heart disease, but in other cases cardiac arrest is unfortunately the first manifestation of cardiac disease. Less commonly, cardiac arrest can occur in the absence of any apparent disease of the heart muscle.

During cardiac arrest, there is no effective pumping of blood by the heart to the brain and other organs. Once cardiac arrest occurs, the likelihood that the patient will survive decreases sharply with each passing minute. The risk of irreversible brain damage also increases markedly with time. Cardiopulmonary resuscitation (CPR, see below) can help protect the brain during cardiac arrest, but in most cases an electric shock is necessary to restore the heart to normal rhythm. In most cities in the United States, if a patient has a cardiac arrest outside the hospital, the likelihood of survival with good neurologic function is less than 5 percent.

CPR and AEDs

It has been known for many years that rhythmic compression of the chest and artificial respiration can circulate some blood and provide some oxygen to the brain and other vital organs during cardiac arrest. The American Heart Association (AHA) offers many courses in CPR and Basic Life Support (BLS); course schedules and

other information are available on the AHA website
(http://www.americanheart.org). An automated external
defibrillator (AED) is a semi-automatic version of the
external defibrillator familiar to fans of medical television dramas. Both AEDs and external defibrillators can
deliver an electric shock across the chest wall to abort
sudden cardiac arrest and restore normal heart rhythm.
Standard external defibrillators require trained medical
professionals to operate. I say AEDs are "semi-automatic"
because one crucial part of the process requires a
bystander's input—attaching the device to the patient in
cardiac arrest. Once the external pads are affixed to the
chest wall (as directed by a diagram on the device), the
AED automatically analyzes the heart rhythm and directs
the bystander as to whether or not a shock should be
delivered (this part has also been manual, though some
newer devices can be programmed to deliver a shock
automatically if appropriate). AEDs can improve out-
comes from cardiac arrest in "high traffic" areas, such as
airports, casinos, and shopping malls. Although many
people assume that an AED will be difficult to operate
properly, after minimal training lay people have no difficulty.[2] In fact, one study showed that untrained sixth-
grade students did remarkably well in using an AED in
a simulated cardiac arrest situation.[3] Another concern

---

[2] The Public Access Defibrillation Investigators. Public-access defibrillation and survival after out-of-hospital cardiac arrest. New Engl J
Med 2004; 351: 637–46.

[3] Gundry JW, Comess KA, DeRook FA, Jorgenson D, Bardy GH.
Comparison of naive sixth-grade children with trained professionals in the use of an automated external defibrillator. Circulation.
1999; 100: 1703–7.

among bystanders is that they might inadvertently hurt the person who is in cardiac arrest. In fact, a person in cardiac arrest is more dead than alive, and prompt action on the part of bystanders can be life-saving. Furthermore, Good Samaritan laws protect bystanders trying to help cardiac arrest victims. Though laws vary from state to state, the federal Cardiac Arrest Survival Act provides additional protection for those trying to help.

Implantable Cardioverter Defibrillators (ICD's)

The ICD is the internal, fully automatic AED. In fact, the original name for the device was the AICD, with the "A" signifying "Automatic." The development and refinement of the ICD is a remarkable tale of inspiration, opposing conventional wisdom, perseverance, and technological triumph.

The ICD was developed by Michel Mirowski, M.D., and Morton Mower, M.D. Mirowski initially conceived of the concept of a fully automatic implantable defibrillator in 1966, after a colleague died suddenly. The initial manuscript discussing the implantable defibrillator was published in 1970 and received harsh criticism, including a scathing editorial written by one of the inventors of the external defibrillator. Mirowski was not dissuaded, and a prototype device was implanted in a research animal in 1975. The first human implant was in 1980, and the device was approved by the U.S. Food and Drug Administration (FDA) in 1985.

Initial devices consisted of epicardial mesh electrodes, which were implanted on the external surface of the heart, and a large pulse generator (or battery pack), which was implanted in the abdominal wall. Thus, implantation of an ICD was fairly substantial surgery. Despite this, it quickly became clear that ICD implantation was a life-saving therapy, even in patients who were quite ill at the time of implant.

The next twenty years were filled with technological developments. Transvenous lead systems essentially eliminated the need for major chest surgery to place mesh electrodes on the surface of the heart. In addition, pulse generators were miniaturized substantially. Thus, nearly all ICD recipients receive their device under the collar bone, just like a pacemaker. Detection and therapy algorithms have grown more sophisticated. Some life threatening arrhythmias (ventricular tachycardia) can be terminated with a painless pacing algorithm, eliminating the need for shocks in many cases. Detection algorithms have become more accurate, so that present-day ICDs deliver therapy for non-life-threatening arrhythmias much less frequently than in previous years.

These dazzling technological advances, however, have been matched by a series of clinical trials documenting the efficacy of the ICD in improving survival. Initial trials focused on patients who had already survived cardiac arrest or ventricular tachycardia. These clinical trials, the largest of which was performed in the United States (AVID Trial), firmly established that these patients should receive an ICD rather than a medicine that tries to prevent recurrent arrhythmia.[4]

---

[4] The Antiarrhythmics versus Implantable Defibrillators (AVID) Investigators. A comparison of antiarrhythmic-drug therapy with implantable defibrillators in patients resuscitated from near-fatal ventricular arrhythmias. New Engl J Med 1997; 337: 1576–83.

Subsequent clinical trials have identified groups of patients who have never manifested ventricular tachycardia or cardiac arrest who nonetheless benefit from ICD implantation. Since the chance of surviving a cardiac arrest is so low, identification of patients at high risk for their first cardiac arrest is of vital importance. Two clinical trials have markedly expanded the pool of patients eligible for prophylactic, or preventative, ICD implantation. The MADIT-II Trial, completed in 2001, demonstrated that patients with prior heart attack and poor heart muscle pumping capacity (left ventricular ejection fraction (LVEF) ≤ 30%) live longer if an ICD is implanted.[5] The SCD-HeFT Trial, completed in 2003, included patients with coronary artery disease as well as other forms of heart muscle weakness.[6] In this trial, patients with mild to moderate heart failure symptoms, and moderately severe heart muscle dysfunction (LVEF ≤ 35%), lived longer with ICD implantation compared to optimal medical therapy.

---

[5] Moss AJ, Zareba W, Hall WJ, Klein H, Wilber DJ, Cannom DS, Daubert JP, Higgins SL, Brown MW, Andrews ML; Multicenter Automatic Defibrillator Implantation Trial II Investigators Prophylactic implantation of a defibrillator in patients with myocardial infarction and reduced ejection fraction. New Engl J Med 2002; 346: 877–83.

[6] Bardy GH, Lee KL, Mark DB, Poole JE, Packer DL, Boineau R, Domanski M, Troutman C, Anderson J, Johnson G, McNulty SE, Clapp-Channing N, Davidson-Ray LD, Fraulo ES, Fishbein DP, Luceri RM, Ip JH; Sudden Cardiac Death in Heart Failure Trial (SCD-HeFT) Investigators. Amiodarone or an implantable cardioverter-defibrillator for congestive heart failure. N Engl J Med. 2005 Jan 20; 352: 225–37.

What More Can You Do?

At a personal level, anything you can do to prevent or slow progression of heart disease will reduce the chance of cardiac arrest. Quitting smoking, controlling diabetes and high blood pressure, losing weight, improving diet, and increasing exercise are all incredibly important. Medical therapy for heart disease as well as its risk factors can also improve survival. If you or someone you know has heart disease, it is important that they know *all* of their important numbers. While the public is aware of the importance of blood pressure and cholesterol measurements, fewer patients realize the importance of LVEF. Many patients who have reduced LVEF will be candidates for preventative ICD implantation. Other patients who should be evaluated for risk of sudden death by cardiac electrophysiologists, specialists in heart rhythm disturbances, are patients with a history of passing out spells or palpitations, or a family history of sudden death or passing out.

At a community level, there is much that everyone can do. Learn CPR and how to use an AED and support community AED programs. The National Center for Early Defibrillation (http://www.early-defib.org/) can help plan and implement these programs. Support the American Heart Association and the Heart Rhythm Society (http://www.hrsonline.org), the professional organization of cardiac electrophysiologists. Lobby government officials to ensure that ICD therapy is available for all patients who stand to benefit from it. Like that emergency medical "something or other" who miraculously arrived for one of Matt's first cardiac arrests, you never know whose life you might save!

Leonard Ganz, M.D., F.A.C.C.
Temple University School of Medicine
The Western Pennsylvania Hospital
Pittsburgh, PA
August 2005

Leonard Ganz, M.D., F.A.C.C. is a cardiac electrophysiologist at the Western Pennsylvania Hospital in Pittsburgh, PA and an Associate Professor of Medicine at Temple University School of Medicine in Philadelphia, PA. Dr. Ganz conducts clinical research and teaches, writes, and lectures widely regarding heart rhythm abnormalities. His passion, though, remains taking care of patients with heart rhythm disturbances. His wife Sue Ellen, and children Rachel, Alana, and Michael keep him in rhythm.

About the Author

Matthew D. Noble lives in Michigan where he is a clinical expert and sales representative for a medical device company selling implantable defibrillators, the devices that prevent sudden cardiac death. He also spends a great deal of time traveling the country speaking at venues ranging from churches to hospitals and everywhere in between. He shares his stories about his life as a way to both encourage others, and increase awareness of Sudden Cardiac Death.

For an update on Matt and his family, or to contact him directly about booking a public appearance, please visit his website at **www.matthewdnoble.com**. You can also write him at:

Matthew D. Noble
C/O Russell Douglas Publishing
13097 Golfside Ct. Suite 103
Clio, MI 48420

Lecture Notes on
Occupational Medicine

Lecture Notes on Occupational Medicine

H.A. WALDRON
Occupational Health Department,
St Mary's Hospital,
London W2 1NY

FOURTH EDITION

OXFORD

BLACKWELL SCIENTIFIC PUBLICATIONS

LONDON EDINBURGH BOSTON

MELBOURNE PARIS BERLIN VIENNA

© 1976, 1979, 1985, 1990 by
Blackwell Scientific Publications
Editorial Offices:
Osney Mead, Oxford OX2 0EL
25 John Street, London WC1N 2BL
23 Ainslie Place, Edinburgh EH3 6AJ
3 Cambridge Center, Suite 208
  Cambridge, Massachusetts 02142, USA
54 University Street, Carlton
  Victoria 3053, Australia

First published 1976
Reprinted 1977
Second edition 1979
Portugese edition 1983
Third edition 1985
Reprinted 1988
Fourth edition 1990

Set by Times Graphics, Singapore
Printed and bound in Great Britain
by The Alden Press, Oxford

DISTRIBUTORS

Marston Book Services Ltd
PO Box 87
Oxford OX2 0DT
(*Orders*: Tel: 0865 791155
        Fax: 0865 791927
        Telex: 837515)

USA
Year Book Medical Publishers
200 North LaSalle Street
Chicago, Illinois 60601
(*Orders*: Tel: (312) 726-9733)

Canada
The C.V. Mosby Company
5240 Finch Avenue East
Scarborough, Ontario
(*Orders*: Tel: (416) 298-1588)

Australia
Blackwell Scientific Publications
(Australia) Pty Ltd
54 University Street
Carlton, Victoria 3053
(*Orders*: Tel: (03) 347-0300)

British Library
Cataloguing in Publication Data

Waldron, H.A. (Harry Arthur)
  Lecture notes on occupational
  medicine.—4th ed.
  1. Industrial medicine
  I. Title
  616.9803

ISBN 0-632-02764-9

Contents

Preface to Fourth Edition

The latest edition of these lecture notes comes after a period of considerable change, both personally and within occupational medicine as a whole. There is great interest in occupational and environmental medicine at present, the latter stimulated to some extent by the development of so-called 'green' politics in this country. Important developments in occupational medicine include the promulgation of the Control of Substances Hazardous to Health Regulations which came into force in October 1989 and which are probably the most important measures since the Health and Safety at Work Act of 1974. The advent of the single European market and the changes which might follow from the Social Charter are also likely to have a profound effect upon occupational health practice in this country. There is thus every reason for practitioners in this country to be as aware of the importance of the interaction between their patient's work and health as their colleagues in Europe and North America seem to be.

I hope that this book will continue to be of help to those who are either starting their careers in occupational health practice or who are still at medical school; it does not, of course, pretend to do more than whet the appetite and perhaps help some of its readers pass their examinations. If it succeeds in creating an interest in occupational medicine where none existed before or of reinforcing an interest already present, then I shall be well satisfied.

Preface to First Edition

The relationship between occupation and health has been recognized for several hundred years, but it is a topic which is still generally under-represented in the medical curriculum. This book presents to the medical student a concise view of the subject in a way which I hope will stimulate him to take more account of the occupation of those patients whom he will see, both in his training and, later, in his professional life. I have particularly stressed the interaction between occupational medicine and other areas of environmental health and suggested that hazards which arise from certain industrial processes are a risk, not merely to those within the walls of the factories in which they are carried out.

There are many excellent texts for the specialist in occupational medicine and I would not expect him to find much here which he did not already know. Others whose field of interest is not primarily with occupational health may find it useful, however, especially those whose work in general practice frequently brings them into contact with illnesses which may have their origins wholly or in part, in their patient's work.

Chapter 1
The Effects of Occupation on Health

The knowledge that one's health can be intimately connected with one's occupation must have become apparent at an early stage of social evolution. The first occupational disease was probably silicosis occurring in the makers of flint tools. Excavations of stone-age sites suggest that the manufacture of flint tools was a specialized occupation and hut floors covered by thousands of pieces of flint debris leave no doubt that the tool markers were heavily exposed to silica. The next most ancient occupational disease might have been farmer's lung which followed the domestication of grain. In general, however, the prevalence of occupational disease would have been low before the introduction of metal working and mining. The ancient physicians, who were extremely acute observers and who recognized that other environmental factors could promote ill health, tended to ignore the effects of occupation. This may have been because the more onerous tasks were undertaken by slaves or prisoners— the lead mines of antiquity were worked by slave labour, for example, and exacted a heavy loss of life—thus placing them beyond the care of the physician. Some texts on the disease of miners appeared during the fifteenth and sixteenth centuries, but no comprehensive treatise on occupational medicine was produced before 1700 when Ramazzini published *De Morbis Artificum*. The modern development of the subject of occupational medicine can be traced directly from Ramazzini's book. His own interest had its origins in a singularly unglamorous event, as he explains:

> The Accident, from which I took occasion to write this Treatise of the Diseases of Tradesmen is as follows. In this City, which is very populous for its Bigness, and is built both close and high, it is usual to have their Houses of Office (cesspits) cleansed every third Year; and, while the Men employed in this Work were cleansing that at my House, I took notice of one of them, who worked with a great deal of Anxiety and Eagerness, and, being moved with Compassion I asked the poor Fellow, Why he did not work more calmly and avoid over-tiring himself with too much Straining? Upon this the poor Wretch lifted up his Eyes from the dismal Vault, and replied, That none but those who have tried it could imagine the Trouble of staying above four Hours in that Place, it being equally troublesome as to be struck blind. After he came out of the Place, I took a narrow View of his Eyes, and found them very red and dim; upon which I asked him, If they had any usual Remedy of that Disorder? He replied, their only Way was to run immediately Home, and confine themselves for a Day to a dark Room, and wash their Eyes now and then with warm Water; by which Means they used to find their Pain somewhat

1

assuaged. Then I asked him, if he felt any Heat in his Throat, and Difficulty of Respiration, or Headache? And whether the Smell affected their Nose, or occasioned a Squeamishness? He answered, That he felt none of those Inconveniences; that the only Parts which suffered were the Eyes, and that if he continued longer at the same Work, without Interruption, he should be blind in a short Time, as it had happened to others. Immediately after he clapt his Hands over his Eyes, and run Home. After this I took notice of several Beggars in the City, who, having been employed in that Work, were either very weak-sighted, or absolutely blind.

Ramazzini it was who suggested that in addition to the questions recommended by Hippocrates, the physician should ask the patient one more, namely what is your occupation? This piece of advice has yet to become properly implemented!

The Industrial Revolution produced an upheaval in the social life of this country the repercussions of which are still being felt. Industry sprawled over the countryside at will, tending to concentrate in the areas where there were readily available sources of energy and raw materials, and in the wake of industry came the squalid towns, hastily built to house the new urban work force. The conditions in the factories and the mines were terrible and resulted in great morbidity and mortality, which in turn had serious economic consequences. During the nineteenth century a series of Acts was passed through Parliament which resulted in a gradual improvement in the lot of the working population. In the beginning, the motivation behind these apparently philanthropic efforts was dictated by the desire of the mill owners to improve efficiency; a sick or dying employee could not work as well as one in reasonable health and was thus uneconomic. To improve the conditions of the workers was, therefore, necessary to ensure the greatest return on capital.

The first Act which related to working conditions was the Health and Morals of Apprentices Act passed in the reign of George III in 1802. This Act stipulated that children in the cotton and woollen mills should work no more than a maximum of 12 hours a day, should do no night work and that their places of work should be ventilated and washed down twice a year! The Act fixed no minimum age for the employment of children. The 1819 Act for the Regulation of Cotton Mills and Factories attempted to remedy this omission by fixing the minimum age of employment at 9, but this Act, like the 1802 Act, failed from the want of an effective mechanism to enforce its provisions. To overcome this defect, another Act was passed in 1825 which required every mill owner to enter into a book the name of any child employed who appeared to be under the age of 9, together with the names of the parents. It was then incumbent upon the parents to sign a document stating that the child *was* over the legal age, thus absolving the mill owner from any blame in the event of subsequent legal proceedings. This somewhat inept law invited abuse so that yet another Act was required to close this loophole. Under the provisions of the Act of 1833 each employed child was required to have a medical certificate stating that it was of the appearance and ordinary strength of a child of 9. This Act was of course as open to abuse as its predecessor but it had the important effect of bringing the medical profession directly into the administration of factory legislation. And what was of greater significance, it established the Factory Inspectorate. The Medical Branch of the Factory Inspectorate was not introduced at this time and it was 1898 before it came into being.

As the nineteenth century progressed many more Acts were passed, designed to improve the conditions of employment and, little by little, conditions for the working population did improve. Improvement is a relative term, however, and many dreadful practices flourished well towards the end of the century; boys were still put up chimneys until 1875, for example, and accounts of the pitiful privations suffered by the working class are to be found in many Victorian novels. Occupational diseases were common and were accepted as the normal consequence of being employed. Many of the occupational diseases were known by colloquial names, a number of which have survived into our own time. This is some indication that they were both common, and of such a gross character that the general public was able to recognize and classify their symptoms.

There is no gainsaying the fact that compared with a generation or two ago, the conditions under which the mass of the population works have improved beyond measure. Largely because of this, doctors have tended to lose sight of the pathogenicity of occupation unless they are confronted with one of the classical industrial diseases, and it is still with these that the major part of occupational medicine is concerned. It is becoming increasingly evident, however, that environmental factors are amongst the major determinants of health. For most people, the environment which has the greatest effect upon their health is to be found at their place of work. About one-third of a man's life is spent at work and a lesser, but still substantial proportion of that of many women. For these reasons alone no practitioners, whatever their speciality, can afford to overlook their patients' job.

Many occupations do appear to carry with them an increased risk of mortality, as reference to Table 1.1, which shows the 20 occupations with the highest SMR*, makes clear. It is not difficult to reconcile some occupations with high SMRs; fishing, steel erecting and coal mining are inherently sufficiently dangerous that it comes as no surprise that the lives of their practitioners may be in jeopardy. The factors which might account for the increased risks amongst electrical engineers, shoe makers and watch repairers are not so immediately obvious, however. Publicans, on the other hand, have been recognized for many years to be following an occupation likely to shorten their lives. William Farr, the first medical commentator in the Registrar General's office wrote in 1861 that the publican has only to abstain from excesses in spirits and other strong

---

* SMR = Standardized mortality ratio. It is the ratio of the observed number of deaths amongst an occupational group compared with the number which would have been expected had the mortality rates of the population at large been experienced, allowing for age correction, i.e. SMR = observed deaths/expected deaths × 100. An SMR greater than 100 indicates that the group under consideration has a greater than usual mortality whilst the converse is true if the SMR is less than 100.

Table 1.1. Twenty occupations with the highest SMRs

Occupation	SMR
Electrical engineers (so described)	317
Bricklayers, etc., labourers, nec	273
Deck and engineroom ratings, barge and boatmen	233
Deck, engineering officers and ship pilots	175
Fishermen	171
Steel erectors; riggers	164
Labourers and unskilled workers nec foundries in engineering and allied trade	160
Coal mine workers above ground	160
Shoemakers and shoe repairers	156
Machine tool operators	156
Publicans, innkeepers	155
Watch and chronometer makers and repairers	154
Leather product makers nec	147
Electronic engineers	145
Printers (so described)	144
Rolling, tube mill operators, metal drawers	144
Brewers, wine makers and related workers	143
Surface workers nec, mines and quarries	141
Coal mine workers underground	141

From Registrar General's *Occupational Mortality Tables*, HMSO, 1978.

drinks to live as long as other people. Farr exemplifies here the British characteristic of disapproving of those who provide them with their pleasures!

On a happier note, there are also a number of occupations which carry with them a decreased mortality and the 20 with the lowest SMRs are listed in Table 1.2. On the whole the list is dominated by those in the professions; the low SMR enjoyed by university teachers is especially gratifying. That Ministers of the Crown and senior government officials are also unduly hearty puts the lie to their frequently expressed belief that theirs is a life of constant stress and toil; if it is, then it certainly does not adversely affect their chances of living to enjoy their pensions.

When interpreting SMRs, however, a number of factors must be borne in mind. One of the most important is to separate out the effects due to occupation from those due to social class (see Table 1.3). One way in which this can be done is by relating the mortality of the husbands in an occupational group to that of their wives, the wives being used as a control for socio-economic factors.

In many cases, the number of deaths within an occupational order may be small and then the SMR becomes misleading. It is necessary, therefore, to apply some statistical test to the SMR in order to determine whether the difference between the number of observed and expected deaths is due to factors other than chance. As a first approximation, and providing the number of deaths is large enough, the chi-squared statistic can be used where

$$\chi^2 = \frac{(\text{observed deaths} - \text{expected deaths})}{(\text{expected deaths})}.$$

Table 1.2. Twenty occupations with lowest SMRs

Occupation	SMR
Trainee craftsmen (engineering and allied trades)	26
Electrical engineers	42
Labourers and unskilled workers nec coke ovens and gas works	46
Foremen (engineering and allied trades)	47
University teachers	49
Paper products makers	50
Technologist nec	52
Managers in building and contracting	54
Physiotherapists	55
Local authority senior officers	57
Teachers nec	57
Mechanical engineers	58
Technical and related workers nec	58
Typists, shorthand writers, secretaries	59
Company secretaries and registrars	60
Ministers of the Crown; MPs nec; senior government officials	61
Printing workers nec	62
Office managers nec	64
Public health inspectors	64
Office machine operators	65

From Registrar General's *Occupational Mortality Tables*, HMSO, 1978.

The probability that a difference is observed and expected numbers of deaths is due to chance can be determined from statistical tables showing the chi-squared distribution with one degree of freedom.

Using this test, it is possible to show that some occupational groups are at a special risk of dying from certain categories of disease due to factors which are associated with their job (Table 1.4).

Another way in which SMRs may be unreliable is due to the introduction of selection factors which tend to bias the results. For example, people who are in poor health are unlikely to take up an occupation which is physically demanding. Similarly, workers who develop a chronic disease will be likely to leave the job in which they became ill if it is taxing and enter a sedentary occupation or alternatively drift into some unskilled labouring job. When a man's relatives are questioned as to his occupation after his death, they may

Table 1.3. SMR by social class, men aged 15–64

Social class	SMR
I	77
II	81
IIIN	99
IIIM	106
IV	114
V	137

From Registrar General's *Occupational Mortality Tables*, HMSO, 1978.

Table 1.4. Occupational groups at special risk of dying from some categories of disease

Disease category	Occupational groups	SMR
Infectious and parasitic diseases	Labourers, nec	206
	Miners and quarrymen	172
	Service, sport and recreation workers	136
Malignant neoplasms	Armed forces	161
	Furnace, forge, foundry and	
	rolling mill workers	135
	Labourers, nec	133
	Construction workers	126
	Painters and decorators	123
Diseases of the nervous system	Miners and quarrymen	149
Diseases of the circulatory system	Armed forces	143
	Miners and quarrymen	137
	Textile workers	121
	Leather workers	120
Diseases of the respiratory system	Miners and quarrymen	244
	Labourers, nec	193
	Furnace, forge, foundry and	
	rolling mill workers	167
	Glass and ceramic makers	163
	Leather workers	134
Diseases of the skin	Farmers, foresters and fishermen	208
	Paper and printing workers	167
	Painters and decorators	166
Diseases of the musculoskeletal system	Clothing workers	319

From Registrar General's *Occupational Mortality Tables*, HMSO, 1978.

well mention the last job which will duly be recorded even though it may not be the one in which the patient was subjected to the hazards which were responsible for his ill health (always supposing the job was of aetiological significance). Conversely, it may happen that the relatives of a dead man will refer back to what they see as a prestigious occupation even though he may not have followed it for many years. Widows of men who have ever been coal miners, for example, will often state that this was their husband's occupation even if he had been away from the pits for many years. This tendency, of course, may artificially enhance the apparent risks of some occupations. Thus it is of the greatest importance, when pursuing a proposed link between occupation and disease to record a full occupational history of the subjects in the group under study, having particular regard to length and time of exposure.

Finally, it must be remembered that the SMR is necessarily a relatively crude index, being composed of the total experience of the particular group to all causes of death. Thus it is possible to find within an occupational group some diseases which are more common than average even though the SMR for all

Table 1.5. Occupations with a high SMR for bronchitis

Occupation	SMR (bronchitis)	SMR (all causes)
Coal miners	1683	62
Glass and ceramic furnacemen	172	100
Rolling tube mill operators	168	104
Metal furnacemen	151	108
Plasterers	146	109
Bus conductors	138	105
Coal, gas and coke oven furnacemen	131	96
Brewers	131	103
Glass formers	130	95
Lorry drivers' mates	129	105

From registrar General's *Occupational Mortality Tables*, HMSO, 1971.

causes may be insignificantly different from 100; it follows in these cases, that there are compensatory low SMRs for other causes of death which average out the overall death rate. For example, Table 1.5 shows 10 occupations in which a high SMR for bronchitis is found but in which the overall SMR is not greatly increased. Some of these occupations clearly carry a risk of respiratory disease. It is really no surprise to find coal miners in their pre-eminent position. Others are unexpected—it is difficult to see how plastering and brewing might contribute to a risk from bronchitis, for example.

Work-related injury and disease

It is difficult to determine accurately the morbidity which can be attached to occupational causes although one suspects that it must be considerable. There is a very great deal of underreporting of occupational diseases largely because doctors are not trained to consider their patients' work as a possible causative agent of their illness. Undergraduate training in occupational medicine takes up a very small part of the curriculum and is often squeezed in with other bits and pieces for which room cannot easily be found amongst the mainstream subjects. I once taught all the occupational medicine to students at a London teaching hospital and for this I was allocated two hours; I was interested to note that chiropody occupied the students for exactly twice as long.

In an attempt to improve the notification of occupational injuries and diseases, the Health and Safety Commission introduced the Reporting of Industrial Diseases and Dangerous Occurrence Regulations (RIDDOR) in 1986 under which all accidents at work resulting in death or serious injury must be reported to the Health and Safety Executive (HSE), as must injuries at work which result in absence from work for more than three days. The diseases which must be reported to HSE under these regulations include all those which are notifiable or prescribed. It is too early to say how successful these regulations will be in providing estimates of the true incidence of occupational morbidity.

Table 1.6. Number of new spells (thousands) of certified absence from work qualifying for sickness or invalidity benefit

	Men	Women
All causes	4450	2530
Industrial injuries	331	65
Prescribed diseases	4.3	2.4

From DHSS, Newcastle upon Tyne.

They will probably improve the estimate of the number of injuries but unless and until doctors become better able to detect and diagnose occupational, or occupationally related disease, the position with respect to them is unlikely to change.

Nevertheless, the data which *are* available demonstrate that many people continue to suffer serious adverse effects as the result of their work. Apart from the 1400 or so deaths a year (650 fatal accidents and 750 from industrial diseases) there are a few thousand dangerous occurrences a year reported to HSE and several thousand newly diagnosed cases of industrial disease (see Tables 1.6—1.8). Nor is the trend downwards as the data in these tables show. Thus, although conditions in industry have certainly improved in recent years there are no grounds for complacency and the importance of occupational health services, both private and governmental, cannot be overemphasized.

Absences from work

Absence from work due to certified sickness results in a staggering number of days lost, by comparison with which the time lost from other causes such as strikes seems relatively trivial. It is generally accepted that little of this has to do with ill health, particularly absences which last for only a few days. Indeed, this is now recognized by the new jargon which does not talk of 'sickness absence' but of 'work withdrawal'.

Relatively little time lost from work is caused by industrial injuries or industrial diseases as Table 1.9 shows. Industrial injuries account for slightly less than 7.5% of new spells of absence in men and about 2.5% in women. This

Table 1.7. Number of dangerous occurrences reported to enforcement agencies (excluding those occurring offshore)

	1981	1982	1983	1984	1985
Dangerous occurrences					
In mines	272	320	338	190	219
In quarries	51	48	32	33	35
On the railways	2	4	4	5	4
In other places of work	3234	2699	2406	2406	2524
Not elsewhere classified	86	82	77	82	118
Totals	3645	3153	2857	2716	2900

From HSE *Health and Safety Statistics*, HMSO, 1988.

Table 1.8. Number of newly prescribed industrial diseases, except those assessed by Special Medical Boards

	1983–84	1984–85	1985–86
Conditions due to:			
Physical agents			
'Tenosynovitis'	337	390	619
Occupational deafness	1468	1492	1179
Vibration induced white finger*		3	641
Others	137	184	229
Biological agents			
Anthrax	0	0	1
Leptospira	2	0	0
Tuberculosis	6	7	3
Brucellosis	3	0	0
Viral hepatitis	3	5	9
Streptococcus suis	1	0	0
Poisoning by lead	0	2	2
Dermatitis	611	619	785
Other conditions	26	19	32
Totals	2594	2721	3500

*Prescribed April 1985.
From HSE *Health and Safety Statistics*, HMSO, 1988.

reflects, of course, that men tend to work more often in jobs which expose them to accidents and injury than women; it is interesting that prescribed diseases account for about the same amount of new spells of absence in both men and women although this is rather less than 0.1% of the total.

There are a number of other interesting features about work withdrawal (Table 1.6). There are, for example marked differences in the number of days

Table 1.9. Number of newly prescribed industrial diseases assessed by Special Medical Boards

	1982	1983	1984	1985	1986
Farmer's lung	11	8	4	6	11
Carcinoma of the bronchus in nickel workers	0	1	5	2	3
Pneumoconiosis	733	670	577	702	747
Byssinosis	133	72	56	37	26
Occupational asthma*	98	183	137	166	166
Lung cancer in asbestos workers[†]				8	34
Bilateral pleural thickening[†]				61	111
Mesothelioma	123	148	201	245	305
Other conditions	9	6	1	2	5
Totals	1104	1088	981	1160	1408

*Prescribed March 1982.
[†]Prescribed April 1985.
From HSE *Health and Safety Statistics*, HMSO, 1988.

lost according to age and region (Tables 1.7 and 1.8). The steady increase in days lost with age might merely be a reminder that those ills to which the flesh is heir become more common as one gets older, and the regional variations might be just a crude reflection of the different types of industry in different parts of the country. It is well known, however, that other factors are also involved.

Most absence from work, and especially that of short duration, is voluntary. Patients, in effect, certify themselves as unfit, although they may require the doctor to act as their agent by signing the appropriate document. Doctors generally are so little acquainted with the demands which their patients' occupations make upon them that they are seldom in a position to evaluate fully an employee's fitness to return to work. The liaison between general practitioners and factory doctors is seldom well enough established for the general practitioners to be able to take their colleagues' advice and so they rely on the patients to tell them whether or not they are fit to work.

Absence from work is frequently the means by which an employee escapes from stress. For example, new employees tend to have more time off work than those with long service and this has been explained by suggesting that the new employee withdraws from work to help him/her adjust to a new environment. Poor relations between employees and management are another cause for high absenteeism. Smaller factories generally have a higher degree of social cohesiveness and as the number of employees increases, so communications become more tortuous, less effective and absenteeism increases (Table 1.8). Monotonous, repetitive work is well recognized to lead to declining morale and a high rate of absenteeism. To some extent the boredom associated with this kind of work can be relieved by putting workers onto shift work and in some studies this has been shown to result in a decrease in the amount of lost time (Table 1.9).

Clearly many of the factors which are associated with absenteeism from work can best be resolved by working towards the elimination of stressful conditions, improving communications and relieving boredom. These are all problems which can be tackled by enlightened management in conjunction with industrial psychologists since these problems are not predominantly medical. Nevertheless, the doctor owes it both to himself and his patient to be aware of the causes of absence from work if only because patients may be more prepared to discuss their problems with their doctor than with management or with colleagues at work.

So far as absence from work for long periods goes, this is usually due to genuine medical or psychiatric conditions and the doctor will help patients best by having at least some knowledge of the patient's occupation and the physical and mental demands which this occupation will impose. Many firms are willing to re-introduce employees back into some form of selective employment until they are fit enough to resume their old job. Some of the more forward thinking companies have special rehabilitation units through which workers can pass to their old job or in which chronically sick or injured employees can work. Doctors outside industry are not likely to become familiar with such arrangements unless they can establish a link with local industrial medical officers or with government agencies such as the Employment Medical Advisory Service (EMAS) in the United Kingdom; it would certainly be in their patients' interest for them to do so, however.

Chapter 2
Industrial Toxicology 1: Metals

Although many of the classic occupational diseases caused by exposure to toxic substances are seen much less frequently now in the fully developed industrialized countries, industrial toxicology is nevertheless one of the key stones for an understanding of occupational medicine. In those countries which are rapidly industrializing, occupational diseases are common and occupational medicine could scarcely be practised in the absence of a sound grounding in toxicology.

The number of potentially toxic materials in use in industry is enormous and so it is possible here to mention only those which are most important and most commonly encountered. In the present chapter, the metals and metalloids (arsenic and phosphorus) are considered; solvents and other organic compounds in Chapters 3 and 4 and the toxic gases in Chapter 5.

Some general considerations of metal toxicology

Within the body, the levels of essential metals are kept within what are referred to as concentration windows. This is because for all these metals there is a concentration below which the signs of deficiency occur and one above which the metal is toxic. The width of the concentration window is thus set by these two extreme levels and in some cases is extremely narrow. In most cases, the metal levels in the body are regulated by uptake from the gut and special absorptive mechanisms have been evolved for this purpose. The general pattern is that metals in the gut bind to a carrier protein in order to become attached to a transport (or storage) protein from which ions are released as required. The activation of the transport mechanism is governed by the metal levels in the body, being stimulated by decreasing and inhibited by increasing levels. There are no specific transport mechanisms for nonessential metals, instead they take advantage of those by which the essential metals are absorbed and their rate of uptake is frequently determined by the concentration of other metals in the gut; some specific examples are given below.

All metals within biological systems are in their ionic state although they all exist in combination with ligands to which they are bound more or less firmly depending on their function. For example, Na^+ and K^+ which are both charge carriers, have a residence time with their ligands (water molecules) of about 10^{10} seconds. Metals which have a predominantly structural function, such as magnesium for example, are very firmly bound and exchange ligands extremely slowly. No metals undergo biotransformation within the body and most are excreted in the urine.

Metals have many functions, but it is possible to recognize some major categories of effect. I have already mentioned that Na^+ and K^+ act as charge carriers and are responsible, *inter alia*, for the propagation of the action potential down the axon. Calcium appears to act as a trigger mechanism for events such as post-synaptic transmission and muscle contraction whilst metals in the first transition series in the period table, which can exist in more than one oxidation state (Fe^{2+}, Fe^{3+}, for example) are involved in redox reactions. Perhaps the most important function of metals, however, is as vital components of metallo-enzymes of which many hundreds are now known. The role of the metal is either to serve as the active site of the enzyme or to maintain the structural integrity of the protein through its binding with amino acid residues.

An important aspect of metal toxicology is the ability of metals to interact with one another. Interactions between metals may occur because they are adjacent to each other in the periodic table or because their ionic radius or electronic configuration is similar. The interactions may be synergistic or antagonistic and it is the ability of toxic metals to interact with those which are essential which underlies many of their harmful effects. For example cadmium and zinc interact and cadmium is thus able to displace zinc in some metallo-enzymes. Lead can displace calcium at any of the sites at which it is active and thus is able, for example, to inhibit post-synaptic transmission.

Lead

Uses
Lead has many uses in industry including the manufacture of pipes, sheet metal and foil. It is also still used in paints, enamels and glazes, although on a smaller scale than a few years ago. An important use has been connected with the development of the motor industry and great quantities of lead have been used in the manufacture of car batteries, and in making the alkyl lead compounds used as anti-knock additives in petrol. In many countries now the use of lead based anti-knock agents is being discontinued because of the supposed behavioural effects of environmental lead on children.

Hazards of use
The predominant hazard in industry arises from the inhalation of dust and fume but the organic compounds may also be absorbed through the skin. Ingestion is a much less serious problem in industry, although in the general environment it is the predominant route of entry.

Metabolism
Inorganic lead is relatively poorly absorbed from the gut, only about 10% of an ingested dose being taken up. The rate of absorption is dependent upon the concentration of other metals in the gut, particularly those of calcium and iron. Lead uptake varies inversely with the concentration of these metals in the gut, a factor which may be of importance when considering exposure to lead in workers in developing countries. Lead which is present in the faeces is mainly that which has been ingested but not absorbed, although there is a small amount in the faeces which has been excreted through the bile. Pulmonary absorption is much more effective, and, depending on the chemical species and the particle

size, about 40% of inhaled lead is absorbed. Organic compounds, including the lead alkyls and lead stearate are absorbed through the skin.

Following absorption, lead is transported bound to the red cell, and considerably less than 10% of the total blood lead concentration represents lead in the plasma. All the soft tissues have their complement of lead, but the skeleton acts as the main depository and more than 90% of the total body burden of lead is in the bones and teeth. Lead displaces calcium in the hydroxyapatite crystal and once within the bone is relatively stable although some exchange does take place between the skeleton and the plasma. Inorganic lead does not normally cross the blood–brain barrier with any ease but organic lead does.

Excretion is almost exclusively via the kidneys but small amounts are lost in addition through the bile and through sweat, and in milk.

Poisoning

The symptons of lead poisoning include abdominal pain, constipation and vomiting. Peripheral neuropathy is seldom seen in industrial cases nowadays, although in the old text books, wrist drop was always given great prominence. Some patients complain of a metallic taste in the mouth and some complain of headache. There may be clinical signs of anaemia, although this is a late manifestation of the disease. A blue line on the gums due to the deposition of lead sulphide in the gingival margin is occasionally seen. This lead line has come to be regarded as one of the classic signs of lead poisoning but students are warned not to hesitate to make the diagnosis in its absence; they are unlikely to see it! Encephalopathy is an uncommon but serious complication in adults with lead poisoning although conversely, it is often the presenting symptom in children.

Organic lead poisoning may result from exposure to tetraethyl lead (TEL); tetramethyl lead (TML) is much less toxic than TEL and cases of poisoning with TML have not been reported. The symptoms of organic lead poisoning differ from those of inorganic poisoning in that psychiatric manifestations are more common presenting symptoms. For comparison, the symptoms of the two conditions are shown in Table 2.1 in order of their frequency of occurrence.

Inorganic lead poisoning may not be easy to diagnose in the absence of biochemical data. When these are to hand, however, the spectrum of abnormalities is virtually pathognomonic (see below). In the past, patients with inorganic lead poisoning have found themselves in a surgical ward having investigations to establish the cause of their acute abdomen and some have come to laparotomy before the true cause of their illness has been discovered, usually by taking a proper occupational history from the patient. Some care needs to be taken in establishing exposure, however, since in most cases of lead poisoning these days, the patient does not work in a 'traditional' lead industry but may be engaged in demolishing bridges or other buildings covered with lead paint, for example. Anyone who takes a flame to old painted structures should be warned about the possibility of lead exposure and protected accordingly.

Table 2.1. Symptoms in inorganic and organic lead poisoning in adults*

Inorganic	Organic
Abdominal pain	Disturbances in sleep pattern
Constipation	Nausea
Vomiting	Anorexia
Non-abdominal pain	Vomiting
Asthenia	Vertigo and headache
Paraesthesiae	Muscular weakness
Psychological symptoms	Weight loss
Diarrhoea	Tremor
	Diarrhoea
	Abdominal pain
	Hyperexcitability
	Mania

*Symptoms are listed in their order of frequency as presenting symptoms.

The psychiatric symptoms of organic lead poisoning have no characteristics by which their origin may easily be discovered. Patients have been known to develop organic lead poisoning by using leaded petrol as a solvent in confined spaces and cases of encephalopathy have been reported in children and adults sniffing petrol. Some cases of congenital malformation have also been reported in children born to women who sniffed leaded petrol during pregnancy.

Lead anaemia

Anaemia is seen only in inorganic poisoning and occurs late in the disease, but disturbances of haem synthesis can be detected almost as soon as exposure to lead has begun. Lead, like many of the other heavy metals, is a powerful inhibitor of enzymes containing a sulphydryl (–SH) group and a number of these enzymes are concerned with haem synthesis. The disturbances produced by the inhibition of these enzymes form the basis of a number of tests by which the effects of lead on those at risk are monitored (Fig. 2.1). The effects include: reduction in the activity of δ-amino laevulinic acid dehydrase (ALA-d) in the circulating red cells; increase in the urinary excretion of δ-amino laevulinic acid (ALA) and coproporphyrin (Cp); and an increase in erythrocyte protoporphyrin (EPP). The increase in EPP occurs because lead inhibits the incorporation of Fe^{2+} into the protoporphyrin molecule and its place may be taken by Zn^{2+} with the formation of zinc protoporphyrin (ZPP). The main elevation of EPP levels occurs about 3 months after the change in exposure since it is only the newly formed red cells which are affected. Since the red cell has a life span of about 120 days it follows that it will take that time to replace the normal red cells with those which are rich in protoporphyrin. It is also obvious that it will take about 3 months for high EPP levels to fall to normal after exposure is discontinued.

There is little or no elevation of the urinary ALA or Cp excretion in organic lead poisoning; nor is the erythrocyte protoporphyrin level much increased; red cell ALA-d activity, however, is significantly decreased.

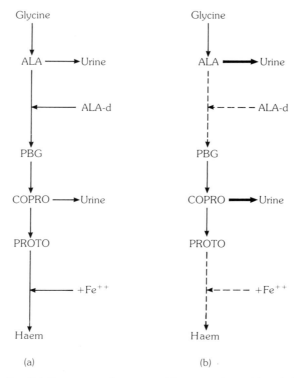

(a)   (b)

Fig 2.1 Diagram to show normal haem synthesis (a) and the effects of lead (b).

A number of enzymes are inhibited, the most important of which is ALA-d. As a result the levels of ALA and COPRO in the urine are increased and the activity of ALA-d in the circulating red cells is decreased. The incorporation of Fe^{2+} into PROTO is also inhibited. If exposure is continued for a long time, frank anaemia will be produced.

Abbreviations: Ala = δ-amino laevulinic acid; PBG = porphobilinogen; COPRO = coproporphyrin; PROTO = protoporphyrin; ALA-d = δ-amino laevulinic acid dehydrase

The inhibition of haem synthesis is one factor in the production of lead anaemia but lead also produces direct effects on the red cell. The permeability of the membrane is altered in such a way as to allow an increased potassium loss from the cell and the life span of the red cell is slightly shortened. There are also alterations in iron metabolism and iron-laden cells (siderocytes) may be found in the peripheral blood and in the bone marrow, and the serum iron may be elevated.

In the older books, great store was given to the presence of basophilic stippled cells in the peripheral blood as an index of lead absorption and lead intoxication. The presence of these cells, however, is not specific for lead poisoning. For example, they are also found after exposure to aniline, benzene and carbon monoxide, and as a test for lead absorption, stippled cell counts have been superseded by more sensitive biochemical tests.

Biochemical indices of lead poisoning

The biochemical features of lead poisoning are so characteristic that, when all are present, a diagnosis may be made with confidence. A raised blood lead concentration is essential for the diagnosis and the urinary lead level will also be raised. There will be a marked elevation of urinary ALA and Cp excretion but only a minimal rise in urinary PBG. The erythrocyte protoporphyrin concentration will be raised and the activity of ALA-d greatly inhibited. There is no other disease in which the combination of effects occurs.

Control and treatment

Medical supervision of certain groups of lead workers is mandatory. Women (because of the high incidence of spontaneous abortion and stillbirth in the past) and young persons are prohibited from working in certain processes connected with lead manufacture.

Biological monitoring of lead workers is based on a test of absorption (the blood lead concentration) and a test which measures metabolic effect, either the urinary ALA concentration or the red cell protoporphyrin concentration. In the control of lead workers, the blood lead concentration is generally given most weight and it is most unlikely that lead poisoning will occur if the level is kept below 80 µg/dl (3.9 µmol/l). Cases of lead poisoning may undoubtedly occur in sensitive individuals when the blood lead is lower than 80 µg/dl but such sensitivity should have been apparent by an unusually great excretion of ALA in the urine or in a markedly elevated EPP. In recent years there has been a tendency to lower the blood lead concentration at which workers should be removed from exposure; in the UK and the other countries of the EEC, the suspension limit is now 70 µg/dl. The frequency with which blood lead estimations will be carried out depends on the concentration found. The UK Code of Practice suggests that when the blood lead is less than 40 µg/dl, the maximum interval between tests shall be 12 months, between 40 and 59 µg/dl the maximum interval shall be 6 months, between 60 and 69 µg/dl, 3 months and over 70 µg/dl, the interval shall be at the discretion of the supervising physician but not more than 3 months. It should be remembered that the commonest cause of an unusually high blood lead concentration in a worker who has been well-controlled is contamination and before any action is taken, a high reading must be confirmed on another sample.

All operations which give rise to dust or fume should be exhaust ventilated and workers should wear appropriate protective clothing. Where one employee in a group, all of whom have approximately the same degree of exposure, shows signs of increased absorption, this may be evidence that local ventilation has failed or that the employee is not complying with safety requirements. Both possibilities ought to be investigated.

The combination of laboratory tests, regular clinical examination and good industrial hygiene should be sufficient to protect workers from developing any significant degree of clinical lead poisoning and severe industrial cases are nowadays a rarity in this country. On a world-wide basis, however, lead poisoning is still the most prevalent industrial disease.

Organic poisoning

The total blood lead concentration is not raised in organic lead poisoning, although the fraction which is lipid-bound is usually elevated. It is technically rather difficult to estimate the lipid-bound fraction, and so biological monitoring of organic lead workers tends to be based on urinary lead analyses; the aim should be to keep the urinary lead concentration below 150 μg/l (0.7 μmol/l).

Treatment

Once lead poisoning is suspected or confirmed, the individual must immediately be removed from exposure and in some cases this is the only treatment which will be required. Where lead colic is a feature of the illness, relief will be gained from an intravenous injection of calcium gluconate. When the blood lead is dangerously high (> 100 μg/dl), when the patient has encephalopathy or when other symptoms are slow to resolve, consideration should be given to treatment with chelating agents. This must only be undertaken in hospital under supervised conditions.

The two most common chelating agents used for treating adult cases are calcium EDTA and penicillamine; lead poisoning in children is usually treated with a combination of Ca-EDTA and dimercapranol (BAL). Treatment is continued until the blood lead concentration has reached acceptable limits; preferably it should be no higher than 40 μg/dl. In some patients it may be necessary to give more than one course of chelation therapy or to use one of the newer chelation agents such as 3-dimercaptopropane sulphonate (DMPS) or dimercaptosuccinic acid (DMSA); both are derivatives of BAL.

In some rare cases it is found that despite removal from exposure and despite treatment, some lead workers continue with blood lead levels which are above those generally considered to be safe. These individuals appear to be unaffected by their high blood lead and no treatment is indicated other than continuous follow up. It seems likely that in these individuals the distribution of lead between the red cells and the plasma is much more in favour of the red cells than is normal, probably because they are able to produce lead binding proteins within the red cells in greater quantity than is usual.

Mercury

Uses

Metallic mercury is used in the manufacture of thermometers and switch-gear; amalgams with copper, tin, silver or gold; and solders containing mercury compounds, but probably its greatest use is in mercury cell rooms for the manufacture of chlorine.

Inorganic mercury compounds which have an industrial use include the nitrate, used in the 'carrotting' of rabbit fur to form felt for hats, the sulphide, which is used as a red pigment (vermillion) and the red oxide used in the manufacture of the anti-fouling paints which are applied to the bottom of ships.

Of the organic compounds, the ethyl, methyl, phenyl and tolyl compounds are used as seed dressings to prevent the spread of fungicidal seed diseases.

They are also used as anti-slime agents in paper making. Mercury fulminate is used in the manufacture of explosives.

Hazards of use

Risks from metallic mercury occur during mining and recovery of the metal from the ore and during the manufacture of compounds from the metal. The risk is from the inhalation of mercury vapour. Since mercury evaporates at room temperature it may be a hazard in laboratories if scientific instruments are broken, thus allowing the metal to escape. Substantial quantities of mercury vapour may also be detected in dentists' surgeries. Although both the inhalation and the ingestion of compounds of mercury may occur in industry, inhalation is the major hazard by far. When handling mercury it should be remembered that it may be absorbed through the unbroken skin. Indeed, mercury used to be administered therapeutically by rubbing mercury ointment on the skin.

Of the organic compounds, only the methyl and ethyl derivatives have been reported to produce systemic toxic effects in humans. The fulminate is a primary skin irritant but does not readily produce systemic poisoning.

Metabolism

Approximately 80% of inhaled mercury vapour will be absorbed from the lungs. The rate of absorption of inhaled mercury compounds will depend upon their particle size and their chemical composition. Absorption of metallic mercury from the gastrointestinal tract is negligible, but by contrast, absorption of methyl mercury is virtually complete. Mercurous mercury salts are virtually insoluble and must be oxidized to the mercuric form before absorption is possible. Less than 15% of ingested inorganic mercury salts are absorbed from the gut; the residue being eliminated in the faeces.

After absorption, elemental mercury is widely distributed through the body and is rapidly oxidized to Hg^{2+} in the tissues. The newly oxidized mercury binds to protein and is distributed as inorganic mercury. Elemental mercury is able to cross the blood–brain barrier easily and it also crosses the placenta. Inorganic compounds do not cross the blood–brain barrier but are widely distributed to the other tissues.

Some organic mercury compounds, particularly the phenyl and alkoxyalkyl derivatives are rapidly converted in the liver to the inorganic form. The conversion of ethyl mercury to the inorganic form is slow and the conversion of methyl mercury is virtually nonexistent. The organic mercury compounds rapidly penetrate the blood–brain barrier and easily cross the placenta.

The kidney contains by far the greatest concentration of mercury, mainly in the cortical and sub-cortical regions, and 50% or more of the total body burden may be in the kidney. The liver also contains a high concentration of mercury, as will the brain following exposure to elemental mercury or the alkylmercury compounds.

Mercury is excreted in the urine following exposure to elemental mercury, inorganic compounds and aryl or alkoxyalkyl mercury. The principal route for the elimination of methyl mercury is via the faeces, but the excretion rate is slow; the half-life of the alkylmercury compounds in humans is estimated to be 70–80 days.

Mercury is also excreted in sweat and in saliva whilst mercury vapour is also eliminated through the lungs.

Methyl mercury passes into breast milk and infants suckling mothers who are heavily exposed may accumulate dangerously high doses; the half-life of alkylmercury compounds in humans is estimated to be 70–80 days and that of inorganic mercury to be about 60 days.

Acute poisoning

In industry acute poisoning has usually occurred when workers have been exposed to mercury which has been heated in a confined space. It is a rare condition. The patient presents with an acute febrile illness, the symptoms of which come on some hours after exposure has terminated. Prominent symptoms include cough, dyspnoea, tachypnoea, fever, nausea, vomiting, lethargy and a feeling of tightness in the chest. Some patients develop rigors and some are cyanosed. In mild cases the symptoms resolve spontaneously, although dyspnoea and tightness in the chest may persist for up to a week, and sometimes longer. Severe cases may require admission to hospital and treatment on a respirator.

Fatal cases show a pathological picture of acute diffuse interstitial fibrosis with a profuse fibrinous exudate and erosion of the lining of the bronchi and bronchioles.

Acute poisoning may also occur from the accidental ingestion of a large quantity of a mercury compound, and in the past cases were reported following the application of mercury for therapeutic purposes. Following ingestion, the symptoms include gastric pain, nausea and vomiting, shock, and in fatal cases, syncope with convulsions, leading to coma.

Chronic poisoning

The most serious effects of chronic mercury poisoning are produced on the nervous system, on behaviour and on the kidney. Symptoms of chronic mercurialism may be caused by both inorganic and organic compounds, but psychiatric symptoms tend to predominate over neurological in inorganic poisoning whereas the converse is true in organic poisoning. The earliest symptoms are vague, and include the development of a sallow complexion, dyspepsia and headaches. Gingivitis and excessive salivation are early symptoms. The teeth may become loose and drop out, leaving those which remain blackened and eroded. A 'mercury line' may be seen rarely on the gums. This resembles the blue 'lead line', but is more often dark brown in colour. Chronic exposure to organic mercury compounds produces skin lesions. The fulminate is particularly notorious in this respect, giving rise to an irritant dermatitis (fulminate itch) and discrete ulcers (powder holes).

Neurological signs
The characteristic disturbance in chronic mercury poisoning is the production of a tremor, which is neither as fine nor as regular as that found in thyrotoxicosis. It begins as an intention tremor in the hands but later affects the eyelids, lips and tongue, finally involving the arms and sometimes also the legs. As it progresses the tremor becomes coarsened and its amplitude is exaggerated if attention is drawn to it. The tremor is known colloquially as the hatters' shakes. Accompanying the tremor there is often a characteristic disturbance of the handwriting which becomes progressively tremulous, irregular and unintelligible. Various speech disorders are found in addition. These include hesitancy in beginning sentences and a difficulty in pronunciation, and both are more severe in organic than in inorganic poisoning.

Motor and sensory nerve disorders are also part of the neurological syndrome. Spastic gait is a feature and cerebellar ataxia may be severe especially in organic poisoning. Hyperactive tendon reflexes, especially the knee jerk, may be elicited and the plantar reflexes may be extensor.

Sensory disturbances include paraesthesiae, alteration in taste and smell, and loss of proprioception in the fingers and toes. Touch and pain modalities, on the other hand, may be normal. Some patients have difficulty in hearing unless the words are spoken slowly and deliberately and actual hearing loss has been found many years after an acute episode of poisoning. In organic poisoning there is a gross peripheral constriction of the visual fields.

The most important pathological lesion found in fatal cases is atrophy of the cerebellar cortex, which accounts for many of the signs and symptoms found during life.

There is some evidence that subclinical neuropsychiatric symptoms can be detected in mercury workers; defects in recent memory have been found in those whose urinary mercury levels have been elevated (> 50 μg/g creatinine) for several months, for example. In one study, speed of foot tapping was found to be inversely related to urinary mercury concentration and when the urinary mercury levels were lowered by removing the workers from exposure, the foot tapping speed returned to normal. Finally, some reports indicate that sensory nerve conduction velocities are low in mercury workers even in the absence of any overt clinical signs.

Erethism
This is a form of toxic organic psychosis which was once common in the hat industry, hence the expression, 'mad as a hatter'. It is described as an abnormal state of timidity and can present as an anxiety neurosis. Later, however, features of an organic syndrome, including irritability, apathy, drowsiness and headaches frequently develop. Less frequently, dementia and psychotic symptoms may point to the organic nature of the syndrome. When first noted, the emotional disorder may be accompanied by signs of vaso-motor disturbance, including blushing, excessive perspiration and dermatographia.

Effects on the kidney
Proteinuria may be found in up to 5% of those chronically exposed to mercury but usually disappears when exposure is discontinued. In a few cases however, it persists and progresses towards chronic renal disease.

The nephrotic syndrome has been reported in workers exposed to mercury and is said to remit completely when exposure is discontinued. It is not certain that this is always the case, however.

Mercurialentis
Examination of the lens with a slit lamp may reveal a brownish coloured reflex from the anterior capsule. This brown colour becomes deeper as exposure is prolonged. It is usually accompanied by fine punctate opacities in the lens but neither these nor the discoloration has any effect on visual acuity. The chief value of this sign is as an indication of prolonged exposure to mercury for forensic purposes, although the sign may appear within a few months of exposure.

Environmental mercury poisoning
There have been a number of large-scale outbreaks of environmental methyl mercury poisoning. The most notorious was the Minamata Bay episode in Japan. A factory manufacturing vinyl chloride using mercuric chloride as a catalyst discharged its effluent into the bay where some of the mercury was methylated by aquatic micro-organisms; the methyl mercury produced entered the food chain and the residents were poisoned through eating contaminated fish. In Iraq, mass poisonings have resulted from the eating of seed grains treated with methyl and ethyl mercury. Grain is treated in this way before planting to guard against disease; it ought never to be eaten, as these tragic episodes amply demonstrate.

Supervision and treatment
The supervision of mercury workers—other than those who are exposed to methyl mercury—is based upon the measurement of urinary mercury concentrations. There is considerable variation in the excretion of mercury and so samples for analysis should be taken at the same time of day and not following a prolonged period free from exposure. The concentration of mercury in the urine should be kept below 50 µg/g creatinine to avoid untoward effects. It is probably useful to test the urine for protein using a simple dipstick method at the same time.

Methyl mercury is excreted mainly in the faeces and urinary mercury concentrations are not helpful in monitoring workers exposed to this compound. Blood mercury levels can be used instead and should not be allowed to exceed 10 µg/dl.

There is no effective treatment for chronic mercury poisoning and it is probable that the symptoms will never completely reverse. BAL has been used in the past but has largely been superseded by penicillamine. BAL is effective in the treatment of acute poisoning with mercuric chloride or in alleviating the symptoms associated with an overdose of mercurial diuretics. The use of BAL in alkyl mercury poisoning is contraindicated since the BAL-alkyl mercury complexes are redistributed to the CNS. DMSA has been used in organic mercury poisoning and is said to be better tolerated than BAL. More recently, mercaptopropionyl glycine has been used to treat organic mercury poisoning. This drug produces a sustained increase in urinary mercury output but seems to have little beneficial effect on the clinical picture.

Cadmium

Uses
Cadmium is a constituent of some alloys used to manufacture bearings for motor car and other engines and the manufacture of these alloys accounts for most of the cadmium used in industry. It is also used as a protective coating for iron, steel and copper in the electroplating industry and it is replacing zinc to some extent as a rust-proofing agent for iron and steel. The negative plates of alkaline storage batteries are made from cadmium and it is incorporated in cadmium vapour lamps. In nuclear reactors it is used as a neutron absorber, either as a coating on graphite or in the form of rods. Cadmium sulphide is used to prepare yellow and orange pigments and cadmium selenosulphide is used to make red pigments. The pigments, in turn, are used for colouring inks, paints and a variety of plastic, rubber, glass and enamel ware.

Hazards of use
The principal industrial hazards arise from the smelting of ores, the welding and melting of cadmium plated metals, the manufacture of alkaline batteries and the preparation of pigments. In all these cases the risk is from inhalation of cadmium (or cadmium oxide) vapour or dust. Ingestion is seldom a hazard in industry.

Metabolism
Following absorption, cadmium induces the formation of metallothionein, a zinc storage protein which contains an unusual mix of amino acids; it contains between 30 and 35% of cysteine, 12% of serine and 13% of lysine or arginine. It has no aromatic amino acids and no histidine in its structure. The very high proportion of sulphur containing amino acids enables it to bind heavy metals and each molecule of metallothionein is able to bind seven divalent cations. Its physiological function is to regulate tissue levels of essential metals, especially zinc and copper. Cadmium is incorporated into metallothionein because its metabolism is similar to that of zinc and about 80–90% of cadmium in the body is bound to metallothionein. The cadmium–metallothionein complex is trans-ported to the kidney and filtered through the glomerulus to be resorbed by the cells of the proximal tubule. In these cells, the protein is broken down by proteases with the release of free cadmium ions. The presence of these free ions induces the cells of the proximal tubule to produce more metallothionein which binds the cadmium ions once more. It is generally considered that kidney

damage occurs when the capacity of the tubular cells to produce metallothionein is surpassed, although, when injected into animals, the cadmium–metallothionein complex itself is nephrotoxic.

The half-life of cadmium in the body is long, of the order of 7–30 years and its excretion is slow. The main route of excretion is through the kidneys but only when the kidney is damaged and its function impaired does cadmium enter the urine in any quantity. Cadmium accumulates preferentially in the kidney and liver and only to a limited degree in the other soft tissues.

Acute poisoning
Following ingestion, symptoms appear suddenly, normally within 2 hours. Symptoms include increased salivation, severe nausea and persistent vomiting sometimes with haematemesis. Shock and collapse may follow and diarrhoea and tenesmus supervene at a later stage. Recovery is also rapid and is usually complete within 24 hours. No treatment is required beyond the replacement of lost fluids.

Following inhalation of cadmium fumes the symptoms are those of acute pulmonary irritation accompanied by dyspnoea. During the time of exposure the patient experiences symptoms which are reminiscent of those of metal fume fever (q.v.). There is some irritation in the throat and a cough but otherwise no ill effects are noted. This 'latent period' may last for up to 10 hours when an influenza-like illness suddenly sets in. In this stage there is severe dyspnoea, cough (which may be controllable), anorexia, nausea, weakness, headaches, diarrhoea, epigastric pain and malaise. There may be a rise in temperature, and proteinuria may be detected. This acute stage lasts anything from 1 day to several weeks and during all this time basal crepitations can be heard in both lungs and there is radiological evidence of bilateral pulmonary infiltration.

Recovery is gradual and complete in most cases. Fatalities may occur as the result of severe pulmonary oedema with central cyanosis, and at post-mortem, proliferative lesions are noted in the alveoli, sometimes completely obliterating the alveolar spaces. An alternative form of death may be due to renal cortical necrosis.

Chronic poisoning
Patients with chronic cadmium poisoning may complain of non-specific symptoms such as fatigue, weight loss, gastrointestinal pain, nausea and persistent cough. Signs of chronic cadmium poisoning include yellow rings on the teeth, anosmia, and a mild hypochromic anaemia due to interference with normal iron and copper metabolism. The major effects of chronic cadmium poisoning, however, are directed against the kidneys and the lungs.

Renal effects
The nephrotoxic effects of cadmium are directed against the renal tubules and the excretion of low molecular weight proteins in the urine is considered to be the earliest sign of cadmium poisoning. The major component of these low molecular weight proteins is β_2-microglobulin (BMG; MW 11 800) which is

freely filtered from the glomerular basement membrane and normally completely resorbed by the proximal tubules. Any damage to the renal tubules will result in the increased excretion of BMG, however, and it should not be considered as characteristic of cadmium poisoning.

The histopathological change in the kidney associated with cadmium poisoning is an increase in the number and the size of lysosomes in the tubular cells. N-acetyl-β-D-glucosaminidase (NAG) is a lysosomal enzyme particularly abundant in the proximal tubules; its large molecular weight (120 000) normally prevents it from being filtered at the glomerulus but it does appear in the urine following cadmium-induced renal damage.

The proteinuria of cadmium poisoning may be accompanied by other evidence of tubular damage such as aminoaciduria, glycosuria and phosphaturia. There may be an increase in urinary calcium concentration and renal stone formation has been reported in some countries. In spite of these changes, however, renal failure is practically unknown but the alteration in calcium metabolism consequent upon the hypercalcuria may, in rare cases, lead to osteomalacia.

Although the effects of cadmium are directed predominantly against the proximal tubule, there is some recent evidence that the distal tubule may also be damaged. Thus, cadmium workers have been found to have a lower than normal urinary concentration of kallikrein, a protease which is produced in the distal tubule.

Renal damage is unlikely to occur until the concentration of cadmium in the renal cortex reaches 200 parts per million (ppm). When it reaches 215 ppm, renal dysfunction is likely to develop in about 10% of those exposed to the metal. Although this notion of a *critical concentration* refers to the total amount of cadmium in the renal cortex, it is only the small amount of the metal which is not bound to metallothionein which is nephrotoxic. The concentration of free cadium which will produce BMG in the urine is about 2 ppm, or 1% of the critical concentration. There is some evidence that ageing may increase the susceptibility of the kidney to damage by cadmium and that some individuals may be at increased risk because their capacity to produce metallothionein is reduced.

Effects on the lungs
Chronic exposure to cadmium results in the development of focal emphysema. Bullae are not formed and bronchitis is not a feature. The effects on the lungs are evident long before renal damage is observed and are manifested by the onset of dyspnoea and by a low gas transfer factor. Cadmium has been shown experimentally to reduce the concentration of α_1-antitrypsin in the plasma and this effect may underlie the production of emphysema in cadmium workers.

Prostatic carcinoma
Cadmium workers were at one time considered to have an enhanced risk of prostatic carcinoma but recent epidemiological surveys have failed to confirm

this. The prevailing view now is that neither prostatic carcinoma nor any other malignant disease is unusually prevalent amongst those exposed to cadmium at work.

Hypertension

Cadmium can induce hypertension in experimental animals and there is some evidence that the absorption of cadmium from the general environment may be aetiologically related to hypertension in humans. This evidence is by no means unequivocal and hypertension is not a risk amongst cadmium workers, nor does it occur in itai-itai disease.

Itai-itai disease

This disease is a painful type of osteomalacia in which multiple fractures and renal dysfunction were features. It occurred amongst elderly multiparous women in Japan and has generally been considered to be due to eating rice contaminated with cadmium from irrigation water which passed through old mining areas. The pathogenesis of the disease is now in some doubt because it has been found in areas where environmental pollution with cadmium does not take place and it has been suggested that it may be a form of vitamin D deficiency.

Control and treatment

The measurement of BMG in the urine is widely used as a means of controlling cadmium exposure. There are some analytical difficulties which result from the instability of BMG in acid urine and these may be overcome by measuring the urinary concentrations of retinol-binding protein (RBP) instead. There is no widely accepted action level for either BMG or RBP. Some authorities consider that the measurement of NAG activity in the urine is a more sensitive control measure but again, action levels are wanting.

Urinary cadmium levels are probably most widely used to control exposure. The excretion of cadmium in the urine is generally low because the amount of cadmium in the kidney is insufficient to saturate all the binding sites. Under these conditions, the amount of cadmium in the urine reflects the amount of cadmium in the body and hence in the renal cortex. When exposure has continued long enough for all the binding sites in the kidney to become saturated, then the amount of cadmium in the urine is related partly to the body burden and partly to recent exposure. In newly exposed cadmium workers there is always a time lag before the cadmium concentration in the urine correlates with exposure. When renal dysfunction becomes established, the amount of cadmium in the urine increases markedly. In order to prevent renal damage the urinary concentration should be kept below 10 µg Cd/g creatinine. Chelating agents such as BAL and Ca-EDTA have been successfully used in acute cadmium poisoning but they have no part to play in treating the chronic disease. Once renal or pulmonary disease has become established there is little which can be done except to ensure that the patient is removed from exposure, followed up and given whatever symptomatic treatment is necessary.

Beryllium

Uses

Beryllium is used as an alloy with copper. The addition of 2–3% of the metal to copper produces an alloy which is hard, corrosion-resistant, nonrusting and nonsparking. This alloy has a much greater tensile strength than copper alone but its electrical conductivity is approximately the same. Alloys with aluminium, magnesium and nickel are also of commercial value.

Beryllium was formerly used as a constituent of the phosphorescent powder used in fluorescent lights and neon lights. The toxic effects of the metal caused its use in fluorescent lights to be abandoned, but elsewhere its use is increasing. The metal has a high modulus of elasticity and is thus able to resist stress. It imparts lightness, hardness and heat resistance to other materials and is becoming widely used in space research, for example in the building of space capsules. In nuclear research it is also a valuable material since it gives off α-particles when bombarded with neutrons and it is widely used for cans and other accessories in nuclear reactors. It is also used as a deoxidizer in steel making and as a refractory in crucible making. Pure beryllium foil is used in the windows of X-ray diffraction tubes.

Hazards of use

A hazard from fume and dust occurs during the processes of crushing and extracting the ore and when the briquettes containing the extracted metal in the form of a copper alloy are crushed and heated. A considerable hazard used to exist in the handling of the powdered beryllium compounds used for making the phosphor for fluorescent lights and in the salvaging of these lamps.

Metabolism

Absorption from the gut is poor and 96% or more of ingested beryllium is eliminated in the faeces. Pulmonary absorption, on the other hand, is efficient and rapid. Once absorbed, the beryllium is protein bound and deposited in the liver, spleen and the skeleton and a small residue remains in the lungs. The rate of urinary excretion depends on how rapidly and in what form the beryllium was absorbed.

Acute poisoning

The symptoms of acute poisoning are those of a chemical pneumonitis. There is a cough with bloodstained sputum, retrosternal pain, anorexia, rapidly increasing fatigue and progressive dyspnoea accompanied by cyanosis. The histological appearances in the lung are those of a lobular pneumonia with the alveoli filled with exudate containing large numbers of plasma cells but few polymorphs. Radiographic changes are minimal in the early stages of the disease but in persistent cases increased linear markings and a diffuse ground-glass appearance may be noted. In addition to the pulmonary manifestations, the patient may have conjunctivitis, rhinitis and pharyngitis. Complete recovery within 1–3 months after removal from exposure is the rule, but fatalities have occurred.

Skin manifestations

Beryllium salts may affect the skin in a number of different ways. They may cause primary irritation, producing a lesion with the appearance of a mild acid burn or they may produce allergic contact dermatitis. The latter is caused mainly by beryllium fluoride and manifests itself in the sudden appearance of intense pruritus and erythema, often accompanied by periorbital oedema. Chemical ulcers develop if beryllium fluoride is allowed to come into contact with broken skin whilst the implantation of beryllium salts under the skin will result in the formation of a subcutaneous granuloma. The implantation of pure beryllium under the skin does not cause granulomata to form.

Not all beryllium compounds affect the skin to an equal degree; beryllium fluoride and sulphate are the most reactive whereas beryllium metal, and the pure oxide and hydroxide are harmless to the skin.

Chronic poisoning

Chronic beryllium poisoning produces a sarcoid-like reaction with the formation of granulomatous lesions in the lungs and other organs. The condition does not occur in those who handle only the pure metal or those whose only exposure is to the ores beryl and bertrandite. There is a latent period ranging from a few weeks to several years between first exposure and the onset of symptoms which develop in an insidious manner. The first sign of anything untoward is a dry, nonproductive cough, accompanied by loss of weight and fatigue. The loss of weight may be dramatic and is often the reason for the patient seeking medical advice. Progressive dyspnoea is the most serious and most distressing symptom of the disease. Tachycardia may be noted on physical examination and the fingers may be clubbed.

The radiological appearances include a fine diffuse granularity with hilar lymph node enlargement. Nodules, varying in size from 1–5 mm are noted and may give a 'snow storm' appearance. The nodules may coalesce to form large opacities, especially in the upper lobes. At a late stage in the disease basal emphysema is noted and this may lead to the development of a small pneumothorax. The signs of cor pulmonale are to be expected as the disease progresses.

Histologically, chronic granulomata are found in the lungs resembling those found in sarcoidosis and similar lesions are also found in the skin, in lymph nodes and in the liver. The granulomata may be well or poorly formed and giant cells are found, as in sarcoid. The predominant cell type is the histiocyte, with lesser numbers of plasma cells and lymphocytes also present. There may be areas of focal calcification, the so-called Schaumann bodies. On the basis of the histological appearance, the lesions can be classified into three groups (Table 2.2). The prognosis seems to be best for patients falling into Group II than for those in either of the sub-groups of Group I.

Table 2.2. Classification of histological changes found in chronic beryllium poisoning

	Interstitial cellular infiltration	Granulomata	Areas of focal calcification
Group I			
A	Moderate to marked	Poorly formed or absent	Frequently present and numerous
B		Well informed.	
Group II	Slight or absent	Numerous and well informed	Few or absent

From D.G. Freiman & H.L. Hardy, *Human Pathology*, **1**, 25, 1970.

Carcinogenicity of beryllium

Beryllium causes sarcomata in the bones and soft tissues of rabbits following intravenous or inhalational exposure and lung cancer has been induced in rats and monkeys following intracheal injections or inhalation of airborne particles. Lung cancer also seems to be a frequent sequel of respiratory disease in beryllium workers and so it is prudent to consider the metal as a human carcinogen and handle it accordingly.

Neighbourhood poisoning

Cases of beryllium poisoning in individuals living in the vicinity of a beryllium-using factory have been reported. This situation is analogous to that which has arisen in connection with asbestos and poses grave problems both to industrial users and to those concerned with environmental health.

Diagnosis and treatment

The diagnosis of beryllium poisoning depends upon a history of exposure to the metal and the demonstration of beryllium in the urine or in some tissue, either the skin or the lung. The presence of beryllium in the urine indicates that exposure has taken place, but because the rate of excretion is variable, does not indicate the degree of exposure. Most patients with the disease have a positive lymphocyte transformation to beryllium, and a positive macrophage inhibition test.

Berylliosis may be differentiated from sarcoidosis by the fact that the latter condition may be accompanied by uveitis, involvement of the salivary and lacrimal glands, erythema nodosum, lupus pernio, cystic changes in the bones and by a positive Kveim test. None of these is seen in berylliosis. Moreover, the radiological changes in sarcoid may resolve spontaneously; this is never the case in beryllium poisoning.

Chelation therapy with EDTA has been successfully tried in some patients with acute poisoning. In chronic poisoning the pulmonary changes are unlikely to be noted until there is severe, irreversible damage, but the disease process can be halted with corticosteroids. The prognosis in chronic beryllium poisoning has improved in recent years. Nowadays deaths from the disease are rare, whereas at one time it carrid a mortality rate of about 33%. Patients are often left with permanent respiratory impairment, however, but most will be able to work although they are often forced to take a light job. Those with established disease should not, of course, be further exposed.

Manganese

Uses

Manganese is used principally in the manufacture of steel alloys, since its addition to steel greatly enhances its hardness and tensile strength. Ferromanganese is added during the process of steel making to prevent the formation of iron oxide and iron sulphide in the finished product. Other alloys are made with copper, zinc and aluminium. Manganese also has a use in the manufacture of dry cell batteries, whilst in the glass and ceramics industries it is used to remove the green and yellow colours due to traces of iron. Manganese pigments are used in the manufacture of paints, varnishes and dyes, especially those used in calico printing, and it is used in glass-making to colour glass violet. Methylcyclopentadienyl manganese tricarbonyl (MMT) is used as a smoke inhibitor in fuel oil and as an anti-knock agent in petrol to supplement lead alkyls.

Hazards of use

The commonest source of hazard arises during the mining and crushing of the ores and the handling of the resultant manganese oxide. Reduction of the dioxide to produce the metal carries a risk of exposure to fume. In the manufacture of batteries and paints the dioxide is handled as a dry dust which presents a hazard in the absence of adequate safety measures.

Metabolism

Manganese is an essential trace mineral. The rate of absorption of inorganic manganese from the gut is very slow and in the trace amounts in which it is present in food, the manganese is probably in the form of organic chelates which are absorbed more avidly. The occupational hazard is thus due to inhaled manganese, although manganese tricarbonyls are absorbed through the skin. Following absorption, plasma clearance is rapid and the metal tends to accumulate in tissues rich in mitochondria, mainly the liver, but also in the kidney; a small amount is present in bone.

The main homeostatic mechanism for regulating the levels of manganese in the body is by biliary excretion and thus elimination is almost exclusively through the faeces. Less than 1% of the daily intake appears in the urine and even after a large intravenous dose, little is excreted through the kidney. MMT, by contrast, is excreted through the urine to a considerable degree.

Acute poisoning

Manganese dioxide fume is irritant to the mucosa of the respiratory tract and may produce pharyngitis or bronchitis. No permanent sequelae are noted although workers exposed to manganese were reported as having an abnormally high risk from pneumonia which does not differ from the usual type except in its slow response to treatment. This view, however, is not generally accepted.

Chronic poisoning

Chronic manganese poisoning is said to pass through three not very distinct stages. In the first there are no specific signs or symptoms but workers may complain of anorexia, lassitude, apathy, headaches, weakness in the legs, cramps, joint pains and irritability. The second stage is characterized by the development of parkinsonian signs such as dysarthria, disturbances of gait and excessive salivation. These may be accompanied or preceded by the appearance of an acute organic psychosis (so-called manganic madness) which usually disappears when true parkinsonian symptoms become established. The final stage of the disease is marked by rigidity, most pronounced in the lower limbs, by muscular pains, paraesthesiae and by disturbances in speech. The tremor present in manganic parkinsonism is frequently an intention tremor and not the resting temor which is seen in idiopathic parkinsonism. There is often some degree of dystonia present in manganic parkinsonism which is not seen in the idiopathic condition. In the early stages, the disease is generally reversible but the development of parkinsonian features denotes permanent damage to the CNS.

In patients with manganic parkinsonism it is the striatum and the pallidum which show most structural damage and the substantia nigra is relatively unaffected; this is the reverse of what is seen in true parkinsonism. The concentration of dopamine in all areas of the basal ganglia is depleted, however.

Manganese pneumonia

Workers engaged in smelting manganese ores or in making potassium permanganate from manganese oxide are reported to be particularly prone to develop lobar pneumonia. The disease does not differ from that seen in other persons except that it is more resistant to treatment with antibiotics. There are no permanent sequelae and fibrotic changes in the lungs are not noted.

Treatment

Removal from exposure leads to recovery from acute poisoning. Mild cases of chronic poisoning may show some resolution of their psychiatric symptoms after exposure is discontinued. The effectiveness of EDTA in treating chronic poisoning is not encouraging, but most patients with parkinsonian symptoms are greatly helped by L-dopa.

Chromium

Uses

Chromium is used for the production of alloys with nickel and molybdenum and in making corrosion-resistant steels. It is also used for chromium plating, as a tanning agent in the leather industry and as a pigment in paints and inks, and in rubber and ceramics.

Hazards of use
These arise from any processes which involve the handling of the metal or its compounds. During the process of chromium plating, a chromic acid mist is produced which is a potential hazard if the local exhaust ventilation on the plating tank is working inefficiently.

Metabolism
Chromium is an essential trace element required for glucose metabolism. Absorption from the gut depends upon the chemical form which is ingested: less than 1% of trivalent chromium is absorbed, whereas for hexavalent compounds, this value rises to 50%. The rate of absorption from the lung is unknown, although considerable quantities are retained there and the lungs are amongst the organs which normally contain the highest concentration of chromium. The metal is rapidly removed from the blood and is excreted predominantly in the urine. At least 80% of chromium is excreted via the kidney, the remainder appears in the faeces.

Poisoning
The trivalent chromium, which binds to organic molecules, is toxic although ironically, workers exposed to hexavalent compounds are most at risk because the hexavalent compounds are much more readily absorbed.

The skin in the organ chiefly affected by chrome and the lesions produced are described in Chapter 7. The nasal mucosa may become ulcerated and this is a hazard which is experienced principally by those engaged in chrome-plating operations. As a rule the ulceration is painless and is discovered during a medical examination. The cartilaginous part of the septum only is affected and it may become perforated. Malignant change does not supervene.

Inflammation of the larynx with ulceration has been described and a pneumonitis can occur with exposure to high concentrations of chromic acid mist. In a few cases, asthmatic symptoms have been described in men exposed to chrome.

Carcinoma of the lung has an increased incidence amongst chromate workers and this association is referred to again in the chapter on occupational cancer.

Zinc

Uses
Zinc is used as a rust-proof coating for iron and steel, in the manufacture of alloys and, in the form of sheet, as a case for batteries, etc. The oxide and the sulphide are used in the dyestuffs and paint industries, and the chloride is used in soldering fluxes. Brass contains copper and from 5–40% of zinc.

Hazards of use
The chief hazard is from the inhalation of zinc oxide fume which is generated when the metal is heated above its melting point. Zinc chloride fumes in heavy concentrations can be toxic, even lethal.

Metabolism

Zinc is an essential metal. It is poorly absorbed from the gut and excreted mainly in the faeces. Just as with iron, the kidneys play little part in regulating body stores. There are a number of zinc-containing enzymes of which the first to be identified was carbonic anhydrase. Zinc is vital for the proper functioning of these enzymes but in addition, it also seems to be necessary in the process of wound healing. It has been suggested that the indolent ulcers on Henry VIII's legs were a consequence of his state of zinc deficiency.

Poisoning

Inhalation of zinc oxide fume gives rise to the syndrome known as metal-fume fever. Other metals can produce the syndrome, including copper and magnesium, which with zinc are the commonest causes, but aluminium, antimony, cadmium, iron, silver and copper are also culpable. The symptoms are recognized in a number of industries, hence the many synonyms for the disease: brassfounders' ague, brass chills, smelter shakes, zinc chills, galvanizers' poisoning, copper fever, foundry fever, Monday fever and the smothers.

The symptoms, which resemble those of influenza, include chills, fever, headaches, nausea, thirst, cough and pain in the limbs. There is usually a leucocytosis of $12.0–16.0 \times 10^9/l$. Recovery is rapid, usually within 24 hours and always within 48 hours. There are no sequelae. Those who work continuously with zinc develop an immunity to attacks which is quickly lost. It is for this reason that the attacks are more prevalent on Mondays after a weekend away from work.

Zinc chloride fumes are toxic in high concentrations, producing dyspnoea, retrosternal and epigastric pain, stridor and cough with expectoration. Fatalities have been recorded.

Zinc stearate

Fatalities following the inhalation of zinc stearate have occurred in infants, and occupational exposure may cause redness and irritation of the mucous membranes of the nose, but the material is generally not regarded as being unduly toxic.

Nickel

Uses

Nickel is used in the production of a number of alloys, including special steels. So-called silver coins are, in fact, made from an alloy of copper and nickel, whilst with zinc and copper, nickel forms the basis of silver-plated tableware, etc.—EPNS. Finely divided nickel is used as a catalyst, especially in the hydrogenation of oils to solid fats. The metal is also used to make enamels and is a constituent of nickel-cadmium batteries. Nickel salts (of which nickel sulphate is the most important) are widely used in electroplating, and all chrome plated products have an under-layer of nickel which is several times the thickness of the chrome finish.

Metabolism
Nickel is an essential element which is required for normal haematopoiesis. It is poorly absorbed from the gut and under normal circumstances it is rapidly excreted in the faeces. When present in excess, however, as occurs following occupational exposure, it is also excreted in the urine with a half-life of between 17 and 39 hours. Nickel carbonyl (qv) is metabolically oxidized to divalent nickel and carbon monoxide.

Hazards of use
All those who handle nickel or its salts are liable to be at risk.

Poisoning
Nickel and its salts are the most potent of skin sensitizers and the so-called nickel itch has been known since 1908 when it was first described by Rambousek. The contact dermatitis which it produces has no special characteristics and it may be found in anyone who comes into contact with the metal in the course of their occupation however it is handled. It may also occur in those who have contact with the metal in items of clothing or jewellery. Nickel dermatitis may at times be so severe that those affected by it are forced into finding alternative employment which does not involve exposure.

The more serious risk resulting from exposure to nickel, however, is the possible development of cancer of the respiratory tract. Studies carried out in several countries have shown that nickel refinery workers have an excess risk of cancer of the nasal sinuses, the lung and the larynx. This risk does not seem to be shared by workers who are exposed to nickel outside refineries.

The most toxic of the nickel compounds is nickel carbonyl which is considered in more detail in Chapter 5.

Vanadium

Uses
Much of the vanadium used in industry goes to the manufacture of special steel alloys, because the addition of small amounts of vanadium greatly increases the tensile strength of steel. It is also a major element in high-strength titanium alloys. Vanadium salts are used also as catalysts in chemical processes, the most important being vanadium pentoxide, in the production of sulphuric acid. Vanadium compounds are also used in the manufacture of dyes, inks, paints and varnishes.

Hazards of use
Hazards may arise during the crushing of the ores when dust may be inhaled. Most cases of poisoning, however, have occurred during the cleaning of oil-fired burners or gas turbines. Vanadium occurs in all fuel oils but the amount of the metal in the ash depends upon the geographical origin of the crude oil. Venezualan oil contains most and there may be as much as 45% vanadium in ash from such oil. Vanadium is a constituent of the blood pigment of sea squirts

and sea cucumbers which pass their life fixed to rocks and the fossilized remains of these creatures account for the vanadium present in crude oil.

Metabolism

Vanadium is an essential element concerned with lipid metabolism. It is poorly absorbed from the gut and even if soluble salts are ingested only about 1% is taken up. In the blood, vanadium is almost entirely bound to transferrin and it is rapidly excreted in the urine; very little appears in the faeces. Although the metal is not stored to any great extent in the body, it has been noted that concentrations in the lung tend to increase with age.

Poisoning

The toxic effects of vanadium are the result of inflammation of the mucous membranes. Thus conjunctivitis, nasal catarrh and bronchitis are prominent initial symptoms. There may be soreness in the throat and chest and the patient has a dry cough. Wheezing and dyspnoea of effort appear at a later stage, usually within 6–24 hours after first exposure. A tremor of the fingers and hands may be present and some patients complain of depression. The characteristic feature of vanadium intoxication is a greenish-black discoloration of the tongue. The colour disappears within 2–3 days after exposure is discontinued.

Eczematous lesions of the skin have been noted and it is suggested that workers should be batch tested with 2% sodium vanadate before being allowed into contact with the metal.

There are no long-term sequelae of vanadium poisoning although it is said that those who inhale the metal have an increased susceptibility to bronchitis and pneumonia.

Treatment

Fortunately none is required since complete, rapid recovery is the rule.

Phosphorous

Phosphorus presents as an industrial hazard in one of four forms, as yellow phosphorous, as tri-ortho-cresyl phosphate, as organic phosphorus insecticides and as phosphine which is discussed in Chapter 5.

Yellow phosphorus

Uses

Yellow phosphorus is one of the three allotropes of phosphorus and the only one which is poisonous. Red phosphorus is made from yellow phosphorus and used in the manufacture of matches and fireworks. Yellow phosphorus is generally banned for the manufacture of all but war goods, where its incendiary properties lend themselves to the manufacture of explosives and so on.

Phosphorus compounds are used in the manufacture of detergents, in paper-making, printing and in the manufacture of soaps and dyes. The fertilizer industry uses vast quantities of phosphorus compounds in producing super-phosphate, and metaphosphates are widely used as water softeners.

Hazards of use

Yellow phosphorus bursts into flame at a temperature of 30°C, burning to form dense white clouds of phosphorus pentoxide. It must never be picked up by the fingers since it will produce painful burns which are slow to heal. In contact with air it oxidizes to form phosphorus trioxide and possibly the pentoxide, the fumes of which are poisonous.

Poisoning

Yellow phosphorus was once widely used to make matches but this practice was banned by the Berne Convention of 1906. Phosphorus sesquisulphide is used as a harmless substitute for 'non-safety' matches. The condition which used to affect those engaged in match dipping was known as 'phossy jaw'.

Phossy jaw was an extensive necrosis, usually of the mandible, which developed after a latent interval of anything up to 5 years after first exposure. The condition was heralded by the onset of toothache in a carious tooth. A dull red spot which could be found on the buccal mucosa at this early stage was pathognomonic of the disease. As the disease progressed, the jaw swelled and became painful. The teeth became loose and sinuses formed from the necrotic cavities in the jaw which often contained large sequestra. The sinuses discharged chronically and the whole jaw was often eventually involved in the disease process. The victim was terribly disfigured and a burden to himself and to others on account of the foul smell of the pus which formed as the necrotic bone became infected. The secondary infection sometimes brought about death by spread to the meninges but septicaemia was the more common terminal event and the overall case mortality rate was about 20%. Excision of the jaw was the only treatment which could be offered to the patient and the operation might entail the removal of the whole mandible. Bones other than the lower jaw were affected and this involvement was frequently brought to light through the development of spontaneous fractures.

Yellow phosphorus continues to be used for making weapons of war and great care is now taken during its handling. Nevertheless, minor cases of phossy jaw still occur, but are detected early and the gross case is more likely to trouble the candidate in a pathology examination than the practising occupational physician.

Organic phosphorus insecticides

These compounds are structurally related to di-iso-propylfluoro phosphate and, like it, are powerful irreversible ChE inhibitors. Since 1945 many new compounds have been elaborated and produced on a large scale. Those which are scheduled under the Agriculture (Poisonous Substances) Act of 1952 are shown in Table 2.3.

Table 2.3. Organo-phosphorus insecticides scheduled under the Agriculture (Poisonous Substances) Act, 1952

Amiton and its salts	Mevinphos
Azinphos-ethyl	Mipafox
Azinphos-methyl	Oxydemeton-methyl
Chlorfenvinphos	Parathion
Demeton	Phenkapton
Demeton-methyl	Phorate
Demeton-s-methyl	Phosphamidon
Dichlorvos	Schradan
Dimefox	Sulfotep
Disulfoten	TEPP
Ethion	Thionazin
Mazidox	Vamidothion
Mecarbam	

Metabolism

Organo-phosphorus compounds are readily absorbed through the skin as well as by inhalation and ingestion. They do not accumulate in the body and most are rapidly degraded and excreted. The degradation products, being water-soluble, are excreted in the urine; very little of the unchanged compounds appear in the urine. In some cases, the process of degradation produces metabolites which are more toxic than the parent compound. For example, malaoxon and paroxon are more toxic than malathion and parathion from which they derive respectively.

Poisoning

The toxic properties of these compounds to humans relate to their anti-ChE activity and depend upon the speed and degree of the ChE inhibition. Toxic symptoms appear when ChE activity is reduced to less than 50% of normal. When parathion was introduced on a large scale its dangers were not fully appreciated and careless use and sloppy handling resulted in several cases of poisoning.

Early signs of poisoning are not specific and include headache, nausea, anorexia and a marked lassitude. Constriction of the pupils may occur and all the symptoms are aggravated by smoking. In a short time following exposure these relatively mild symptoms are superseded by vomiting, diarrhoea, abdominal pain and muscle twitching. Incontinence of urine and faeces is common. Pulmonary oedema is a frequent finding. The onset of convulsions usually signifies that the patient is about to pass into a coma which may lead to death. The complete course from exposure to death may take as little as an hour so that speed is of the essence if treatment is to be successful.

Treatment with atropine should be given immediately and the patient supported with mechanical respiration if necessary. Cholinesterase activity can be restored by compounds which split the enzyme from its attachment to the phosphate group of the insecticide. Pralidoxime (P2S of P2AM) is satisfactory for this purpose, and a number of hospitals hold supplies of this drug and maintain a 24-hour service.

Late sequelae of poisoning with organo-phosphorus compounds have been noted. The patient recovers from the acute phase but about 3 weeks later notes progressive muscular weakness and fatigue with vomiting and diarrhoea. Marked muscle wasting may follow. The symptoms are similar to those of TOCP poisoning.

To avoid these late complications, all patients who have an attack of acute poisoning should be kept under observation until their blood cholinesterase activity has returned to normal.

Chronic effects

Neuromuscular function and nerve conduction velocities are altered in some workers with prolonged exposure to organo-phosphorus compounds but the significance of these findings is uncertain. There is also some evidence to suggest that prolonged exposure may impair renal tubular function.

Prevention

Those using organo-phosphorus insecticides scheduled under the 1952 Act are obliged by law to be issued with and to wear protective clothing. No one is allowed to work with them for more than 10 hours in one day or 60 hours in seven days. No one under the age of 18 may work with them at all.

Those at risk should have periodic tests of their blood cholinesterase activity, or alternatively have nerve conduction velocities measured. There is a good correlation between urinary excretion of *p*-nitrophenol and exposure to parathion and this fact may also be made use of in screening programmes. It is also helpful to conduct periodic clinical or radiological examinations of the chest, since the finding of pulmonary oedema without any evidence of cardiac enlargement in an otherwise fit agricultural worker should raise the possibility of intoxication.

Arsenic

Uses

Arsenical compounds are used in the manufacture of agricultural insecticides and weed killers, one of which, cacodylic acid (dimethyl arsonic acid) is quite commonly used by foresters in the United States. Some fungicides and wood preservations contain arsenic and so do some sheep and cattle dips. In the glass industry it is used to remove the green tint produced by iron oxide. Anti-fouling compounds for ships may contain arsenic and they are also used in dyes and soaps. Arsenic is added to some alloys in small amounts (0.3–0.5%) to increase hardening and heat resistance and similar amounts added to molten lead make the metal harder and assist in the formation of truly spherical pellets of lead shot. A number of organic arsenical compounds are still in therapeutic use.

Arsenical pigments were once widely used, and they resulted in a considerable morbidity. Cupric arsenite (Scheele's green) enjoyed great popularity in the nineteenth century as a colouring for wallpaper and was capable of releasing dimethyl arsine through the action of a mould growing in the paste, which it is said could prove fatal. These compounds are seldom met nowadays.

Hazards of use

Industrial risks mainly result from the inhalation of the very light dust of the arsenical compound during handling processes, but some vapour may be encountered during the smelting and refining of ores.

Crop sprayers are at risk from arsenic which comes into contact with the skin. They might also, of course, inhale the spray if not properly protected.

Metabolism

Inorganic arsenic compounds are absorbed by inhalation, ingestion and through the intact skin. Over 95% of arsenic in the blood is bound to the protein of haemoglobin. It is stored in the tissues, and tends to accumulate in the muscles and liver, and to a lesser extent in the other viscera, and particularly in hair and nails. The affinity of arsenic for the protein in hair is the basis of forensic tests for detecting arsenical poisoning.

Excretion takes place predominantly through the kidney. In the urine arsenic is mainly in the organic, methylated form. The concentration of arsenic in the urine is a reasonable indication of the degree of exposure and is the most widely used form of biological monitoring.

Acute poisoning

Acute poisoning in industry is rare but when it is seen, it is the result of inhaling high concentrations of dust. The first symptoms are those of severe respiratory irritation with cough, inspiratory chest pain and dyspnoea. These early symptoms are followed by headache, vertigo and lassitude and those gastrointestinal symptoms such as are seen after the ingestion of arsenic or its compounds.

Acute poisoning by ingestion is the more common presentation and is usually the result of arsenic administered for suicidal or homicidal purposes. If the dose is large enough, the victim may collapse and die within 20 minutes. More often, however, smaller doses are ingested which produce vomiting, diarrhoea, abdominal pain and muscle cramps. If the patient survives there are usually no sequelae although a few cases are known in which exfoliative dermatitis and peripheral neuropathy have developed.

Chronic poisoning

Chronic intoxication particularly affects the skin and is discussed in Chapter 6. Peripheral neuropathy appears in some cases and is usually accompanied by pain, burning and tenderness, and difficulty in walking. The presence of broad white striae on the finger nails (Mees lines) is said to be diagnostic.

Gastrointestinal symptoms, including nausea, vomiting and abdominal pain occur, but none is common.

Arsenic dust has a local action on the mucous membranes producing conjunctivitis, blepharitis, rhinitis, pharyngitis, laryngitis and bronchitis. Hoarseness may be a prominent symptom and painless perforation of the cartilaginous part of the nasal septum is sometimes observed. Arsenic dust in the glass industry produces a well-recognized rash on the skin. The carcinogenic action of arsenic is considered in Chapter 8.

Organic arsenic compounds

The organic arsenic compounds are powerful vesicants and lung irritants and exposure to these compounds is restricted to the chemists who synthesize them and to those who are concerned with their development as war gases. BAL (British anti-Lewisite), was developed specifically to counter the action of the arsenical war gas, Lewisite (chlorovinyl dichlorarsine). It is a dithiol compound, 2, 3, -dimercapto propanol, and owes its efficacy to the high affinity which arsenic has for sulphydryl (–SH) groups. BAL was later used in the treatment of lead and mercury poisoning on the basis of their known affinity for –SH groups, but it has now been largely replaced by EDTA and penicillamine.

Aluminium

Aluminium is very widely used both alone and in combination with other metals in the manufacture of household utensils, laboratory equipment, cables and wires, packaging materials, foils and reflectors and powder for use in paints.

Aluminium is extremely poorly absorbed and under normal circumstances the lungs, skin and gastrointestinal tract act as almost complete barriers to its uptake. In states of iron deficiency, when plasma ferritin levels are low, the rate of uptake from the gut may be enhanced, however. Because of its poor uptake, the body burden of aluminium is very low, probably not more than 30–40 mg. The lungs contain the highest level of aluminium and levels increase with age; this is because insoluble compounds are trapped and retained there. Aluminium is found in the brain and in this organ too, levels increase with age. The only route for the elimination of aluminium from the body is via the kidney.

Such toxic effects as there are from aluminium are directed against the lung. There is some evidence that men who work in the potroom in aluminium smelters may develop an asthma-like condition with wheeze and shortness of breath but by no means all those who have investigated this problem are convinced that potroom asthma exists as a specific entity.

A respiratory disease was described by Shaver in workers manufacturing corundum, a commonly used abrasive which consists mainly of aluminium oxide. The main symptoms of this condition were shortness of breath, wheeze and cough. An acute form characterized by cough, fever, tachypnoea and cyanosis was also described. There were a number of abnormalities on the chest X-ray which resembled those seen in silicosis. Shaver's disease has now been consigned to history, no new cases having been reported since 1950.

Exposure to pure aluminium powder may produce a form of interstitial pulmonary fibrosis. Patients may complain of breathlessness and a dry, nonproductive cough. Chest pain is common due most often to the development of a spontaneous pneumothorax. Pulmonary function tests show a restrictive impairment often with an abormal diffusing capacity. Nowadays, when aluminium powder is stamped out the surface is covered with stearates and in this protected form it is not dangerous.

The neurotoxic effects of aluminium have been much investigated in recent years. Dialysis dementia was reported first in 1972 in patients who had received long-term haemodialysis for renal failure. A variety of neurological symptoms was noted, including dyspraxia, asterixis, tremor, myoclonus, loss of memory and changes in personality. All were preceded by changes in the EEG. Later in the disease patients developed loss of speech and motor co-ordination and seizures occurred, frequently followed by death. The concentration of aluminium in the brains of those who died from dialysis dementia was elevated and there seems little reason to doubt that the metal was the causative agent.

More recently, consideration has been given to the possible role of aluminium in the production of Alzheimer's disease. Certainly aluminium levels increase in the brain in old age and aluminium silicates can be found in the plaques found in affected neurones. There is no evidence to date, however, which unequivocally links aluminium with the aetiology of Alzheimer's disease and the cry to abandon aluminium pots and pans in order to reduce the incidence of the disease seems more than a little premature.

Antimony

Antimony is used industrially in several metallurgical processes, in the ceramic and glass industries, as a pigment in paints, and in the rubber and plastics industries. Antimony compounds are also used in the manufacture of semiconductors to 'dope' crystals in much the same way as arsine is used (see p. 84). Although it is known to be toxic, cases of poisoning usually arise from mishaps outside industry, often through overdosage with compounds such as potassium antimony tartarate (tartar emetic) used to treat schistosomiasis or from the preparation and storage of food in vessels with an antimony glaze.

The symptoms of acute poisoning are similar to those of acute arsenical poisoning although vomiting is more severe and continuous and accompanied by watery diarrhoea. Cardiac arrhythmias have been frequently noted as toxic manifestations of antimony poisoning and the mortality rate from this complication may be considerable. Mild jaundice has also been noted, whilst in a number of cases, a maculopapular rash has been observed.

The antimony used in industry is frequently contaminated with arsenic and toxic symptoms noted in workers handling antimony ores have often been attributed to the arsenic present. In some cases, however, it seems likely that antimony was producing adverse reactions in those exposed to dust and fume, including such symptoms as vomiting, diarrhoea, vertigo and headaches. Electrocardiographic changes have been reported in some workers, the most common being abnormalities of the T-wave. On the skin, antimony may produce punched out ulcers, 'antimony pocks' which usually appear on the forearms and are slow to heal.

Osmium

Osmium is not itself toxic, but osmium tetroxide, used as an histological stain, is irritant to the mucous membranes of the eyes, nose, pharynx and bronchus. In high concentrations it produces a constriction of the chest, an inability to breathe and, rarely, a fatal bronchiolitis. Osmium tetroxide vapour is so irritant that the risk of inhaling a lethal quantity is slight. Continued inhalation of small amounts, however, is said to predispose to bronchitis and chemical pneumonitis. Headache is sometimes a feature of mild intoxication and characteristically, a halo is seen around light sources.

Platinum

Platinum salts give rise to a pronounced irritation of the nose and upper respiratory tract, which in turn produces a running nose and a cough. Platinum asthma is a common and important condition arising in those exposed to chloroplatinic acid or one of its salts and normally results only after prolonged exposure. This is not an invariable rule however. Skin lesions are also produced, consisting of a dry scaly dermatitis which cracks and bleeds. This combination of respiratory and dermatological disorders is sometimes called platinosis.

Platinum metal (in those who can afford it) may give rise to a contact dermatitis.

Selenium and tellurium

Selenium is one of the essential elements, its function being related to the detoxification of free radicals. It is also antagonistic to the toxic effects of mercury. Soluble selenium compounds are rapidly absorbed from the lung and the gut and methylated in the liver to form the trimethylselenonium ion which is rapidly excreted in the urine. Under conditions of high exposure the volatile metabolite dimethylselenide is formed and this is eliminated through the lungs where it gives the breath the smell of garlic.

Selenium dioxide is met as a by-product of a number of processes including copper and nickel smelting, during silver refining or when selenium alloys are welded or heated. Selenium dioxide dusts are highly irritant to mucous membranes and the inhalation of high concentrations may produce pulmonary oedema. In its liquid form, selenium dioxide is highly vesicant and can cause serious skin burns which should be treated with 10% sodium thiosulphate. Continued contact with selenium dioxide may result in a local or generalized dermatitis and some workers exposed to it may develop conjunctivitis referred to in the trade as 'rose eye'.

The antioxidant properties of selenium are sometimes said to be protective against the development of cancer but the evidence in support of this view is somewhat tenuous.

Not much is known about the metabolism of tellurium except that it too produces a dimethyl compound which gives a garlic smell to the breath. Much smaller amounts of tellurium than selenium are required to produce this effect; the administration of ascorbic acid is reputed to be effective in preventing this unfortunate metabolic reaction.

Long-term exposure to tellurium may reduce the ability to sweat but this does not seem to cause heat stress in those working in hot environments. In experimental animals tellurium is teratogenic and it may cause testicular damage; neither effect has been reported amongst those exposed to it in their course of their work.

Silver

Although silver produces no constitutional symptoms, absorbed silver is precipitated in the tissues where it is fixed and becomes dissolved, producing either local or generalized argyria. Local argyria is more common, resulting from the impregnation of the skin with small particles of silver. These are converted first to silver albuminate and then to silver sulphide which produces discrete areas of grey-blue pigmentation. Local lesions may be found in the eyes, confined to the conjunctiva.

In the more rare generalized argyria, the uncovered areas of skin are a uniform dark, slate-grey colour. Affected men are known as 'blue men'. The finger-nails are chocolate brown and the buccal mucosa is grey or blue in colour. The covered parts of the skin are as a rule unaffected or at most only faintly pigmented. The conjunctiva are discoloured grey to deep brown and examination of the lens with a slit lamp shows a grey pigmentation of Decemet's membrane. There is usually no disturbance of vision.

In cases of generalized argyria which come to autopsy, silver granules can be found in the internal organs and in the mucosa of the respiratory tract. The granules are also seen in the internal elastic laminae of the arterioles, in the elastic fibres of connective tissue, in the connective tissue between myocardial fibrils, and in the basement membranes of sweat glands, renal tubule cells and the ependymal cells of the choroid plexus. The testes may appear black, but here as elsewhere, no interference with function is recorded as a result of the silver impregnation.

Thallium

Thallium is an extremely toxic substance, more toxic than lead, but less toxic than arsenic. Industrial poisoning is rare despite its great potential for harm: it is absorbed via every route, cutaneous, pulmonary and gastrointestinal. Excretion is slow and the metal is cumulative.

Acute poisoning may result from the deliberate or accidental ingestion of a thallium containing rat poison. The initial effects are hypotension and bradycardia which result from the direct action of thallium on the sinus node and on the contractility of the cardiac muscle. The early effects are followed by hypertension and tachycardia thought to be due to degeneration of the vagus.

Chronic thallium poisoning presents a very characteristic pattern comprising peripheral neuropathy, gastroenteritis and loss of hair. The neuropathy resembles that seen in riboflavin deficiency and the mechanism is the same, a disruption in the transport of electrons during intracellular respiration. Clinically the neuropathy may resemble a Guillain–Barré syndrome except that the deep tendon reflexes are lost relatively late in the course of thallium poisoning. In many cases the presenting symptoms of the disease are abdominal pain and bloody diarrhoea. Hepatic and renal necrosis may develop; the hair loss occurs late in the disease although a dark line can be seen at the base of the hair shaft within a few days of the ingestion of a large dose of the metal.

Thallium poisoning is treated with Prussian blue given twice daily through a stomach tube. Thallium displaces potassium from the Prussian blue molecule and the thallium ions are thus sequestered in the gut and their absorption is hindered. The concurrent intravenous administration of potassium sufficient to maintain plasma potassium levels between 4.0 and 4.5 mmol/l will enhance the excretion of thallium into the gut and speed up its elimination.

Tin

In industry, tin is met in both its inorganic and its organic forms. Inorganic tin compounds are poorly absorbed from the gut although the divalent form is taken up rather more readily than the tetravalent. Absorbed tin is preferentially deposited in the lung, kidney, liver and bone and is excreted mainly through the urine.

Organotin compounds are absorbed much more effectively from the gut and tri-alkyl tin is well absorbed through intact skin. The highest concentration of organotin compounds is generally found in the liver. Most organotin compounds undergo biotransformation in the liver although the dealkylation of diethyl tin compounds appear also to take place in the gut. One important reaction is the conversion of tetra-alkyl tin compounds into their more toxic tri-forms. Ethyl tin compounds are excreted in the urine whereas diethyl tin is excreted in the urine and in the bile. In many cases, organotin compounds have long half-lives in the body and are slow to clear.

Inorganic tin compounds do not cause toxic effects in humans although prolonged exposure to tin oxide dust and fumes produces a benign form of pneumoconiosis known as stannosis (qv).

Of the organic compounds, the mono-organic and di-organic forms are less toxic than the tri-organic, and the toxicity of the tri-alkyl tin compounds decreases as the number of carbon atoms in the alkyl chain decreases. Some of the organotin compounds are irritant but the alkyl and aromatic compounds are also neurotoxic. Workers handling dibutyl and tributyl tin have experienced burns which heal without scarring; splashes of tributyl tin in the eye may cause permanent damage and the inhalation of this compound may produce intense respiratory irritation. Triethyl tin intoxication produces widespread damage to the white matter in the CNS with symptoms such as vertigo, nausea, vomiting and visual disturbances. These symptoms may be accompanied by signs of raised intracranial pressure and focal EEG changes.

Chapter 3
Industrial Toxicology 2: Organic Solvents

Many thousands of organic compounds are used in industry and large numbers of new compounds are introduced each year. Many of the organic compounds are used as solvents and hence exposure to solvents is widespread. As with the metals, it will be possible here to mention only the most important of the selection available, and a few general considerations of some of the metabolic and toxicological properties of solvents may be helpful in understanding what follows.

General considerations of solvent metabolism and toxicology

Organic solvents—by which one simply means any compound used to carry another in solution—may be either fat or water soluble and they may undergo biotransformation in the body or circulate unchanged. Their solubility determines their distribution within the body. Fat soluble solvents tend to accumulate selectively in the organs rich in lipids, including the nervous system. Water soluble solvents, on the other hand, enter the body water compartment and have the potential to become much more widely distributed. All solvents are readily absorbed through the lung in their vapour phase, but fat soluble solvents may also be absorbed through the skin.

Solvents which are not biotransformed are excreted either in exhaled air or unchanged in the urine. From the solvents which are biotransformed (and these are the majority), metabolites appear in the urine and their rate of excretion may be used to monitor exposure at work. For all solvents, biological monitoring may also include estimations of the concentration of the unchanged compound in the exhaled air or in the blood.[*]

Just as with metals, interactions are important in determining the metabolic and toxic consequences of solvent exposure. Many organic compounds interfere with the metabolism of others, mainly through competition for common pathways. Thus the rate of metabolism of two (or more) benzene analogues will be slower when given together than when administered separately; the co-administration of two chemically unrelated species such as trichloroethylene and benzene may also result in metabolic interference due to competition for co-factors.

One interesting interaction is that between ethanol and some solvents. The biotransformation of the benzene analogues, for example, follows a common pathway, the first step of which is an oxidation to form the alcohol derivative.

---

[*]It should be noted that it is more accurate to talk of biotransformation than detoxification when considering the metabolism of organic compounds, because in a number of cases, the daughter compounds are more toxic than their parents.

This is followed by a reduction reaction brought about by alcohol dehydrogenase using NADP as co-factor. In acute experiments it can be shown that when alcohol is co-administered with a benzene analogue the biotransformation of the solvent is considerably delayed. Under experimental conditions, when the molar dose of ethanol far exceeds that of the solvent the ethanol is able to compete successfully for the enzyme and thus delay the biotransformation of the solvent. The solvent will be metabolized again when the relative solvent/ethanol concentrations are in favour of the solvent.

The effects of alcohol on solvent metabolism, however, are not as simple as acute exposure chamber studies would lead one to believe. Ethanol is an enzyme inducer and continuous exposure leads to an increase in the activity of the P-450 mixed function oxidazes which catalyse the initial oxidation of many solvents. Thus animals given ethanol over a long time may be able to biotransform solvents at a rate which is quicker than normal and there is also some suggestion that amongst workers, consistently heavy drinkers get rid of solvents faster than their more abstemious colleagues.

So far as toxic effects are concerned, there is good reason to suppose that alcohol will add to any central nervous system effects induced by exposure to solvents but there is so far precious little evidence that psychotropic drugs interact with solvents. There is good evidence also that the neurotoxic effects of solvents are affected by co-exposure. For example, the weak neurotoxicity of a material such as methyl ethyl ketone may be enhanced by other solvents in a mixture whereas the neurotoxicity of n-hexane is diminished by co-administration of toluene.

The practical significance of these interactions becomes apparent when one realizes that exposures at work are often to mixtures of solvents rather than to single compounds and this must be taken into account when setting safety standards or devising programmes for biological monitoring.

Aromatic solvents

Benzene

Uses
Benzene is the starting point for a great many synthetic processes in the chemical industry, it was formerly used on a grand scale as a solvent but its toxicity is such that it has been banned from general use if present in a concentration greater than 1% in any solvent. It may be a component of motor fuel. In essential processes in this country it is used entirely in closed systems so that exposures are low. In less developed countries, however, benzene is used as a solvent in the manufacture of rubber or plastic shoes and in photogravure printing; exposures amongst those who use benzene for these purposes may be extremely high.

Hazards of use

Closed systems present little hazard and the only possibility of excessive exposure arises when the systems are maintained or repaired. Operators undertaking such work must be adequately equipped with protective clothing. Where benzene is used as a solvent there is an ever-present danger particularly if it is used in a poorly ventilated workshop.

Metabolism

Benzene is absorbed through the lungs and through the skin. It is lipid soluble and so accumulates in the fatty tissues which act as a reservoir. A large amount of absorbed benzene is exhaled unchanged but between 15 and 60% is biotransformed. The biotransformation of benzene is complex but the preliminary step is oxidation to benzene epoxide which, like all epoxides, is highly reactive and may combine with proteins or with nucleic acids. Benzene epoxide may undergo spontaneous transformation to phenol or it may be hydrated and reduced to catechol or condensed with glutathione to form mercapturic acid. The biological half-life is about 12 hours.

Acute poisoning

This is the more uncommon form of poisoning encountered in industry and is due to accidental exposure to very high concentrations of vapour. The early symptoms include euphoria, giddiness, headache and vomiting. If the victim is not rescued from this exposure unconsciousness and death from respiratory failure may follow.

Chronic poisoning

Benzene is outstanding amongst the industrial poisons in having its principal effects on the bone marrow. There are usually no symptoms in the early stages of chronic intoxication and those which are present tend to be vague and nonspecific and do not correspond in any degree with the severity of the damage inflicted upon the bone marrow. Symptoms of tiredness, mild gastrointestinal disturbance and giddiness are usually first noted and these are followed by haemorrhages from mucous membranes and the development of skin rashes. Anaemia is a common finding in workers with chronic benzene poisoning and this may be accompanied by macrocytosis and thrombocytopaenia. Myelocytes and nucleated red cells may be seen in the peripheral blood film and the red cells show basophilic stippling. Leucopaenia is a frequent finding, with a relative and absolute lymphopaenia. In the early stages the bone marrow may be hyperplastic but if exposure is not discontinued, a true aplastic anaemia may develop with the destruction of all the cellular elements. Aplastic anaemia is the most feared consequence of exposure to benzene and it is thought that the toxic agent is a metabolite which interferes with DNA synthesis; increased rates of chromosome aberrations are seen in workers exposed to benzene and in experimental animals.

Exposure to benzene is also associated with the development of acute leukaemia. Most cases are of the acute myeloblastic type but a few cases of erythroleukaemia have also been described. Leukaemia most often occurs in patients who already have a hypoplastic marrow and a history of heavy exposure is invariable. There may be an interval of several years between the end of last exposure and the development of the leukaemia. It should be noted in passing that not all authorities are convinced that benzene can cause leukaemia but the majority of opinion is against them.

Treatment
Patients with acute poisoning must be removed from exposure and respiratory support given where necessary; this is the case, of course, whatever solvent is involved. There are usually no serious late sequelae.

For those who develop aplastic anaemia or leukaemia following benzene exposure the prognosis is the same as in any other form of these diseases, that is, not outstandingly hopeful. On this account, all those who are exposed to benzene should have regular haematological examinations and those showing any abnormalities should be removed from exposure. Urinary phenol estimations are a useful adjunct to biological monitoring as they correlate reasonably well with exposure; with exposures at the current TLV of 10 ppm, urinary phenol concentrations at the end of the day would not be expected to exceed about 20 mgm/l.

Toluene

Uses
Toluene is one of the most widely used solvents in industry. It is found in paints, resins and glues, as a solvent for rubber and in photogravure printing. It is also an important raw material for synthetic reactions.

Hazards of use
All processes in which toluene are used should be properly ventilated in order to minimize exposure and care should be taken when handling drums to avoid spillage. Toluene is one of the solvents which is commonly sniffed and although sniffing seems to be mainly an out of work pastime, attention should be given to the identification of sniffers in the work force. At normal temperatures toluene gives off highly inflammable vapours and great care must be taken to minimize the risk of fire and explosion. If a vessel which has contained toluene is to be welded or cut with a flame all traces of vapour must be removed by purging.

Metabolism
Toluene is absorbed through the lung and, to a limited degree only, through the skin. Being lipid soluble it accumulates in fatty organs. The biological half-life is 3–4 hours so that it is rapidly excreted once exposure is discontinued. Less than 10% of an absorbed dose is exhaled unchanged, the remainder being biotransformed, mainly to hippuric acid (see Fig. 3.1); small amounts of o-cresol and p-cresol are also formed.

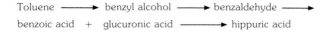

Toluene ⟶ benzyl alcohol ⟶ benzaldehyde ⟶
benzoic acid + glucuronic acid ⟶ hippuric acid

Fig. 3.1 Metabolism of toluene in humans

Toxic effects
All solvents have narcotic properties which many solvent workers experience
from time to time. The concentration at which these properties manifest
themselves obviously varies from solvent to solvent and their narcotic powers
also differ; those which are most narcotic are, or have been, used as
anaesthetics. Above about 1000 ppm, toluene causes vertigo and an intense
headache, higher concentrations may induce coma. High concentrations are
also hallucinogenic and it is for this reason that glues containing toluene are
sniffed. At much lower concentrations, it is usual to find some evidence of
undue tiredness, and vague feelings of ill health which have recovered by the
start of the next working shift. Toluene does not depress the bone marrow and
it is not notably hepatotoxic.

Toluene does not affect the peripheral nervous system and under normal
conditions of exposure there is no unequivocal evidence that it causes organic
brain damage. Experience in this country would also suggest that permanent
neuropsychiatric sequelae are not a consequence of exposure to toluene
although evidence to the contrary has come from elsewhere, most notably from
the Nordic countries. In glue sniffers, on the other hand, there have been well
documented cases of cerebellar degeneration and more recently cases of
dementia have been reported. Sudden deaths in glue sniffers have been ascribed
to ventricular arrhythmias due to sensitization of the myocardium to circulating
catecholamines but the cause is probably more complex than this since the
technique used to sniff glues frequently results in hypercapnia and acidosis.

Xylene

Uses
Xylene is much less commonly encountered than toluene but it is used as a
thinner for paints and varnishes, in the synthesis of dyes and as an additive to
aviation fuels. It is also used in histology laboratories as a solvent for paraffin.

Metabolism
Pulmonary retention of xylene is high, between 60 and 65% of an inhaled dose
being absorbed. It is also well absorbed through the skin and dermal absorption
is a significant route of entry in industry. Virtually all the xylene which is
absorbed is excreted in the form of metabolites, less than 5% being exhaled
unchanged. The route of biotransformation is similar to that of toluene with the
formation of methylhippuric acid which appears in the urine (Fig. 3.2).

Poisoning
The symptoms of acute poisoning are similar to those of toluene poisoning but
xylene is, in addition, an irritant with an unpleasant smell and workers may

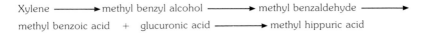

Xylene ⟶ methyl benzyl alcohol ⟶ methyl benzaldehyde ⟶

methyl benzoic acid + glucuronic acid ⟶ methyl hippuric acid

Fig. 3.2 Metabolism of xylene in humans

notice effects on the eyes and the upper respiratory tract. There is no well recognized symptom of chronic intoxication although it may cause an irritant dermatitis and some workers complain of a sweetish taste in the mouth. It is not hepatotoxic or neurotoxic.

Styrene

Uses
Styrene is a highly reactive compound because of the vinyl group which it has in its molecule, and it readily undergoes polymerization, oxidation, hydration or halogenation. It is common to add 3% hydroquinone to styrene to inhibit its polymerization during storage or transport. Its principal uses are in the manufacture of polystyrene and of synthetic rubbers and it is used to carry the resin used in making glass reinforced plastics.

Metabolism
Styrene is avidly absorbed through the lungs and it is also readily absorbed through the skin. A small fraction only (<5%) is excreted unchanged and in humans, the principal metabolic route leads to the formation of mandelic and phenylglyoxylic acids which are excreted in the urine. The biological half-life of phenylglyoxylic acid in the urine is longer than that of mandelic acid and so is excreted for a longer time when exposure is discontinued. The first stage in the process is oxidation to form styrene oxide which is a highly reactive compound with mutagenic properties. It is for this reason that the carcinogenicity of styrene has been investigated. Styrene oxide is very short lived, however, and is rapidly reduced to styrene glycol (Fig. 3.3). In some animals mandelic acid is converted to benzyl alcohol with subsequent formation of hippuric acid which is the main breakdown product. Less than 1% of the styrene absorbed is oxidized on the aromatic ring to form styrene 3,4 oxide which is then converted to vinylphenol; this is of academic rather than practical interest.

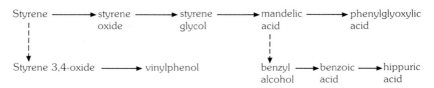

Fig. 3.3 Metabolism of styrene in humans

Toxicity
Styrene has all the narcotic potential of other solvents and produces feelings of lassitude and vague ill health at the end of the day. In addition it has an irritant vapour which may affect the eyes, nose and upper respiratory tract and the skin. It also produces an unpleasant metallic taste in the mouth. It is not neurotoxic and not notably hepatotoxic although there are some reports of elevated levels of bile acids in the blood of solvent workers with otherwise normal liver function; the significance of these findings waits to be clarified. There are some largely anecdotal accounts that styrene workers are unusually short-tempered and argumentative late in a day on which they have been heavily exposed but formal proof of this assertion is wanting.

Ethylbenzene
This compound is chemically similar to styrene (except that it lacks the vinyl group) and is used in the manufacture of styrene and cellulose acetate; it has virtually the same metabolic pathway as styrene, being broken down to mandelic and phenylglyoxylic acids. Lacking the reactive double bond, it is less irritant than styrene but is more volatile and so more likely to produce narcotic symptoms.

Chlorinated hydrocarbons

The chlorinated hydrocarbons are noninflammable, noncombustible and non-explosive and thus find extensive use through industry as degreasing agents, rubber and plastic solvents, paint solvents, refrigerants and dry cleaning fluids and some are used as fungicides and in fire extinguishers.

The introduction of chlorine into a hydrocarbon molecule generally enhances its toxicity and this toxicity increases with increasing molecular weight. As a rule the toxicity of chlorinated hydrocarbons is a function of the instability of the halogen ion and the more volatile the compound, the greater its toxicity.

Although they do not combust, at high temperatures, halogenated hydrocarbons are decomposed in the presence of air to produce highly toxic compounds including the free halide, hydrogen halides and carbonylhalides of which phosgene ($COCl_2$) is a particularly unpleasant example.

Carbon tetrachloride

Uses
Carbon tetrachloride is used in the production of freons but it was formerly much used as a solvent, as a fumigant, in fire extinguishers and as a dry cleaning agent for both domestic and industrial use. Because of its high toxicity, it has been superseded where possible by other compounds.

Metabolism
Carbon tetrachloride is readily absorbed through the lungs and it concentrates in the fatty tissues. About half of an absorbed dose is excreted unchanged in exhaled air and about 5% is eliminated as carbon dioxide. The remainder is

excreted in the urine but the precise nature of the metabolite (or metabolites) has not been determined. Carbon tetrachloride is also metabolized by ribosomal enzymes to the highly reactive CCl_3 radical through a series of hydroxylation reactions. This radical is the putative toxic agent and only those cells which contain the appropriate enzyme system are sensitive to its effects.

The toxic effects of carbon tetrachloride are enhanced by enzyme inducers such as phenobarbitone and alcohol; in addition, alcohol enhances the uptake of carbon tetrachloride from the gut.

Poisoning

In rapidly fatal cases of carbon tetrachloride poisoning, the narcotic effect produces unconsciousness which is preceded by signs of central nervous system disturbance. Such cases are extremely rare now. In severe but not immediately fatal cases, the symptoms are predominantly those due to liver or renal damage. Usually renal symptoms are more striking than hepatic symptoms. Initially the patient will complain of a persistent headache, nausea and vomiting, colic and diarrhoea, and hepatic tenderness. Signs of renal or hepatic damage appear after a variable latent interval. Renal signs include oliguria with albumin, casts and red cells in the urine and a raised blood urea. Total anuria may point to a fatal outcome. Hepatic damage is indicated by the development of jaundice and alterations in liver function tests. Cardiac arrhythmias and ventricular fibrillation have also been recorded. Pathological changes include centrilobular necrosis and fatty degeneration in the liver and proximal tubular necrosis in the kidney.

Carbon tetrachloride is a highly potent experimental carcinogen and it has been widely used to induce hepatic tumours in rats and mice. There is no evidence that it has this effect in humans.

Tetrachloroethane

Uses

Tetrachloroethane is now used only as an intermediate in the manufacture of tetrachloroethylene and trichloroethylene. It was formerly used to a much greater extent but on account of its great toxicity, it has been replaced by other solvents.

Metabolism

It is absorbed through the lung and skin and is eliminated slowly from the body. Its metabolism is complex; some is converted to trichloroethylene and dichloroacetaldehyde which are subsequently broken down to trichloroethanol and trichloroacetic acid, and glyoxalic acid and glycine respectively. Tetrachloroethane is itself broken down to form trichloroacetic acid and oxalic acid.

Poisoning

Tetrachloroethane is the most toxic of the chlorinated hydrocarbons; it has a smell which resembles that of chloroform but it has two or three times the narcotic effect of chloroform. There are two principal syndromes of tetrachloroethane poisoning, the neurological and the hepatic. A toxic polyneuropathy was first noted amongst women working to make artificial pearls and in other workers, signs of central nervous system effects have been noted, including tremor, vertigo and headaches. Four stages in the hepatic syndrome have been described, the end result being toxic jaundice and death.

1,1,1-Trichloroethane (methyl chloroform)

Uses
Trichloroethane is one of the most widely used solvents especially for the degreasing of metal. It is inflammable and does not support combustion but at 260°C it decomposes to form hydrochloric acid and traces of phosgene.

Metabolism
Trichloroethane is rapidly absorbed through the lung and to a small extent through the skin. It is mainly excreted unchanged in expired air, less than 10% being metabolized. Some of that which is metabolized is converted to carbon dioxide but the majority is converted to trichloroethanol.

Poisoning
There are no serious ill effects following exposure to trichloroethane at the concentrations usual in industry; contact with the skin will produce a mild irritant dermatitis (as will all degreasing agents) and conjunctivitis is to be expected if a splash gets in the eyes. It has the usual narcotic effects at high concentrations and was briefly used as an anaesthetic with no accounts of hepatic or renal damage or of cardiac dysfunction.

A few fatalities have occurred following exposure to extremely high concentrations usually as the result of using the solvent in a confined space so that an anaesthetic concentration was generated. Death resulted from respiratory depression or cardiac arrhythmia.

Trichloroethylene

Uses
Trichloroethylene is nonexplosive, noninflammable, very volatile and cheap so that it comes as no surprise to find it is one of the most successful solvents ever put on the market. It is still widely used as a degreasing agent and for organic synthesis in the chemical industry. At one time it was extensively used as a dry cleaning agent and as a refrigerant but it has generally been replaced by other solvents for these purposes. It is still used on a limited scale as an anaesthetic in obstetric practice.

Metabolism
Trichloroethylene is rapidly absorbed from the lungs, the retention rate ranging from 45 to 75%; it can also penetrate the skin. Very little is eliminated

Trichloroethylene ⟶ trichloroacetaldehyde ⟶ chloral hydrate ⟶
trichloroethanol + trichloroacetic acid

Fig. 3.4 Metabolism of trichloroethylene in humans

unchanged on the breath, the majority being broken down to trichloroethanol
and trichloroacetic acid (see Fig. 3.4).

The formation of trichloroethanol from chloral hydrate is the result of a
rapid reduction whereas trichloroacetic acid is formed by a slow oxidation. The
half lives of the two compounds differ; for trichloroacetic acid it is between 70
and 100 hours because it binds to plasma proteins, whereas for trichloroethanol
the half life is only 10–15 hours. There appears to be a sex difference in the
metabolism of trichloroethylene. In men, the excretion of trichloroethanol is
greater than in women whereas the converse is true for trichloroacetic acid.

Poisoning

Trichloroethylene is a powerful narcotic which, of course, makes it a good
anaesthetic. It also produces a pleasant euphoria which may lead to addiction.
Mild narcotic effects will be noted following exposures to moderately high
concentrations but these are short lasting and of no long term consequence. It
is not nearly as hepatotoxic as chloroform, carbon tetrachloride or tetrachloroethane, but liver damage has been reported in a number of fatal cases due to
acute poisoning.

There is some debate as to whether a syndrome of chronic poisoning really
exists. Some authorities report that lassitude, giddiness, irritability, headache
and gastrointestinal disturbances follow repeated exposures and that they may
persist for several weeks or months after the cessation of exposure. There is not
much support for this view in this country.

Although trichloroethylene does not cause peripheral neuropathy, there
have been a few undoubted cases of cranial nerve damage both following
anaesthetic use and exposure at work. The Vth, VIth, VIIIth, IXth and XIIth
cranial nerves may all be affected but the Vth suffers most; in a fatal case, gross
degeneration of the nerve and its nuclei was found at autopsy. The proximate
toxic substance is not known with certainty but is thought to be dichloro-
acetylene.

Trichloroethylene is one of the solvents most likely to account for the
so-called sudden death syndrome. Characteristically, death occurs in a young
person who has been heavily exposed to the solvent following some sudden
exertion such as running up stairs. Death is thought to be due to ventricular
fibrillation brought about by sensitization of the myocardium to catecholamines.
The effect can be induced in experimental animals and prevented by the
co-administration of calcium.

One interesting effect of trichloroethylene is to produce a facial vasodilation
in response to drinking alcohol; the effect is known as degreasers' flush, a
syndrome much favoured by examiners. The vasodilation is thought to be
brought about by circulating trichloroacetaldehyde, the metabolism of which is
inhibited by alcohol.

Tetrachloroethylene (perchloroethylene)

Uses
Tetrachloroethylene has replaced trichloroethylene to a large extent as a dry cleaning fluid and as a degreasing agent.

Metabolism
The vapour is absorbed through the lungs and skin absorption occurs following contact with the liquid. It is stored for long periods in fatty tissues and there tends to be an accumulation of the solvent with repeated exposures. The solvent is released slowly from fat and this dictates the rate of elimination. Almost no tetrachloroethylene is metabolized and it is mainly excreted through the lung unchanged; the 3% or so which is broken down is excreted in the urine as trichloroacetic acid.

Poisoning
Apart from the usual narcotic effects, tetrachloroethylene has few untoward characteristics. In common with most other chlorinated hydrocarbon solvents, it has been found to be teratogenic to the chick by Russian workers; there are no indications that it is teratogenic to humans.

Methylene chloride (dichloromethane)

Uses
Methylene chloride is a highly volatile solvent used in the manufacture of cellulose acetate film and it is a component of some paint strippers.

Metabolism
This solvent is absorbed through the lungs and probably through the skin. Methylene chloride is metabolized predominantly to carbon dioxide but a substantial proportion (about a third) is converted to carbon monoxide which combines with haemoglobin to form carboxyhaemoglobin. An 8-hour exposure to about 150 ppm of methylene chloride produces an equivalent amount of carboxyhaemoglobin as exposure to 35 ppm of carbon monoxide for the same time; in both cases the COHb level increases to about 5%. For an equivalent exposure, smokers will have a greater COHb concentration than non-smokers.

Poisoning
Methylene chloride has—as you should by now expect—narcotic properties against which workers ought to be able to protect themselves, for, at about 300 ppm, a sweet smell can be detected and this will alert employees to the fact that they are being exposed above the TLV. The discovery that methylene chloride was converted to carbon monoxide led to much speculation about the likelihood that exposure might cause cardiovascular or cerebrovascular disease. There have indeed been a small number of case reports of both occurring in workers

who have been unusually heavily exposed but there is no evidence to suggest that at the levels commonly encountered in industry, there is any increased risk of vascular disease.

Irritation of the skin and eyes may follow direct contact. In severe cases there may be skin or corneal burns; contamination with liquid methyl bromide is more likely to produce these effects than either the gas or the vapour.

Other solvents

Carbon disulphide

Uses

Carbon disulphide has a long and inglorious part to play in the history of occupational medicine. It was introduced into use in the 1850s as a rubber solvent and it was also used in the manufacture of matches in which process it acted as the solvent for phosphorus. Far and away the most important use of carbon disulphide now is in the production of viscose rayon fibres. Carbon disulphide is introduced into the process during xanthation of the alkali cellulose; sodium cellulose xanthate is formed which is dissolved in caustic soda to form viscose which can be spun into fibres or cast into cellophane. The xanthation process is enclosed so as to minimize exposure but carbon disulphide is liberated during all the spinning and casting processes and whenever the fibres break or are cut. Hydrogen sulphide is emitted at the same time.

Metabolism

Inhalation is the main route of entry but skin absorption also occurs. Between 70 and 90% is metabolized, the remainder being excreted unchanged through the lungs. The compound is extremely reactive and has a high affinity for organic ligands and binds to amino acids, peptides and proteins in blood and tissues. It is oxidatively metabolized to carbon dioxide with the release of the sulphene radical which forms a ligand complex with cytochrome P-450. This results in the generation of oxygen free radicals and the destruction of the cytochrome. A number of sulphur compounds appear in the urine of exposed workers incuding thiourea, mercaptothiazolinone and 2-thio-thiazolidine-4-carboxylic acid (usually known as TTCA).

Poisoning

Carbon disulphide is a multi-system poison and many toxic effects have been described. The most important are the neurological and cardiovascular effects but in addition it is a skin irritant, it may induce gastrointestinal disorders, and it has been shown to cause abnormalities in thyroid and adreno-cortical function. It may also, of course, induce acute narcosis.

Neurological effects

Both the central and the peripheral nervous systems may be affected. Exposure to high concentrations of carbon disulphide may induce a toxic organic psychosis which was first recognized in Paris in the 1850s by August Delpech, amongst the workers engaged in the cold vulcanization of rubber. The symptoms include extreme irritability, uncontrollable anger, insomnia, terrifying nightmares, loss of memory, delirium and headache. Later the patient may become depressed and paranoid and is at great danger of taking his own life. Clinically, it may be possible to detect both diffuse and focal neurological signs. The picture may be further complicated by the appearance of typical parkin-sonian features. The pathological correlates of this psychopathy are not clear; it has been suggested that it may be due to disturbances in the cerebral circulation, to the binding of free sulphur to neurofilaments, which interferes with normal axonal function, to the inhibition of dopamine-β-hydroxylase, or to disturbances in vitamin B_6 metabolism. Such a plethora of explanations suggests that none is sufficient fully to explain the condition.

The florid symptoms seen in the early days of carbon disulphide use are not encountered nowadays, indeed it would be a positive disgrace if they were. However, carbon disulphide is about the only solvent for which there is good evidence for subclinical neuropsychological effects. Carbon disulphide workers have a higher prevalence of abnormal EEGs than control subjects and they also perform less well in psychological tests than controls.

In the peripheral nervous system, carbon disulphide produces a mixed neuropathy which is pathologically identical with that produced by n-hexane and methyl-butyl-ketone (MBK). Nerve conduction velocities are slowed and this is an early indication of axonal damage; the conduction velocities return to normal if exposure is discontinued. The cardinal pathological sign is the appearance of swellings within the axon. These swellings first appear proximal to the node of Ranvier and the myelin overlying the swelling is absent or considerably thinned. (It is this which accounts for the slowing in nerve conduction.) Under the electron microscope it can be seen that the axonal swellings are due to the accumulation of 10 nm microfilaments and other intracellular organelles. This accumulation of debris interferes with the normal flow of material along the axon and the distal ends of the nerve fibres begin to die back. Similar changes can be seen within the brain stem. In carbon disulphide neuropathy the toxic agent is thought to be the carbon disulphide itself but it is not clear how it causes the neurofilamentous accumulations. It may be because it has a high affinity for –SH groups and is thus able to inhibit enzyme function or it may be that it is able to induce crosslinkage between proteins in the neurofilaments. Once exposure is discontinued there is a slow return to normal.

Cardiovascular effects
Carbon disulphide induces sclerotic changes in the arterial system the clinical effects of which depend upon the vessels most affected. Renal changes have been reported following unusually heavy exposure and cerebral arteriosclerosis has been postulated as causing some of the CNS effects. Perhaps the most significant effects, however, are those on the coronary arteries, and it has become clear in recent years that long term exposure to carbon disulphide is

associated with a greatly increased prevalence of ischaemic heart disease, up to as much as five times greater than in a control population. When exposure is controlled it can be shown that the risk returns towards normal again.

Susceptibility to carbon disulphide
The compound tetraethylthiuram disulphide (TETD, disulfiram, Antabuse) contains two CS_2 groups in its molecule and is broken down to diethyldithio-carbamate (DDC). The rate at which DDC appears in the urine after a dose of TETD is a measure of the subject's ability to handle sulphur-containing compounds and it has been suggested that susceptibility to carbon disulphide poisoning is inversely related to the amount of DDC excreted. It has been further suggested that prospective carbon disulphide workers should all undergo this test and only accepted if their excretion of DDC is in excess of 150 mg/g creatinine within 4 hours of a dose of 0.5 g of TETD.

n-Hexane and methyl-butyl-ketone
It is appropriate to consider these solvents together since their metabolism and their toxic effects are similar.

Uses
n-Hexane is widely used as a solvent in glues and adhesives and in paints and dyes. MBK, and the other commonly used ketones, are used as a solvent for dyes, resins, gums, tars, waxes and fats and as an extractant in a range of synthetic processes.

Metabolism
n-Hexane is mainly taken up through the lungs and only about 15% is retained. Skin absorption is extremely poor. MBK, by contrast, is readily absorbed by any route. The biotransformation of these compounds is interconnected and both produce a toxic metabolite, 2,5-hexanedione (see Fig. 3.5).

Poisoning
The principal toxic effect of these compounds is the production of a filamentous peripheral neuropathy similar to that produced by carbon disulphide. Both motor and sensory disturbances are noted but there is no interference with higher cerebral function. The proximate toxic agent is the common metabolite 2,5-hexanedione and it is the γ-diketone spacing in the molecule which is

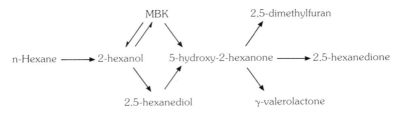

Fig. 3.5 Metabolism of n-hexane and methyl-butyl-ketone (MBK) in humans

essential for its toxic effect. Neither methyl-ethyl-ketone (MEK) nor methyl-isobutyl-ketone (MiBK) is neurotoxic since neither is metabolized to a compound containing the γ-diketone spacing within its molecule. It is of interest, however, that both MEK and MiBK are thought to be able to enhance the neurotoxicity of MBK so that solvents containing mixtures of ketones may be more neurotoxic than at first supposed.

The mechanism whereby 2,5-hexandione induces the striking changes in the neurones is not clear. *In vitro,* it can be shown to inhibit some of the enzymes involved in the gylcolytic pathway and it may also produce crosslinking of the neurofilaments by forming Schiff bases with amino groups.

Acetone

Acetone is one of the most safe of all solvents although it should not be forgotten that it is highly flammable and explosive. It is water soluble and enters the body mainly through inhalation. It appears unchanged in exhaled air and in the urine; it is also metabolized to formic acid.

Glycols and their derivatives

The glycols that are used commercially are colourless liquids which contain two hydroxyl groups per molecule which makes them chemically active and important as intermediates in synthetic processes. They are also completely water soluble and they are widely used as solvents for resins, lacquers, paints, dyes and inks. They are also used as antifreeze agents. The two in most common use are ethylene glycol and diethylene glycol.

Metabolism
Both compounds have a low volatility; inhalation is not an important route of entry and neither penetrates the skin. They are absorbed from the gut, however, and biotransformed to oxalic acid by alcohol dehydrogenase.

Poisoning
In normal use, neither of these compounds presents a serious hazard to health. If large quantities are ingested, however, either with the deliberate intention of self harm or in mistake for ethanol, there may be a deposition of calcium oxalate crystals within the renal tubules. Acute tubular necrosis and anuria will quickly follow and the patient will die unless treated promptly. Since ethanol is a better substrate than ethylene glycol for alcohol dehydrogenase, it is often advocated that patients with ethylene glycol poisoning should be given ethanol in order to slow down the breakdown of the glycol; haemodialysis should also form part of an effective treatment regime.

Glycol ethers

The glycol ethers are a large group of over 30 compounds. They are more volatile than the parent compounds and are miscible with water and most organic compounds and they are thus widely used as dispersants in industry. They are used as solvents for resins, paints and inks and they are important solvents for cellulose ester and mitrocellulose. The most important of the group are ethylene glycol monomethyl ether (methyl cellosolve), ethylene glycol monoethyl ether (cellosolve) and ethylene glycol iso-propyl ether, ethylene glycol n-butyl ether and propylene glycol monomethyl ether. Fortunately, these compounds are generally referred to by their abbreviated form, EGME, EGEE, EGiPE, EGBE and PGME.

Metabolism
Since they are more volatile than their parent compounds all the glycol ethers are inhaled through the lung and they may also be absorbed through the skin. Their subsequent metabolism largely determines their toxicity. Those compounds which contain a primary alcohol are good substrates for ADH and are oxidized to the corresponding alkoxyacids which have a high toxicity. Thus, methoxyacetic acid is formed from EGME, butoxyacetic acid is formed from EGBE and, by analogy, one would expect ethyoxyacetic acid to be formed from EGEE. From EGiPE, isopropoxyacetic acid has been recovered in dogs and rats. As an alternative route, the ether linkage may be cleaved with the production of oxalic acid and carbon dioxide; about 14% of the total dose may be excreted as CO_2. By contrast, PGME is not a good substrate for ADH since it contains a secondary alcohol group and so it is mainly broken down to carbon dioxide and to PGME-glucuronide and sulphates which appear in the urine; these compounds account for 10–20% of the total metabolites.

Poisoning
The glycol ethers and the ethylene derivatives are more toxic than the propylene derivatives and EGME is probably the most toxic of the group in common use. During the early days of its use, it was found to cause a toxic encephalopathy which is not seen under present conditions of use. It also affected the bone marrow, causing anaemia and the appearance of immature leucocytes in the peripheral blood. EGBE has been found to cause a haemolytic anaemia in animals but this does not seem to be the case in humans. The isopropyl and n-propyl glycol ethers may, in addition, cause liver and kidney damage. Splashes into the eye of any of the ethylene glycol ethers cause an irritant conjunctivitis with corneal clouding which may last for several days. Splashes of PGME cause a mild irritation only.

Some of the ethylene glycol ethers have been shown to be both fetotoxic and teratogenic and to cause testicular changes in animals with alterions in sperm morphology. The degree of toxicity to the reproductive system is inversely related to the size of the alkoxy group—as are the effects of the bone marrow. Thus, the order of toxicity is EGME > EGEE > EGBE. It may be noted that the reverse is the case so far as haemolytic effects are concerned.

The reproductive effects of glycol ethers have been noted in several species of animals but there is no good evidence for their occurrence in humans. Nevertheless, there is now a trend away from the use of the ethylene glycol ethers in favour of PGME wherever possible; PGME has no teratogenic effects, it exerts only weak fetotoxicity at high doses and it has no effects on the testis.

Dioxane

Dioxane, diethylene ether, is a ring compound, and has been in use for over half a century. It is a solvent for waxes, fat, greases and mineral oils and a cellulose and nitrocellulose solvent. At room temperatures liquid dioxane can produce explosive air/vapour mixtures.

Metabolism

Dioxane is volatile and well absorbed through the lungs and probably also through the skin. Its main metabolic by-product is β-hydroxyethoxyacetic acid and almost none of an absorbed dose escapes biotransformation.

Poisoning

The vapour has the expected narcotic effect in excess and it also causes irritation of the eyes, nose and throat at concentrations in the range 200 to 300 ppm. Liver and kidney damage may follow excessive exposures and in fatal cases in which death resulted from renal failure, hepatic enlargement and haemorrhagic kidneys have been noted at autopsy. Dioxane produces tumours in experimental animals but such epidemiological studies as have been carried out on populations exposed at work have not demonstrated any excess risk.

White spirit

White spirit is one of the most commonly used of all solvents; in the USA it is also known as Stoddard solvent. It is a mongrel of a solvent containing many straight and branched paraffins and aromatic hydrocarbons; the aliphatic/aromatic ratio is generally about 4 : 1 but variations are common. White spirit is an important paint solvent and few home decorators can fail to have noted some of its effects. The metabolism of white spirit is complex. The major components will tend to be broken down in the normal way but the presence of so many other—often related—compounds will produce interactions, the degree of which cannot always be accurately predicted. White spirit has a vapour which has an unpleasant smell and which is mildly irritant; after a few minutes exposure, however, olfactory fatigue occurs and the smell is not noted. It may cause mild conjunctivitis and painters will generally admit to feelings of tiredness and general ill health which are greater than those experienced by other workers. In the Scandinavian countries there is a strong belief that exposure to white spirit may cause presenile dementia and in Finland and Denmark this is now a compensatable disease. Our recent studies of painters in the UK have shown that they have a higher than expected morbidity from minor psychiatric symptoms but there is no relationship between length of employment or degree of exposure (so far as this could be assessed). This would tend to suggest that the effects which were noted were more likely to be the results of acute exposure. If this is so, then the expectation is that they are reversible although the time course for this may be rather long. There was nothing to suggest that the effects were the result of organic brain damage. It is interesting to note that follow-up studies of Swedish patients who have been given a diagnosis of chronic organic solvent syndrome have shown them either to have improved or to have remained functioning at the same level as when the diagnosis was made. There was no evidence for the kind of relentless deterioration which would have been likely to have been the consequence of a dementing illness.

The evidence to date suggests that exposure to solvents for prolonged periods and at high concentrations may induce some nonspecific neuropsychiatric symptoms in a small proportion of exposed workers. There is no good evidence that any kind of dementing illness is produced and it is likely that most symptoms are reversible when exposure is discontinued; at worst, patients do not seem to deteriorate further and the continuation of symptoms may be more related to other factors than to solvent exposure.

Chapter 4
Industrial Toxicology 3: Miscellaneous Organic Compounds

Vinyl chloride

Vinyl chloride is a colourless gas which is used in the synthesis of polyvinyl chloride (PVC) as plastic without which modern life is almost unthinkable. It is flammable and when mixed with air in proportions between 4 and 22% by volume is explosive.

Metabolism

The gas is rapidly absorbed through the lung and it also passes through the skin. It is quickly eliminated, either unchanged or as metabolites in the urine. The first step in its metabolism is oxidation to chloroethylene oxide which spontaneously rearranges to form chloro-acetaldehyde. This compound may be further oxidized to form monochloracetic acid. The main urinary metabolites are hydroxyethyl cysteine, carboxyethyl cysteine, monochloroacetic acid and thio-diglycolic acid.

Poisoning

Acute effects such as a feeling of elation followed by lethargy are well recognized; at concentrations above 10 000 vertigo may be noted whilst hearing and vision are impaired when the concentration is greater than 16 000 ppm; loss of consciousness occurs with concentrations in excess of 70 000 ppm.

Constant exposure to high concentrations of the vapour may give rise to a chronic condition which is known as vinyl chloride disease. The major components of this syndrome are Raynaud's phenomenon, skin changes akin to scleroderma, acro-osteolysis, hepatosplenal fibrosis and haemangiosarcoma of the liver.

The Raynaud's phenomenon is caused by diffuse degenerative changes in the small blood vessels leading to occlusion of the capillaries and arterioles. Complete obliteration of the palmar arch may sometimes be noted at angiography. In association with the Raynaud's phenomenon, the skin of the hands and forearms may be inelastic and thinned; occasionally skin on other parts of the body may also be affected. The acro-osteolysis is generally localized to the distal phalanges of the hands and is due to an aseptic necrosis caused by ischaemia. The bony changes (Fig. 4.1) may progress to produce a transverse defect which subsequently heals to give a blunt, wide phalanx. Re-calcification may occur once exposure is discontinued.

The liver is affected in all cases of VCM poisoning. The liver may become enlarged but liver function tests are usually normal. If exposure is not discontinued at this stage, hepatosplenal fibrosis may supervene. There may be some elevation of transaminase levels but the diagnosis can be made only with

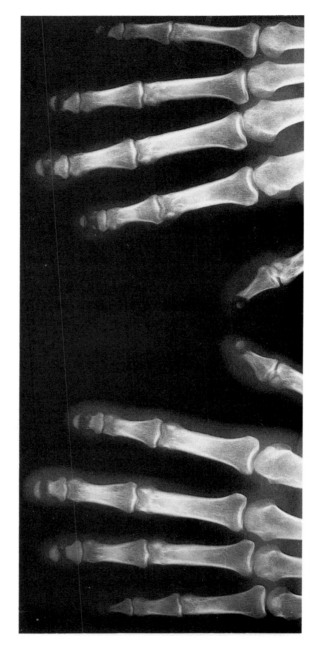

Fig. 4.1 Radiography showing the changes of acro-osteolysis in the fingers of both hands

an adequate liver biopsy. The parenchymal cells show relatively little change; a few swollen cells may be seen and some may be necrotic but fibrotic tissue can be seen in the portal spaces and extending between the parenchymal cells. When exposure is discontinued the hepatosplenomegaly and the parenchymal changes reverse but the fibrosis may deteriorate further.

The most serious of the components of vinyl chloride disease is angiosarcoma of the liver; this is rare and confined to workers with extremely high exposures and one would not expect to see it in future with the advent of much more rigorous control limits.

It is clear from this account that vinyl chloride disease is a multi-system disorder, most likely with an immunological basis. Workers exposed to VCM have been found to have circulating immune complexes and immunofluorescent studies have shown that these complexes are deposited on the vascular endothelium. Other features which suggest that workers exposed to VCM suffer from an immune complex disorder include the finding of hyperimmunoglobulinaemia, cryoglobulinaemia together with *in vivo* complement activation via the classical pathway.

Acrylamide

Uses
Acrylamide is another vinyl monomer which will readily undergo polymerization and co-polymerization. It is used in the manufacture of flocculators which are substances which aid the separation of suspended solids from aqueous systems. As such they are useful in mining, soil stabilization and in the disposal of industrial wastes. Acrylamide is used also in the manufacture of paper, adhesives, fibres, dyes, pigments and leather substitutes and in the preparation of plastics and rubber.

Hazards of use
Only the monomer is toxic. Any process involving the handling of the monomer is potentially hazardous and workers should wear protective clothing to avoid getting it into contact with the skin.

Metabolism
Acrylamide may be absorbed by inhalation, ingestion or through the skin, but the last seems to be the most common path of entry. The fate of the substance in the body does not seem to have been reported.

Poisoning
The most serious effects are on the nervous system and two distinct lesions are produced, a peripheral neuropathy and a disturbance in the midbrain. Patients complain mainly of numbness and paraesthesiae in both upper and lower limbs with marked weakness, especially in the legs. Reflexes may be diminished or absent and there may be wasting of the muscles. Patients often have difficulty with their balance and they may be found to have an absence of vibration sense

and a positive Romberg sign. In some the speech is slurred. Tiredness and lethargy are common, and there may be, in addition, generalized tremors, weight loss and impairment of bladder function. Increased sweating of the hands and feet are also noted. The palms may be erythematous, with peeling skin.

The condition invariably improves once exposure has been discontinued although the time required for the signs and symptoms to abate is variable. As with other industrial toxins, simple protective measures will safeguard those handling the monomer.

The substance has what has been called an anamnestic effect. That is to say, if acrylamide is administered to an animal which has recovered from the effects of acute intoxication, then the same symptoms will be produced by a lower dose of the drug. For this reason, workers who have shown signs of intoxication are best not re-exposed.

Nitro and amino derivatives of benzene

The most important of these compounds are nitrobenzene, dinitrobenzene (DNB), trinitrotoluene (TNT), aniline, dinitrophenol and dinitroortho cresol (DNOC).

Uses

These nitro and amino derivates of benzene are intermediates used in the synthesis of more complex, but less toxic, molecules, the majority of which are used as dyes or explosives.

Hazards of use

All these substances can be absorbed through the skin and the lungs and the hazard associated with their use is dependent to a large extent on their physical state and their volatility. For this reason, aniline and nitrobenzene, which are bitter liquids, are regarded as more toxic than the solid DNB and TNT.

Metabolism

Absorption is possible through the lungs, the skin and the gastrointestinal tract, but the first two routes are of greatest significance to industrial toxicology. Phenol derivatives are excreted in the urine, although DNB and TNT are also excreted unchanged.

Being lipid soluble, fatty tissues contain higher concentrations than do other tissues.

In the urine they are excreted mainly as phenol or nitro derivatives although DNB and TNT may be present unchanged.

Poisoning

All these compounds are capable of producing anaemia and toxic jaundice in varying degrees. The metabolites, notably p-amino phenol, oxidize the ferrous iron in haemoglobin to the ferric state forming methaemoglobin which binds oxygen much more firmly than does haemoglobin and some degree of tissue anoxia results, depending on the concentration in the blood. Methaemoglobin has a dark colour and when present in concentrations in excess of about 3 gm/100 ml produces a blue-grey discoloration of the skin sometimes referred to as 'toxic cyanosis'. This discoloration is most noticeable on the cheeks, ears, nose and finger-nails. The term anilism is applied to cases in which methaemo-globinaemia results from exposure to this class of chemicals and workers sometimes refer to themselves as being blued up.

The methaemoglobinaemia is accompanied by morphological changes in the circulating red cells. Examination of a peripheral blood film shows the presence of polychromasia, punctate basophilia and red cells containing Heinz bodies. Some of the amino-compounds have an irritant on the bladder producing a haemorrhage cystitis. Bladder cancer in workers handling these compounds is discussed further in Chapter 8.

Nitrobenzene

Nitrobenzene is an oily liquid known commercially as oil of mirbane. Acute poisoning most often follows the absorption of large amounts through the skin after the working clothes have become accidentally splashed. The symptoms of acute poisoning include fatigue, headache, vomiting and vertigo. In serious cases, unconsciousness supervenes and there are signs of circulatory collapse. The respiratory rate is first quickened, but slows if the patient becomes unconscious. The characteristic cyanosis is present and pronounced anaemia may follow. By about the third day jaundice and splenomegaly are noted on clinical examination.

The symptoms of acute poisoning may persist for many days and they may later be replaced or augmented by signs and symptoms due to excessive blood destruction. There are no late sequelae in those who survive.

Chronic poisoning follows long-term exposure to low concentrations and anaemia is the leading feature, with or without a mild haemolytic jaundice and albuminuria. Cyanosis, if present at all, is slight. Fatigue, headache, loss of appetite and cachexia are all found as a result of exposure and there may be erythema of exposed skin. Recovery may take several weeks and may not be complete.

Dinitrobenzene

DNB is a solid which is well absorbed through the skin. It is less toxic than nitrobenzene. Acute poisoning is manifested by the rapid onset of headache, vertigo and vomiting, and then by exhaustion, numbness in the legs and a staggering gait. The patient may become unconscious and cyanosed and death may result from central respiratory paralysis. In those who survive, the cyanosis exhaustion and vertigo are likely to persist for several days or weeks.

Chronic poisoning gives rise to weakness, fatigue, headaches and vomiting, and evening fever. Cyanosis and pallor are usually present. The usual blood changes will be found and albuminuria and porphyrinuria are occasionally present.

In many cases, those exposed to DNB become increasingly sensitive to its effects, so that the time interval between exposure and the development of cyanosis shortens. Acute exacerbations of symptoms has been known to occur following exposure to sunlight and after drinking alcohol. In each case, this is due to the liberation of DNB from fatty tissues in which it has been stored.

Trinitrotoluene
The skin is the important portal of entry for this solid material and absorption is greater in hot weather since TNT dust on the skin is dissolved in sweat. It is often used mixed with oxygen donors such as ammonium nitrate (amatol, ammonal) and barium nitrate (baratol).

Cyanosis and the usual blood changes indicate poisoning and in addition the hands and feet are sometimes stained orange. Symptoms of intoxication include a very irritant dermatitis and toxic gastritis. The patient has anorexia, nausea and vomiting and is constipated. The liver is usually enlarged and tender and the level of urinary coproporphyrin excretion is raised.

Treatment should be given in hospital. The skin must be thoroughly washed down with ether until there is no longer a pink reaction with alkaline ether. Recovery is usually complete but patients with toxic gastritis should not be re-exposed.

Toxic jaundice following exposure to TNT is rare but since it has a mortality rate of 30% it is to be taken very seriously. Symptoms may occur within a few weeks of first exposure but there is sometimes a latent period between removal from exposure and their onset. Prodromal symptoms such as drowsiness and vertigo are sometimes noted or alternatively the condition may be a progression from toxic gastritis. It can also occur with no warning. The degree of jaundice is variable, but hepatic enlargement is unusual until late in the illness. Fatalities are the result of hepatic necrosis.

Aplastic anaemia is less common than toxic jaundice but invariably fatal. Like the toxic jaundice, it may occur some time after exposure has been discontinued.

Aniline
Aniline is colourless oily liquid which turns brown on exposure to the light. It is readily absorbed through the skin and most cases of industrial poisoning are the result of accidental contamination of working clothes. Pulmonary absorption is a risk, particularly if workers enter confined spaces in which the vapour is present. The closely related nitro-anilines are also absorbed through the skin. Paraphenyline diamine is considered more toxic than aniline.

Mild symptoms of intoxication take the form of flushing, a throbbing sensation in the head, burning in the throat and tightness in the chest. These are followed in turn, by the onset of a violent headache and cyanosis. It is important that exposure should cease when these early symptoms are noted. The removal of all clothing and any aniline on the skin is vital. The prognosis depends upon how much aniline has been absorbed, but in mild cases complete relief of symptoms may be expected within 24 hours. At the end of this time, the patient will no longer be cyanosed. As with the other compounds in this section, the cyanosis is due to methaemoglobinaemia. The appearance of punctate basophilia in the peripheral blood is said to be a delicate measure of increased absorption.

In severe cases of aniline poisoning there is deep cyanosis, nausea and vomiting and circulatory collapse. The patient lapses into coma and the appearance of convulsions presages death. Characteristically, the attack occurs after the employee has left work.

Chronic absorption of aniline will produce a low-grade anaemia with cyanosis which resolves when the employee leaves work at the end of the day. The manifestation of symptoms will depend upon the degree of anaemia.

Aliphatic nitrates

The most important of these compounds are ethylene glycol dinitrate (EGDN) and nitroglycerin (NG) which are used to produce dynamite, a mixture of about 60% ammonium and sodium nitrate, 20% EGDN, 5% NG, 3% nitrocellulose and a variable amount of sawdust, chalk and rhodamin.

Both NG and EGDN are readily absorbed through the skin and the dust is also absorbed through the lungs. Both compounds are highly reactive and rapidly disappear from the blood. NG is metabolized to inorganic nitrates and nitrites which appear in the urine; the principal metabolites of EGDN are 1,2- and 1,3-glyceryl dinitrate.

Both NG and EGDN are potent vasodilators and the acute effects which follow exposure are the result of this property. The symptoms include throbbing headache, tachycardia, palpitation, nausea and vomiting. Most workers become habituated to these effects so that they are noted only on return to work after 1 or 2 days' absence. Sudden deaths have also been noted amongst dynamite workers. These occur typically on a Monday morning and may be preceded by symptoms which mimic those of angina pectoris. Whether dynamite workers are at risk from chronic effects is less clear. They may certainly develop hypotension at work but this appears to be a reversible phenomenon with no untoward sequelae; a few workers may also be found with a high incidence of ectopic beats on ambulatory monitoring. Epidemiological studies tend to suggest that, with present levels of exposure, the risk of death from cardiovascular disease is not substantially greater than in the general population.

Pesticides

Hundreds of organic compounds are used as pesticides but they can conveniently be grouped together for discussion into organochlorines, organophosphorus derivatives, carbamates and compounds related to pyrethrum.

Organochlorines

This group includes DDT, lindane (hexachlorocyclohexane), dieldrin and related chlorinated cyclodienes and hexachlorobenzene. All the organochlorine pesticides are lipid soluble and are easily absorbed by all routes. They are extremely persistent in the environment and may produce adverse effects on animals at the top of the food chain, with the general exception of humans. In recent years attempts have been made to replace these compounds with others which are more readily broken down. Residues of organochlorine compounds can be measured in fat but relatively little is known about urinary metabolites.

DDT

DDT (dichloro-diphenyl trichloroethane) is an organochlorine compound and a most effective insecticide. It is a very stable chemical and its widespread use has resulted in a considerable accumulation in the environment which has given rise to fears that it might somehow disturb the delicate ecological balance.

The compound is absorbed through the gut and through intact skin. Once in the body, DDT undergoes a slow series of metabolic changes, the principle products of which are DDE, stored in fatty tissues and DDA, which is excreted in the urine.

In high doses, DDT affects the central nervous system, and symptoms of intoxication include paraesthesiae, tremors and convulsions. Untoward effects are not generally observed with doses less than 10 mg/kg body weight, hence cases of acute poisoning are confined to those who ingest large amounts accidentally or with suicidal intent. In fact, few fatalities have been recorded and complete recovery is the rule.

Occupational exposure is not sufficiently great to produce symptoms of acute intoxication although peripheral neuropathy has been ascribed to chronic occupational exposure. Some induction of liver enzymes can be demonstrated to have taken place in workers occupationally exposed to DDT but there is no evidence of liver dysfunction of the kind which has been demonstrated in experimental animals.

Lindane

Lindane (hexachlorocyclohexane) exists in five isomeric forms. The γ-isomer is a powerful insecticide and goes under a variety of trade names of which gammexane and BHC are probably the best known. It is more toxic to insects than DDT but does not have such a long activity and on this account is sometimes used in combination with DDT.

Toxic effects are noted only in those who use BHC carelessly or improperly and although skin rashes have been observed in employees working with BHC, these were probably due to impurities present in the compound. Individuals have poisoned themselves by taking BHC as a vermifuge, or by using the powder or a solution in poorly ventilated spaces, or by splashing their skin with the solution. Those who have been poisoned develop colic, diarrhoea, headaches, lassitude and vertigo. Neurological symptoms are prominent including ataxia, tremor and convulsions. Bone marrow depression has been recorded and some cases have ended fatally.

Users of BHC should be warned not to spray it in confined spaces, not to get it on their skin and not to take it for the therapeutic purposes.

Chlorinated cyclodienes

Dieldrin is the most commonly used of the chlorinated cyclodiene pesticides. Others in this group include endrin, aldin and isodrin. Dieldrin and endrin are the most stable of the group; aldin is readily changed to dieldrin and isodrin to endrin.

All four compounds are readily absorbed through intact skin and this is the usual route of absorption for those occupationally exposed. The compounds, or their metabolites, are stored in fatty tissues but clearance from the body is accelerated by microsomal enzyme inducers such as phenobarbitone or DDT.

The most serious manifestation of acute intoxication is the production of epileptiform fits which can be well controlled with anticonvulsants. Long-term exposure to subtoxic levels does not seem to have any untoward effects.

Hexachlorobenzene

Hexachlorobenzene is used as a fungicidal dressing for seed grain, especially wheat. It is relatively little used in Britain and no cases of occupational poisoning are known, but episodes of cutaneous porphyria have been reported from Turkey amongst villagers who have eaten seed dressed with hexachlorobenzene.

Organo-phosphorous compounds

These compounds are structurally related to di-iso-propyl fluoro phosphate and, like it, are powerful irreversible inhibitors of cholinesterase.

Metabolism

Organo-phosphorus compounds are readily absorbed through the skin as well as by ingestion and inhalation. They do not accumulate in the body and most are rapidly degraded and excreted. The principal urinary metabolites are alkyl phosphates, for example, dimethylphosphate (formed from dimethylparathion), diethylphosphate (from parathion, disulphoton and phorate), diethylphorothiolate (from disulphoton and phorate) and diethylthiophosphate (from disulphoton and phorate). In addition, p-nitrophenol is formed from parathion.

Poisoning

The toxic properties of these compounds to humans lie in their ability to inhibit cholinesterase; symptoms will begin to appear when the ChE activity is reduced to less than 50% of normal. Early signs of poisoning are nonspecific and include headache, nausea, anorexia and marked lassitude. There may be constriction of the pupils. In a short time following exposure these relatively mild symptoms are superseded by vomiting, diarrhoea, abdominal pain and muscle twitching. Incontinence of urine and faeces is common as is pulmonary oedema. The onset of convulsions usually signifies that the patient is about to pass into a coma which may lead to death. The complete course from exposure to death may take as little as an hour so that speed is of the essence if treatment is to be successful.

Treatment with atropine should be given immediately and the patient supported with mechanical respiration if necessary. Cholinesterase activity can be restored by compounds which split the enzyme from its attachment to the phosphate group of the insecticide. Pralidoxime is satisfactory for this purpose and a number of hospitals hold supplies of this drug for emergency purposes.

Late sequelae of organo-phosphorus poisoning have been noted. The patient may recover from the acute phase but about 3 weeks later note progressive muscular weakness and fatigue with vomiting and diarrhoea. Marked muscle wasting may follow. These symptoms are similar to those of TOCP poisoning (q.v).

To avoid these late complications, all patients who have an attack of acute poisoning should be kept under close observation until their cholinesterase activity (in either the plasma or the red cell) has returned to normal.

Carbamates

The most important of this group is carbaryl (l-napthyl-N-methyl-carbamate) which is absorbed by all routes. It is rapidly metabolized to free and conjugate l-naphthol which appears in the urine. The carbamates are also ChE inhibitors and produce the same kinds of symptoms as the organo-phosphorus insecticides. Their inhibition is rapidly reversible, however, so that they do not pose as serious a threat to health as the organo-phosphorus compounds.

Pyrethrum

Pyrethrum is an insecticide derived from plants. There are six active compounds, esters of two acids and three alcohols; they are known as pyrethrin I and II, cinerin I and II and jasmolin I and II. Pyrethrum may be absorbed through the gut and through the lungs but not through the skin. It is rapidly metabolized and excreted in the urine; the precise nature of its metabolites is unknown. Pyrethrum is a sensitizer and most of its untoward effects in humans result from this property. Contact dermatitis is well known and it is often made worse by exposure to sunlight; signs and symptoms like those of hayfever may also be induced and there have been occasional reports of effects on the lung (see Chapter 6).

Herbicides

Phenoxy acid derivatives

These include 2,4-dichlorophenoxyacetic acid (2,4-D) and 2,4,5-trichlorophenoxy acetic acid (2,4,5-T) both of which have excited a great deal of alarm and despondency in recent years, particularly since 2,4,5-T has been found to be contaminated with minute traces of dioxin (2,3,7,8-tetradibenzo p-dioxin). The phenoxy acid compounds are rapidly absorbed through skin, lungs and gut and rapidly eliminated unchanged in the gut. They are remarkably nontoxic to humans but fears have been raised that they are teratogenic, fears which appear to be groundless. There is some epidemiological evidence that people who are exposed to them have a higher than expected incidence of lymphomas but this is still somewhat equivocal.

Dioxin is not used commercially and is a byproduct of the formation of 2,4,5-T. It is extraordinarily toxic to experimental animals but humans do not share this exquisite sensitivity which is fortunate when one considers the number of industrial accidents which have resulted in environmental contamination. The most recent was at Seveso, in northern Italy in 1976. The most consistent finding in men and women exposed either at work or in the environment is chloracne and enlargement of the liver with biochemical signs of impaired liver function. There may also be an increased excretion of ALA and uroporphyrin in the urine. In humans, dioxin does not seem to be notably teratogenic nor does it induce malignant disease; studies of exposed workers have been unable to demonstrate any increased prevalence of chromosomal aberrations.

Pentachlorophenol

Pentachlorophenol is used mainly as a fungicide and it can be absorbed through the skin and the gut. Fine dusts and sprays cause an intense irritation of the eyes and upper respiratory tract and provide an indication to the worker that he is over-exposing himself. The compound is excreted in the urine in free and conjugated forms.

The signs of severe intoxication include loss of appetite, respiratory distress, hyperpyrexia, sweating, anaesthesia, coma and death.

Dinitroortho cresol (DNOC)

This is a homologue of 4-dinitrophenol (DNP) which is also used as a fungicide and pesticide. It is absorbed by all routes and it is extremely toxic. Symptoms of poisoning are similar to those of pentachlorophenol and are likely to occur when the blood concentration is in excess of 4 mg/dl. Thirst may be an important early symptom but the most serious effects are due to interference with normal temperature regulating mechanisms; in severe cases of poisoning the patient may develop hyperpyrexia and death will supervene unless adequate treatment is quickly given.

Paraquat

Paraquat achieved a considerable notoriety at one time because of the cases of poisoning which were recorded in people who drank the concentrated solution by accident, mistaking it for soft drinks, or with suicidal intent. Gramoxone, the 20% concentrate, is available only to farmers and horticulturalists and in its working strength (about 20 ppm) it is not dangerous. The form in which it is available to the public (as Weedol, a mixture of paraquat and diquat) is also harmless when used correctly. The lethal dose in humans is 6 g paraquat ion (about 30 ml of gramoxone) and no one who has taken a dose in excess of this has been known to survive.

Following ingestion the patient experiences a burning sensation in the mouth and throat and has abdominal pain accompanied by nausea and vomiting. These early symptoms are followed by hepatic and renal failure, the last being due to proximal tubular damage.

The patient often survives the acute phase but after 5–10 days of apparently good health begins to show signs of respiratory distress. This progresses rapidly and death from respiratory failure ensues. The pathological lesion in the lungs is one of the pulmonary fibrosis with an exuberant fibrotic reaction which obliterates the alveoli. The fibrotic reaction is thought to develop in response to a metabolite produced in the liver.

In order for the patient to have any chance of survival treatment must be instigated with the greatest speed. Absorption from the gut is slow and in the first 24 hours only about 10% of an ingested dose is taken up; the first stage of treatment, therefore, is to perform gastric lavage using absorbents such as Fuller's earth in saline. After lavage is complete, 500 ml of a 30% solution should be left in the stomach to absorb any paraquat which remains. Haemoperfusion and haemodialysis have all been tried and treatment with steroids or immunosuppressive drugs may be given.

The prognosis in an individual case can be given on the basis of a simple examination of the urine. Paraquat is reduced to a free blue radical by alkaline sodium dithionite. If 2 ml of the reagent (freshly prepared by adding 10 ml of 1M sodium hydroxide to 100 mg of sodium dithionite) is added to 10 ml of clear urine, the colour produced may be compared with that obtained from test solutions (containing 1,5 and 10 mg/l of paraquat). The test is sensitive enough to detect about 1 mg/l of paraquat in urine. If there is no colour reaction it is safe to assume that a toxic amount of paraquat has been ingested, whereas a colour change indicates the need for urgent treatment. Under the same test conditions, diquat is reduced to a green free radical so that a greeny-blue discoloration in the urine indicates that Weedol has been ingested.

Other organic compounds

Methyl bromide

Uses
Methyl bromide is an extremely volatile liquid which is in gaseous form at temperatures above 4.5°C. It is used as a fire extinguisher (sometimes mixed with carbon tetrachloride), as a refrigerant, as an insecticide and a fumigant.

Hazards of use
The danger comes from the leakage of gas from storage vessels or from faults in delivery pipes and so on. Its great volatility enables a large volume of gas to escape from even a trivial leak and its high density relative to air (it is 3.3 times as heavy as air) adds to the danger. Any process involving methyl bromide which is carried out indoors is potentially dangerous.

Metabolism

The gas is absorbed through the lungs and the skin and stored in tissues rich in fat. It is slowly broken down with the release of free bromide and measurements of the level of bromide in the blood are useful as a guide to exposure, although they do not correlate absolutely with the degree of toxicity. There are two phases of excretion; unchanged gas is excreted rapidly through the lungs, whereas bromide is excreted slowly through the kidney.

Poisoning

Methyl bromide is highly toxic but there is a latent period between exposure and the declarations of symptoms which can be as long as 48 hours. At high concentrations the gas has a slightly sweet smell.

The major effect which is noted immediately upon exposure to the gas is an irritation of the respiratory tract. Individuals thus quickly remove themselves from further exposure. There is little narcotic action by contrast with the chlorinated hydrocarbons. After the latent interval, the patient is suddenly seized with nausea and vomiting, headaches, watering of the eyes, cough, anorexia and abdominal pain. The vision becomes blurred and the patient may have diplopia. At this stage he appears to be drunk having a staggering gait, slurred speech and vertigo. In severe cases pulmonary oedema and oliguria may occur and epileptiform convulsions may develop.

The prognosis depends upon the length of exposure and the concentration of the gas to which the patient was exposed. Mild forms of poisoning usually recover but it may be up to 18 months before recovery is complete. Sequelae include lassitude, peripheral neuropathy, tremor, uraemia and a variety of psychiatric symptoms such as depression, hallucinations, amnesia and insomnia.

Fatalities occur when pulmonary oedema is severe or where there is oliguria. Pathological changes in such cases include haemorrhages in the brain, liver, kidneys and lungs with small bloodstained pleural effusions. Degenerative changes are seen in the liver and kidney.

Splashes of methyl bromide on the skin produce a characteristic pattern of events. The skin is first cooled by evaporation and then a tingling, burning sensation is noted. The skin then becomes red and after several hours, small vesicles appear. The vesicles are extremely distended by straw-coloured fluid but they do not refill if they are punctured. The vesicles may coalesce. Healing takes place after a few days and is followed by a considerable desquamation.

If the degree of exposure is insufficient to produce vesicles, a dry eczematous reaction may be produced.

Treatment

No specific treatment is available and supportive measures are all that can be offered.

Tri-ortho-cresyl phosphate

Uses
Tri-ortho-cresyl phosphate (TOCP) is used in the plastics industry in great quantities as a plasticizer, i.e. a substance which renders the plastic material more pliable. It is also used in oils.

Hazards of use
The material, which is an oil with a pungent aroma, is absorbed through the skin, so all those handling it are potentially at risk. Special protective clothing, including gloves, must be worn. The oil is not very volatile and has a low vapour pressure at normal working temperatures, so inhalation is less of a risk than skin absorption. Cases of poisoning due to inhalation of the vapour have been recorded, however.

Metabolism
The compound is absorbed through the skin and becomes distributed via the blood throughout the body. The liver and spleen retain most of the absorbed material, followed by the voluntary muscles, brain and bone. Excretion takes place through the kidney.

TOCP is a potent inhibitor of pseudo-cholinesterase but has less effect on acetylcholinesterase (ChE).

Poisoning
Poisoning with TOCP develops in three stages. Initially the patient experiences mild gastrointestinal symptoms, including nausea, vomiting, abdominal pain and diarrhoea but these subside and the patient remains well for between 1 and 3 weeks. After this interval, the distal muscles become painful and there is numbness of the fingers and toes. Bilateral foot-drop develops. There follows another interval of approximately 10 days when bilateral wrist-drop is noted. The weakness in the hands is not usually so severe as in the legs and feet, and there is no paralysis above the elbows. The signs of peripheral neuritis may be complicated by those of lower motor neurone involvement and in advanced cases the muscles of the lower limbs may be completely flaccid with absent ankle jerks. Sensory changes are not noted and loss of sphincter control is rare.

Many patients recover completely in due course but some go on to develop upper motor neurone signs with spasticity, exaggerated reflexes and marked muscle wasting. Clinically, these cases resemble those of motor neurone disease.

Cases of nonoccupational origin have been recorded due to adulteration of cooking oil with TOCP.

Resins
A vast number of resins are in industrial use as constituents of paints and varnishes, as adhesives, as sand bonders in foundry work and for making

moulds. There are a great many formulations, the most common of which, arranged in order of risk, are shown in Table 4.1.

The principal risks from the use of resins are skin sensitization, with the production of an eczematous reaction, and respiratory irritation. The epoxy resins are the most active in producing skin lesions whilst the isocyanates used in polyurethane resins are the most potent producers of respiratory symptoms. The hardeners used in epoxy resins have been potent skin sensitizers and their fumes have caused asthma. Some of the constituents of other resin systems may also produce untoward effects. For example, styrene and formaldehyde used in

Table 4.1. Formulation of some common resin systems

System	Resins and formers	Catalyst	Curers and hardeners	Principal risks to health
High risk				
Epoxy	Epichlorhidrin aducts	Organic peroxides	Butyl glycidil ether Maleic anhydride Bisphenol polyamides	Skin sensitization
Medium risk				
Phenolic	Phenolformaldehyde	Phosphoric acid Toluene sulphonic acid	Formaldehyde	Dermatitis, conjunctivitis and respiratory irritation from formaldehyde
Polyester	Polyesters of adipic acid and styrene monomer	Organic cobalt compounds	Organic peroxides	Dermatitis and conjunctivitis from styrene
Polyurethane	Polyesters	Amines	Isocyanates	Dermatitis and respiratory symptoms especially from TDI
Low risk				
Acrylic	Acrylic acid Acrylamide Acrylonitrile	Organic peroxides	Heat	Respiratory irritation from unreacted acrylic compounds
Alkyd	Phthalic anhydride Glycerol		Air drying	
Furane	Furfural alcohol	Phosphoric acid Toluene sulphonic acid	Other resins	Furfural alcohol causes CNS depression

polyester and phenolic resins respectively, both produce dermatitis and conjunctivitis and, in addition, the inhalation of formaldehyde may produce irritation of the upper respiratory tract. The conjunctivitis caused by formaldehyde may be severe and be complicated by extensive corneal damage.

Anaesthetics

The two anaesthetics in most common use are nitrous oxide and halothane. It goes without saying that if medical or nursing staff are over-exposed in the theatre, then they will suffer the same effects, in kind if not in degree, as those of their patients. And there is good evidence that anaesthetists and other operating theatre staff suffer some behavioural effects at the end of the day. These behavioural changes are related to a depression of arousal and result, for example, in prolonged reaction times which may in turn lead to an increased tendency to have an accident. The other effect which has been much discussed is the possibility that exposure to anaesthetic gases may cause an increased incidence of stillbirth or congenital malformation. Some US studies have showed that female operating staff have a somewhat greater relative risk for these events than other nursing or medical staff but these results have not been confirmed in the UK. Nevertheless, it is prudent to minimize exposure and modern operating suites have scrubbers to remove waste gases.

Various urinary metabolites of halothane can be detected of which trifluoracetic acid is the major one. Trifluoracetic acid can also be detected in the blood and its half-life is between 50 and 70 hours. Increased plasma bromide concentrations have also been found after exposure to halothane.

Drugs

Some of the effects of drugs on those who manufacture or handle them are well known. Gynaecomastia has been documented in men manufacturing synthetic oestrogens and progestogens, depression in adrenocortical function has been noted in those manufacturing steroids and sensitization has been found to a number of antibiotics. In general, however, this is not well explored territory. Some concern has recently been expressed about the hazards of handling cytotoxic drugs. The urine of nurses working on oncology wards has been found to contain mutagenic substances and also to contain a higher concentration of thioethers than nurses working in other departments. The significance of these findings to the long term health of nurses is not at all clear but there seems no reason to doubt that those who handle cytotoxic drugs will absorb a certain amount and since the drugs are mutagenic a code of practice should be followed which will minimize exposure.

Chapter 5
Industrial Toxicology 4: Gases

The toxic gases may be classified into one of the three following categories:
1   Simple asphyxiants.
2   Chemical asphyxiants.
3   Irritants.

Simple asphyxiants

These gases are dangerous only when they are present in the air in a volume sufficient to diminish the partial pressure of oxygen below that which can support respiration. Nitrogen, methane and carbon dioxide are the three most important gases in this category.

Nitrogen

Nitrogen is the main constituent of chokedamp of mines, but it has industrial uses in the manufacture of ammonia and it is also used to produce an inert atmosphere for the prevention of oxidation in some metallurgical processes.

Blackdamp, which consists of about 88% nitrogen and 12% carbon dioxide is formed by the oxidation of the iron pyrites and calcite found in coal. It was formerly a hazard when ventilation in deep mines was inadequate and was recognized by the extinguishing of the miner's safety lamp. This occurred when the concentration of blackdamp in the air was in excess of 17.7%. With good ventilation in mines, blackdamp should no longer be a hazard.

Methane

Methane is known as firedamp in the mines and it became a hazard when deep shafts were first dug into the coal seams during the early part of the seventeenth century. The gas was formed in pockets in the seam and escaped when the coal was being mined. It presented two hazards to the miners, one of death from asphyxiation and one of death from the explosive mixture it formed with air. The latter danger was greatly alleviated by the introduction of the Davy Lamp in 1816, which has continued in modified form to the present day. Davy found that by interposing a metal gauze between a flame and an explosive mixture, the heat was diffused and dispersed by the gauze, so allowing the flame to burn without fear of explosion. With modern lamps the percentage of methane in the air can be estimated roughly by the height of the pale blue cap above the luminous part of the flame. In 1844 Faraday discovered that the hazard of firedamp explosion was increased by the ignition of mixtures of coal dust and air, which carried the explosion deep underground. Wet working and good ventilation have considerably reduced the hazards from firedamp.

Carbon dioxide

Carbon dioxide has a wide variety of industrial uses from the manufacture of fizzy drinks to the manufacture of freezing mixtures. It is readily liquified and is used in this form for fire extinguishers and to make carbon dioxide 'snow'. Dangerous concentrations of the gas may be encountered in mines, in fermenting vats, in breweries and mineral water factories, in coke ovens and blast furnaces and in agricultural silos and silage pits. If solid carbon dioxide is allowed to evaporate in a confined space, a dangerous concentration may build up.

Unlike the two previous asphyxiants, carbon dioxide has a powerful physiological effect and produces an increase in the respiratory rate through its action on the respiratory centre in the medulla. The symptoms produced can be related to the proportion of carbon dioxide in the atmosphere. Thus a concentration in excess of 3% will produce dyspnoea which becomes pronounced when the concentration is over 5%. With concentrations greater than 10%, loss of consciousness supervenes after a minute or so.

The treatment of carbon dioxide poisoning consists of removing the affected person from exposure and administering oxygen.

In situations where it can be presumed that a risk from carbon dioxide might exist, the extinction of a lighted candle introduced into the oven, silo or whatever, indicates a dangerous atmosphere. Work must then only be permitted with the use of breathing apparatus. In potentially hazardous situations, men should always work in pairs.

Solid carbon dioxide can produce burns which are slow to heal. Consequently no one should be so unwise or foolhardy as to attempt to handle this substance without wearing gloves.

Chemical asphyxiants

Gases in this class produce their toxic effects through some sort of chemical combination with metabolically important proteins. The most important of these gases are carbon monoxide, nickel carbonyl, hydrogen sulphide, hydrogen cyanide, arsine, stibene and phosphine

Carbon monoxide

Carbon monoxide is produced by the incomplete combustion of carbon compounds. As many of the gases used in industry contain carbon monoxide in varying proportions, there is an ever present hazard wherever they are used. The one exception is North Sea Gas which consists of methane with small amounts of butane and propane (Table 5.1). The exhaust gases of petrol and diesel engines also produce carbon monoxide and dangerous quantities may be generated in confined spaces.

In mines, carbon monoxide is the dangerous constituent of afterdamp, the gas produced during underground explosions from methane and coal dust.

Carbon monoxide is colourless and odourless and the early signs of intoxication are insidious, factors which combine to make it especially dangerous. The initial symptoms include giddiness and headache and then the patient

Table 5.1. Chemical composition of some gases used in industry

	Carbon monoxide	Carbon dioxide	Methane	Hydrogen	Nitrogen
Coal gas	16%	2%	20%	55%	Trace
Producer gas	30%	10%	Trace	10%	50% +
Water gas	40%	5%	Trace	50%	3%
Blast furnace gas	27%	15%	Trace	2%	55%
Coke oven gas	9%	3%	25%	55%	6%
Natural gas (North Sea and Petroleum gas)	Nil	Nil	85%	Nil	Nil

loses the power in his/her legs and becomes unconscious. Concentrations of 3500 parts/10^6 are immediately hazardous to life.

Carbon monoxide has a greater affinity for haemoglobin than oxygen and combines with it to form carboxyhaemoglobin. This is a stable pigment which only slowly becomes dissociated. The symptoms of intoxication can be correlated with the carboxyhaemoglobin concentration as shown in Table 5.2. Death occurs when the blood is 60–80% saturated with carboxyhaemoglobin. No cyanosis is produced, despite the profound tissue anoxia, and the patient is classically described as being cherry pink.

All those likely to be exposed to carbon monoxide should wear respirators and know how to provide first aid measures in cases of poisoning. Treatment consists of giving artificial respiration and of keeping the patient warm. The patient should be made to rest. A mixture of 95% oxygen and 5% carbon dioxide should be given; this is more effective in reducing the carboxyhaemoglobin saturation than oxygen alone. The carboxyhaemoglobin level should also be measured and if it is found to be greater than 50% consideration should be given to the use of hyperbaric oxygen.

After recovery from carbon monoxide poisoning the patient may experience severe headache. If asphyxiation has been prolonged, organic brain damage may result, with the production of lesions in the basal ganglia, dementia or depression. The elderly are more likely to be left with permanent neurological deficits than the young.

Table 5.2. Correlation between carboxyhaemoglobin concentrations and symptoms of carbon monoxide poisoning

Carboxyhaemoglobin concentrate	Symptoms of intoxication
<20%	None except slight breathlessness on exertion.
20%–30%	Flushing, slight headache. Some breathlessness on exertion.
30%–40%	Severe headache, vertigo, nausea and vomiting, irritability and impaired judgement.
40%–50%	Symptoms as above but more severe. Fainting on exertion.
50%–60%	Loss of consciousness.
>60%	Depression of respiratory centre leading to death.

Carbon monoxide is not a cumulative poison and any gas which is absorbed during exposure to low concentrations will be excreted via the lungs when exposure has been discontinued. Many authorities dispute the existence of chronic carbon monoxide poisoning on these grounds. Nevertheless, exposure to low concentrations has been shown to impair performance in some psychological tests, and in animals it hastens the development of arteriosclerosis and produces myocardial damage.

Nickel carbonyl

Nickel carbonyl is used principally in the refining of nickel ores by the Mond process. Poisoning with this gas has two phases. Initially there is headache, nausea, vomiting and dizziness, and unconsciousness may supervene. These symptoms are very like those of carbon monoxide poisoning and in fact, carbon monoxide is always encountered with nickel carbonyl in industry.

The initial symptoms rapidly pass, to be followed in 8–36 hours by dyspnoea, cyanosis, weakness and pulmonary oedema. There is at first a dry cough which soon becomes worse and is accompanied by the production of bloodstained sputum. The respiratory symptoms increase in severity for about 6 days and signs of cardiac failure may be noted. Most of those affected recover with no permanent disability. In fatal cases, death occurs within 2 weeks. The final outcome depends upon the degree of damage sustained by the alveolar epithelium. At autopsy, areas of external haemorrhage are found together with atelectasis and necrosis. Haemorrhages may also be found on the brain and meninges. Those who suffer from nickel carbonyl poisoning should be given oxygen and ventilation as required and the use of bronchodilators may be indicated. All urine samples should be monitored for their nickel content since this gives a guide to the severity of the intoxication. Disulfiram can be given as an antidote in a starting dose of 800 mg followed by a second dose of 400 mg 6 hours later. Further doses may be indicated, depending on the severity of the illness. The patient should be advised to avoid alcohol for a week following the last dose of disulfiram.

To rule out the possibility of concommitant carbon monoxide poisoning, carboxyhaemoglobin levels should also be measured.

Repeated exposure to low concentrations of nickel carbonyl may give rise to a sensitivity to nickel which may in turn lead to the development of asthmatic attacks and pulmonary eosinophilia which manifests itself as patchy opacities on a chest X-ray.

Hydrogen sulphide

Hydrogen sulphide is met wherever sulphur and its compounds are worked. In mines it is called stinkdamp, for the good reason that it smells like rotting eggs. The gas is also found in gasworks, in sewers where organic matter is putrifying and in a number of chemical processes involving the manufacture of sulphur compounds.

It is at least as poisonous as hydrogen cyanide, and like HCN inhibits cytochrome oxidase by binding with ferric ions. Symptoms of intoxication will be produced when the concentration is in excess of 200 parts/10^6; above 600 parts/10^6 it is rapidly fatal.

Although the gas has such an unpleasant smell and can be detected at concentrations as low as 0.3 parts/10^6 above about 30 parts/10^6 there is a rapid accommodation to the smell which therefore increases the danger of exposure.

Once the gas is absorbed it is oxidized to a limited extent but a build up of free hydrogen sulphide occurs. The gas can combine with methaemoglobin to form a green pigment sulphmethaemoglobin, but this does not affect tissue oxygenation.

Exposure to low concentrations causes lacrimation, photophobia, and irritation of the nasal mucosa and the pharynx. Headache, vertigo and collapse may follow. Hydrogen sulphide has a profoundly irritant effect on the cornea due to the formation of sodium sulphide, and in addition to producing pain, photophobia and lacrimation, it also causes blurring of vision and keratitis. It may cause vesicles to form on the cornea, which eventually rupture. The cornea usually recovers completely upon removal from exposure and ulceration and scarring are rare. There are no cumulative effects.

Anyone exposed to a high concentration of hydrogen sulphide will die immediately from the paralytic effect which the free hydrogen sulphide has on the respiratory centre in the medulla.

Treatment consists in removing the affected persons from exposure and giving oxygen. It is also worth administering amyl or sodium nitrite; the nitrite converts haemoglobin to methaemoglobin which then combines with the hydrogen sulphide to form sulphmethaemoglobin. Amyl nitrite can be given by breaking a capsule into a handkerchief which is then held over the patient's nose; sodium nitrite is given as 10 ml of a 3% solution intravenously over 2–3 minutes, with a further 5 ml if necessary. The amount of hydrogen sulphide in workplaces can be tested with lead acetate paper. At concentrations greater than 34 parts/10^6 the paper darkens immediately, at 4 parts/10^6 it will take 1 or 2 seconds to do so. Respirators should be worn by all those who are likely to be exposed to concentrations greater than 10 parts/10^6.

Hydrogen cyanide

The toxicity of this gas resides in the cyanide ion, so that all its soluble inorganic salts become hazardous under conditions which favour the release of the cyanide ion. Hydrogen cyanide in the form of potassium or sodium cyanide is used in some heat treatment or hardening processes of steel, in electroplating in the chemical industry and as a fumigant. The gas is also produced by the combustion of polyurethane foams. The poisonous properties of cyanide are well known. From time to time cyanide has enjoyed considerable popularity amongst would-be poisoners and some executioners.

Cyanide produces its action by inhibiting cytochrome oxidase thus interfering with tissue oxygenation. There is no interference with oxygen transport as is the case in the carbon monoxide poisoning.

The symptoms of poisoning occur rapidly after inhalation, but if small amounts of cyanide are ingested, death may not ensue for hours. Symptoms include headache, rapid weak respirations, vomiting, excitability, tachycardia, hypotension, convulsions and coma leading to death. Pulmonary oedema and lactic acidosis may also be prominent features.

If any treatment is to be effective in a patient who is unconscious following exposure to cyanide, it must be given with all possible speed. Hypoxia is treated with oxygen and ventilation and an injection of 300 mg dicobalt edetate in 20 ml glucose solution should be given by slow intravenous injection. The treatment is dangerous when administered in the absence of serious cyanide poisoning. If there are no signs of recovery within a very short time following the administration of dicobalt-EDTA (say a minute), a further 300 mg may be given. During the administration of this compound the patient may become hypotensive and vomiting is common. Rarely, anaphylactic reactions occur.

The symptoms of excitement and tachycardia will readily develop in anyone who supposes that he or she has been exposed to cyanide—understandably. However, since the poison works so rapidly, if there is an appreciable delay between presumed exposure and the development of serious symptoms, particularly drowsiness or unconsciousness, then it is most unlikely that a harmful dose has been taken. Reassurance under those circumstances may completely alleviate all symptoms.

In most cases of poisoning, the effects are so rapid that emergency treatment must be given on the spot. The patient must be removed from exposure and any contaminated clothing taken off and the skin washed. Oxygen should be given if available and capsules of amyl nitrite broken into a handkerchief which is held over the patient's nose.

All personnel working in areas where cyanide is used must be instructed in its dangers and great care must be taken in the storage and handling of cyanide salts. They must not be kept where they can come into contact with acids, for example! Workers should be trained in emergency first-aid and treatment kits, containing di-cobalt EDTA must be readily available for all.

Arsine

Arsine is formed when nascent hydrogen is produced in the presence of arsenic or arsenic-containing materials. Arsenic is a contaminant of many ores including aluminium, antimony, copper, gold, lead, silver, tin and zinc, and so the formation of arsine is a hazard in the metal-working industries, especially from the action of acid on arsenic-bearing metals. The main risks are probably connected with aluminium.

The only commercial use of arsine is in the manufacture of semiconductors in the electronics industry. The arsine is used in a carrier gas such as nitrogen in a concentration of about 100 ppm. This so-called doping mixture is passed over silica crystals in a furnace where it is decomposed to form arsine which diffuses into the crystals. Excess arsine is converted to other arsenic compounds and removed by a scrubber. Other doping mixtures used in the electronics industry employ stibene, phosphine and diborane.

Arsine gradually decomposes to form pure arsenic. If cylinders of the gas are being stored or transported slight leakages of gas may result in arsenic being deposited on surfaces which could present a hazard to those handling the cylinder.

The gas is a powerful haemolytic agent and the signs and symptoms of poisoning are the result of its action on the blood. In mild cases there may be an interval of up to a day between exposure and the development of the premonitory symptoms, nausea, headache, shivering and epigastric pain. Haemoglobinuria of a high level of free haemoglobin in the plasma denote a serious degree of haemolysis. Jaundice shows on the second or third day. (It is worth noting that arsine is one of the commonest causes of toxic jaundice of occupational origin.) The jaundice is accompanied by hepatic pain and tenderness. The kidneys are severely damaged and albumin and casts are present in the urine, and anuria may be a fatal complication. The degree of anaemia clearly depends upon the extent of the haemolysis and red cell counts as low as one million/cm^3 have been recorded.

There is a considerable mortality from arsine poisoning as the result of myocardial failure. Those who survive the initial catastrophe can expect to recover fully although in some cases a peripheral neuropathy may develop which is slow to resolve. There is no specific treatment and in this respect poisoning with arsine differs from poisoning with other arsenic compounds where BAL is beneficial. Supportive measures including blood transfusion and dialysis should be given as required.

Continued exposure to very low concentrations may give rise to the development of anaemia, the true cause of which may be often unrecognized. Those who may be especially susceptible to haemolytic agents, workers with a deficiency of red cell glutathione, for example, must not be exposed at all to arsine.

Stibene

Stibene (antimony hydride) is formed accidentally when nascent hydrogen comes into contact with antimony or its compounds, when antimony alloys, or ores containing antimony are treated with acid and by wet treatment of slags or drosses contaminated with antimony.

The gas is highly toxic, colourless, but with an unpleasant smell. It rapidly decomposes at temperatures above 150°C and by contact with most oxidizing substances.

The toxic effects of stibene closely resemble those of arsine with which it may be encountered. Like arsine, it is a powerful haemolytic agent and the treatment of acute poisoning requires prompt, vigorous treatment including, when necessary, exchange transfusions and renal dialysis. There is no state of chronic poisoning.

Phosphine

Phosphine has no great commercial use and is usually met as it is evolved during manufacturing processes. It has an odour of decaying fish and is detectable in a concentration as low as 0.2 ppm. At a concentration of 20 ppm it will rapidly cause death.

The gas is evolved during the preparation and use of calcium phosphide, in the manufacture of acetylene from impure calcium carbide and when zinc phosphide (sometimes used as a rat-killer) or aluminium phosphide (used to fumigate grain) are accidentally wetted. Quenching metal alloys with water may also generate the gas. Probably the main production of phosphine, however, is in the making of spheroidal graphite.

Symptoms of poisoning include abdominal pain, nausea and vomiting. Ataxia, convulsions, coma and death may supervene within 24 hours. In milder cases, the gas may produce signs of respiratory irritation and recovery is complete.

Chronic poisoning, in which neurological symptoms predominate, is said to occur in those who are continuously exposed to very low concentrations.

Those who suffer from phosphine poisoning should be treated with oxygen and ventilation as indicated. The early administration of up to 30 mg/kg of methylprednisolone by intravenous injection is advocated by some authorities. Patients should be monitored in order to detect any secondary effects on the liver or kidney and treated accordingly.

Irritant gases

The irritant gases are irrespirable except at very low concentrations. Their action on the respiratory tract depends upon their solubility. Those, such as ammonia, which are readily soluble, dissolve out of the inhaled air in the upper respiratory tract and so have little effect on the lungs. Conversely, insoluble gases, such as nitrogen dioxide, penetrate the lungs and are much more injurious, causing severe pulmonary oedema.

A number of gases will be considered here: ammonia, ethylene oxide, formaldehyde and glutaraldehyde, sulphur dioxide, nitrous fumes, chlorine, phosgene and fluorine.

Ammonia

Ammonia is used in great quantities in the manufacture of agricultural fertilizers. It is also used as a refrigerant, to produce an anti-oxidant atmosphere in metal furnaces and in a number of synthetic processes in the chemical industry.

The toxic effects of ammonia are due to its caustic action. If splashed on the skin it will cause a burn and enough may be absorbed to produce systemic symptoms. The vapour will cause conjunctival irritation and if splashed in the eye, conjunctivitis and keratitis will follow. More serious effects may include ulceration of the cornea and the conjunctivae which may lead to the formation of scar tissue, corneal opacities and perhaps blindness. Ammonia will rapidly penetrate the anterior chamber of the eye and it has been known to produce opacities in the lens.

Inhalation of the vapour causes a chemical bronchitis with dyspnoea, pulmonary oedema, a cough with a frothy, sometimes bloodstained sputum, tachycardia and pyrexia. In addition, ammonia vapour causes pain and oedema in the mouth and throat, with ulceration of the mucosa. Hoarseness, conjunctivitis and lacrimation are also prominent effects.

Mild cases will recover promptly on removal from exposure, although some will relapse with pulmonary oedema. Burns on the skin should be treated by copious washing with water and a buffered phosphate solution. Splashes in the eyes are treated by irrigation and corticosteroid drugs. Severe systemic effects will require hospitalization.

People whose work involves contact with ammonia must be pre-warned of its dangers and wear gloves and goggles to prevent effects from splashing. Adequate ventilation of the work place is essential. Those who are required to repair plant where the concentration of ammonia may be high, should wear respirators.

Ethylene oxide

Ethylene oxide is a highly reactive gas which is easily liquefied and polymerized. It is an important starting point in the manufacture of ethylene glycol and some higher alcohols. It is also used as a fumigant and a sterilizing agent when it is usually mixed with carbon dioxide.

Exposure to high concentrations results in irritation of the mucous membranes and of the respiratory tract, perhaps with the production of pulmonary oedema. Prolonged exposure to low concentrations tends to impair the sense of smell. Liquid ethylene oxide may produce severe chemical burns if not immediately washed off the skin; there may be some delay in doing this since skin contact produces no immediate effects. The cold liquid can induce frostbite and great care should be taken to ensure that it does not get into boots or shoes or under gloves, cuffs or collars.

There is presently a great deal of interest in the toxicology of ethylene oxide because of the suggestion that it may induce leukaemia. Chromosome breaks have been reported by some authors in workers exposed at low levels but not by others. The evidence regarding its leukaemogenic potential is equally confusing although the bulk of recent studies have tended to absolve it from blame. Nevertheless, it is subject to a maximum exposure limit which is 5 ppm in this country; in the USA a more stringent standard of 1 ppm is in force.

Formaldehyde and glutaraldehyde

These aldehydes are close cousins and share a number of family characteristics; on this account they can conveniently be considered together.

Formaldehyde is used widely (in aqueous solutions as formaldehyde) in laboratories for fixing specimens and it is widely used in the production of resins used in particle boards and laminates. It is also used in the textile industry for finishing fabrics by the application of polymers and resins which give the fabric body, and flame resistant qualities. Glutaraldehyde is a sterilizing agent which is widely used in hospitals to sterilize endoscopes and other items.

Both these aldehydes are potent irritants to mucous membranes. They are also sensitizers and those exposed to them may develop contact dermatitis or occupational asthma. There is also some concern about the potential carcinogenicity of formaldehyde since it is both mutagenic and teratogenic in experimental systems. There is no strong evidence for either of these effects in man, however.

Formaldehyde is partially metabolized to formic acid in humans and urinary levels can be used to monitor exposure; there does not seem to be an analagous metabolite by which to measure exposure to glutaraldehyde.

Sulphur dioxide

Sulphur dioxide is produced by the combustion of sulphur compounds. It is used in the production of sulphuric acid, as a preservative of food and wine, as a fumigant and it was used in the past as a refrigerant. More commonly, however, it is encountered as a contaminant, both inside and outside industry. In industry it is an important contaminant in magnesium foundries, whilst in the general environment it is a notable constituent of fog and smog.

The gas has a characteristically pungent smell which can be detected when the concentration is about 3 ppm. It is highly irritant to the mucous membranes of the eye and the respiratory tract. In low concentrations the vapour produces lacrimation, sneezing and coughing. Serious poisoning is rare because the gas is so irritant that those exposed rapidly run away. When escape is difficult, the patient will develop severe respiratory distress, collapse and die. Workers continuously exposed to low concentrations will develop some tolerance to its effects and be able to work in a concentration containing up to 10 ppm, whereas those who are unacclimatized develop symptoms when the concentration is of the order of 3 ppm. Mild cases will recover with no treatment beyond removal from exposure, and the conjunctivitis heals with no sequelae. Serious cases of poisoning require treatment in hospital.

Continuous exposure to low concentrations tends to produce upper respiratory disease and partial loss of taste and smell. Abrupt increases in the concentration of sulphur dioxide to levels greater than 0.25 parts/10^6 in the atmosphere of cities is associated with a slight increase in general mortality, if at the same time smoke concentrations are also increased. Levels of sulphur dioxide greater than 0.5 parts/10^6 are associated with a 20% increase in mortality compared with 'normal' mortality, but only if smoke levels are greater than 200 $\mu g/m^3$. Those who suffer most are patients with chronic pulmonary disease.

Liquid sulphur dioxide

This was widely used as a refrigerant and severe injuries to the eyes have been caused as the result of accidental splashing. The corneal epithelium swells and is shed after a few days to reveal infiltration of the stroma and interstitial vascularization. Corneal scarring, overgrowth of the cornea by conjunctival epithelium and permanent defects of vision are all late results. Prolonged irrigation of the eye with water must be undertaken as quickly as possible after liquid sulphur dioxide has gone into the eye.

Nitrous fumes

Nitrous fumes are an equilibrium mixture of the two dioxides of nitrogen, nitogen oxide (NO_2) and dinitrogen tetroxide (N_2O_4) in the ratio of approximately $3:7$; the equilibrium between the two, however, is temperature dependent. The other oxides of nitrogen are nontoxic and nitrous oxide (N_2O) is used as an anaesthetic; despite some fears to the contrary, there is no evidence that it has any neuropsychological effects at low concentrations. Nitrous fumes take the form of reddish-brown fumes, slightly heavier than air and they are produced whenever nitric acid is exposed to the air or whenever it reacts with organic material. They are also produced during the combustion of material such as celluloid, which contains a nitrous radical, by the combination of nitrogen and oxygen during such processes as oxyacetylene, carbon-arc or electric-arc welding and in mining when dynamite is used for blasting and burns quietly instead of exploding. During the fermentation of silage the fumes may also be given off as the result of the reduction of nitrogen, and those working in silos may be affected by the fumes and get what is known as silo-fillers' disease.

Of all the irritant gases, nitrous fumes are the most insidious and since the margin between concentrations which will provoke mild symptoms and those which will produce fatal results is small, the gas is a serious danger. Moreover, workers may inhale potentially lethal amounts without the ill effects being noted for anything from 2 to 24 hours. Fortunately, workers are easily trained to take great care when they see the distinctive coloured fumes and thus avoid any ill effects.

There are three more or less distinct syndromes of poisoning with nitrous fumes. Exposure to concentrations in the range of 100 to 500 ppm may cause sudden bronchospasm and death from respiratory failure. The most typical consequence of exposure, however, is the development of a chemical alveolitis with severe pulmonary oedema. Upper respiratory irritation is generally mild. As a rule, the immediate symptoms which follow exposure are so mild as to escape notice, but some irritation of the eyes and throat may be noted together with a cough and some tightness in the chest. As the pulmonary oedema develops the patient will become dsypnoeic and develop a cough with much bloodstained sputum. In severe cases, cyanosis, circulatory failure and death may follow. Treatment of these cases is as for any other cause of severe pulmonary oedema and complete recovery should be expected.

The third syndrome of poisoning with nitrous fumes is associated with an inflammatory response in the lungs thought to be due to an autoimmune reaction. The condition is sometimes referred to as bronchiolitis fibrosa obliterans. It is not clear whether this condition is a late sequel of acute intoxication or whether it is caused by repeated exposure to concentrations in the range 20–50 ppm.

The hazards of nitrous fumes must be made known to all who work where they are liable to be generated and measures must be taken to prevent the escape of the fumes into the general working environment. Welding processes must be carried out with adequate ventilation and oxygen must not be used to sweeten the air in confined spaces where welding is in operation. It is important to warn workers of the dangers of putting sawdust or wood shavings or any other organic material onto spilt nitric acid: it should be hosed away with large quantities of water by workers wearing suitable respirators.

Chlorine

Chlorine is used for the manufacture of chlorine compounds, for bleaching paper and man-made fibres and as a disinfectant for water supplies, swimming pools and sewage. It has the doubtful distinction of being the first war gas.

The gas has a pungent, irritating odour and this usually causes those exposed to take prompt evasive action. Immediate symptoms of intoxication are choking, a retrosternal burning pain, coughing, irritation of the eyes and mouth, and excessive salivation and lacrimation. An intense headache and severe epigastric pain are common. Nausea and vomiting may follow. The patient appears acutely ill and becomes cyanosed. He or she may develop pulmonary oedema if the concentration of gas is high (greater than 40 ppm).

Complete rest with supportive treatment is essential and can best be given in hospital. Respiratory distress can persist for up to 2 weeks but recovery is complete.

A high standard of safety is called for in those industries using chlorine and respirators must be worn for hazardous jobs. Adequate ventilation in the general working area is essential.

It is perhaps worth remembering also that chlorine may be liberated from domestic hypochlorite bleaches if they are reacted with ammonia, acids or sodium bisulphate, as may occur when bleaches of different composition are mixed.

Phosgene

Phosgene (carbonyl chloride) is used in the synthesis of several organic compounds and as an agent for direct chlorination. It may also be liberated when halogenated hydrocarbons are heated, so that welding and smoking should not be allowed where degreasing agents such as trichlorethylene or carbon tetrachloride are in use. For the same reason, portable fire extinguishers which contain carbon tetrachloride should not be provided for use in enclosed spaces since there is a risk that the carbon tetrachloride will decompose on contact with hot metal. The use of phosgene as a war gas provided the opportunity to study the toxic effects on a wide scale: 80% or more of the fatalities due to gas in the 1914–18 war were caused by phosgene.

The gas has a sweet smell, said to resemble that of green corn or geraniums. It is much more toxic than chlorine. There are no immediate symptoms following exposure to low concentrations beyond a slight irritation of the eyes and upper respiratory tract. After 24–48 hours, however, severe pulmonary oedema may develop, with circulatory collapse.

After exposure to high concentrations, the patient will notice tightness in the chest, with nausea and vomiting a few minutes after he or she has begun to inhale the gas. Upper respiratory tract irritation is noted and conjunctivitis develops. Pulmonary oedema with cough, cyanosis and collapse all follow suit. Any activity enhances the symptoms so complete rest is mandatory. Treatment is only practicable in hospital, bearing in mind that acute pulmonary oedema may develop after an interval as late as 48 hours.

Chest X-rays show the presence of multiple, ill-rounded shadows, and the area of the opacities correlates reasonably well with the degree of exposure.

Recovery is slow and effort syndrome is a common sequel to an attack of gassing. Repeated acute episodes can lead to chronic pulmonary disease.

Fluorine and compounds of fluorine

Fluorine is one of the most chemically active elements known. In the free state it is a green-yellow gas with a pungent smell which can be detected at low concentrations. Compounds of fluorine including fluorspar (calcium fluoride) and cryolite (sodium aluminium fluoride) are used as fluxes in the metal industry and they are also used in the chemical industry. Clays containing calcium fluoride are used in the pottery industry and when these clays are fired, fluorosilicates are produced. These substances constitute a serious hazard. Uranium hexafluoride is used to separate uranium isotopes, whilst hydrofluoric acid is used in the manufacture of aluminium fluoride. It is also used to etch glass and in the pottery industry, to etch china prior to gold decoration. Organic fluorine compounds such as dichlorodifluoromethane (freon) are used in refrigeration and in vast amounts as propellants in aerosol cans. Teflon, widely used as a nonstick lining for pans, is polytetrafluoroethylene.

Hydrofluoric acid

In addition to its industrial uses, hydrofluoric acid is evolved in the manufacture of super-phosphates by treating bones with sulphuric acid.

Anhydrous hydrofluoric acid is a colourless liquid, which gives off an irritant vapour. Fluorine gas is invariably converted to hydrofluoric acid by combining with the water in the atmosphere or on wet mucosal surfaces.

On the skin hydrofluoric acid produces an effect which varies from mild erythema to a severe burn, depending on the concentration and length of exposure. The burn is characterized by an intense throbbing pain which may be delayed several hours. A tough white coagulum forms over the area of damage, under which progressive destruction of all tissues continues. Burns under the fingernails are notable in this respect because of the difficulties of treatment.

Fluoride ions rapidly penetrate the skin and their effect on subcutaneous nerve endings produces severe pain as a result of the decrease in the concentration of calcium ions which are taken up by fluoride. Hypocalcaemia and cardiovascular collapse can occur after liquid HF has been in contact with even a relatively small surface area of skin and even if treatment has been prompt and efficient; tetany may also occur as plasma calcium levels fall. There may also be a fall in the concentration of other electrolytes, for example, potassium.

If the vapour is inhaled the larynx and the trachea are affected; there is severe retrosternal pain and cough, with sputum and perhaps haemoptysis. Pulmonary oedema may also result. Should the liquid be swallowed, the mouth and pharynx are burned and there is nausea, vomiting and collapse. Slow ulceration of all sites in contact with the liquid or vapour is the ultimate result.

Treatment
Those who have inhaled the vapour should be given oxygen and their respiration supported if necessary. Bronchodilators may be indicated and some authorities advocate the early administration of up to 30 mg/kg of methyl prednisolone. Serum calcium levels should be measured and the patient observed for signs of tetany. Calcium gluconate (10%) can be administered as necessary.

Burns must be given immediate first aid. Contaminated clothing is removed and the area washed with copious amounts of water for 1 minute. A gel containing 2.5% calcium gluconate should be applied and massaged into the burnt area and this should be continued until 15 minutes after the pain in the burn is relieved or until the patient is removed to hospital.

Great care must be taken by all those handling hydrofluoric acid. The liquid attacks glass and so is transported and stored in tarred barrels or metal containers. Workers must wear protective clothing and be taught to examine their gloves regularly for small holes. Face masks must be worn and good exhaust ventilation is required. Running water must be available in areas where hydrofluoric acid is handled for drenching the skin in case of burns. All workers should be instructed in the dangers of hydrofluoric acid and in how to give first aid.

Fluorosis

The chronic absorption of relatively high concentrations of fluoride ion can produce pathological changes which are largely confined to skeletal tissues. Such changes have been found in workers handling fluorspar, fluorapatite and cryolite. In addition, the condition has been found in some members of the general public living near foundries using iron ore and coal containing fluoride, and near factories manufacturing aluminium. Fluorosis has also been reported to occur in animals grazing near factories which emit fluoride, aluminium factories for example, and fertilizer and brick and ceramics factories.

The skeletal changes include the coarsening of the spongy trabeculae, periosteal new bone deposition with the formation of osteophytes, and ossification of ligaments and tendons. Bone which is severely affected is chalky-white and easily cut with a knife. Symptoms are not apparent in the early stages of the disease, but gradually vague pains are noted in the small joints of the hands and the feet. As the changes progress the patient may develop kyphosis together with limitation of spinal movement and flexion contractions of the hips and knees. Ultimately, compression of the nerve roots and spinal cord may cause the development of paraesthesiae, weakness and paralysis.

The teeth become mottled even when the intake of fluoride is relatively low, and in some parts of the world, the condition is almost unavoidable because of the high concentration of fluoride in the drinking water. Tooth mottling is a very sensitive index of chronic fluorine poisoning. The teeth show chalky-white streaks and blotches and are dotted with irregular defects in the enamel which is discoloured a light brown or black. All the permanent teeth are affected and changes in the deciduous teeth have also been recorded. Children born to some female cryolite workers have developed dental mottling as the result of absorbing fluoride excreted in their mother's milk.

Fluorides are avid bone seekers and they produce their effects by depressing collagen formation and bone resorption and by increasing bone crystal formation. There is some evidence that a high dietary intake of calcium will reduce the toxicity of ingested fluoride compounds, presumably through the formation of the relatively insoluble calcium fluoride.

At low levels, fluoride in drinking water (<1 mg/l) is said actually to be of benefit in dental hygiene, reducing the rate of decay and the incidence of caried teeth. A number of local authorities have introduced schemes for the fluoridation of public water supplies, but clearly such schemes must be rigidly controlled to prevent concentrations in excess of 1 mg/l being presented to the general public.

Treatment

There is no specific treatment and so there is a great need to protect workers from absorbing the dust generated during smelting of fluoride ores. Such processes should be exhaust ventilated and as much of the handling as possible carried out mechanically. Masks should be worn by those likely to be in contact with the dust.

Polytetrafluorethylene

Polytetrafluorethylene (PTFE) begins to decompose when heated to temperatures of about 250°C, producing hydrogen fluoride and a range of aliphatic and cyclic saturated and unsaturated compounds. At higher temperatures, sulphur dioxide, carbon monoxide, chlorine, phosgene and perfluoroisobutylene may all be evolved, the last being extremely toxic.

Inhalation of these breakdown products produces an illness known as polymer fume fever which resembles metal fume fever. Smoking cigarettes contaminated with PTFE is the common cause of the illness, the cigarettes becoming contaminated either from the workers' hands or from specks of PTFE powder which settle onto the lighted end of the cigarettes from the air.

The symptoms of the illness include fever and shivering, and a cough with tightness in the chest. In rare cases pulmonary oedema has been recorded.

The symptoms subside within 24–48 hours and there are no sequelae. No syndrome of chronic poisoning is known.

Chapter 6
Occupational Lung Diseases

Obstructive airways disease

Occupational asthma

Occupational asthma is a disease characterized by reversible airways obstruction which is causally related to exposure of a variety of agents in the workplace. It is a disease which is becoming increasingly prevalent. There are in excess of 200 agents which have been reported to cause occupational asthma; the most important are shown in Table 6.1. In some cases (shown in the table), sufferers from occupational asthma are entitled to compensation. The prevalence of occupational asthma amongst groups at risk is not known with certainty but such studies as have been carried out suggest that it may be high. For example, up to a third of new entrants to platinum refining leave within 18 months because they develop asthma and a similar proportion of those using colophony resin in the electronics industry may be affected. Between 5 and 10% of those handling laboratory animals may develop asthma and be forced to find other work and up to half of those who handle locusts are affected; this might be a case of the animals fighting back.

There is always a variable interval between first exposure and the development of symptoms which may vary from a few weeks to several years. The symptoms of an attack may develop within minutes of exposure (the immediate type) or some hours after first exposure, perhaps long after the patient has left work (non-immediate type). In the immediate type of attack the symptoms tend to be maximal within 10–20 minutes of onset and last for up to 2 hours. In the nonimmediate type, the symptoms are maximal within 4–8 hours and often recover within 24 hours. It should not be thought that the differentiation is always clear cut, however, and intermediate types occur. Nor does the occurrence of immediate symptoms exclude the possibility of late symptoms for, in some unfortunate individuals, both occur. In some cases there is a tendency for symptoms to recur at about the same time on a number of successive nights following a single exposure. This is sometimes referred to as late recurrent asthma or recurrent nocturnal asthma and seems to occur particularly in those whose symptoms are due to TDI or Western red cedar.

The diagnosis of occupational asthma depends to a large degree on the examining physician bearing the possibility in mind. It should always be considered when asthma first comes on in adult life but must be differentiated from the type of bronchial hyperreactivity which can follow exposure to agents such as cold, exercise or cigarette smoke, for example. It must also be differentiated from an exacerbation of symptoms in an individual with long standing idiopathic asthma.

Table 6.1. Some common causes of occupational asthma

Low molecular weight compounds
Biological agents
    Colophony
    Iroko
    Mahogany
    Western red cedar

Chemical agents
    Amino-ethyl-ethanolamine
    Antibiotics
    Cobalt
    Di-isocyanates
    Nickel
    Platinum (soluble salts)
    Trimellitic anhydride
    Vanadium

High molecular weight compounds
Animal and insect proteins
Enzyme detergents (*Bacillus subtilis*)
Coffee beans
Flour (wheat and rye)
Grains
Gum acacia
Papain
Tea

Wheeze is not always the most prominent symptom and in many cases all the patient will complain of is a cough or a little breathlessness. Those who are affected, however, will often appreciate that their symptoms develop at work and may increase in severity as work progresses; the cardinal feature to elicit from the history is that—in the early stages at least—the symptoms improve away from work, over the weekend or on holiday.

Although a genetic or hereditary predisposition is sometimes invoked to explain why some individuals develop occupational asthma, only in the asthma caused by soluble platinum salts, enzyme detergents and by high molecular weight compounds such as animal proteins does this hold true. Genetic factors play little or no part in the development of isocyanate asthma or that induced by other low molecular weight compounds. Therefore a history of atopy is no criterion for excluding an individual from work involving exposure to sensitizers other than those referred to above. Because the results of skin prick tests may be negative, many cases of occupational asthma are diagnosed as having intrinsic asthma; others who smoke may be mistakenly said to have chronic bronchitis, especially if a productive cough is prominent amongst the symptoms.

The most helpful aid to diagnosis is self-measurement of the peak expiratory flow rate (PEFR) at 2-hour intervals throughout the day using a simple peak flow meter. Routine measurement of lung function before and after a working shift is often exceedingly unhelpful and may be downright misleading. The patient is asked to read his or her PEFR for several days including a weekend and preferably a longer period away from work. Two weeks is generally the minimum for which readings should be taken. The patient must be carefully instructed in the test procedure and must continue with his or her normal work whilst taking measurements; a note should be made of any bronchodilators which are taken, and their dose should not be varied throughout the period of observation. Drugs which would block the changes in the airways in response to sensitizers (corticosteroids or sodium cromoglycate) should be withheld.

In non-asthmatics the diurnal variation in PEFR will generally be less than 10% whereas in asthmatics it is usually greater than 20%. Depending on the time taken for lung function to recover, four patterns may be seen in PEFR records.

1   There may be progressive deterioration throughout the working week in which case the reduction in lung function is greater at the end than the beginning of the week and recovery may take up to 3 days. If recovery takes only 1 or 2 days and is substantial, then the weekly pattern is regular. If it takes the full 3 days and a late reaction occurs on the first day at work, the lung function on that day is the best of the week and it may be reduced throughout the weekend.

2   If deterioration is more or less the same on each day and recovery after leaving work is rapid, then the pattern will be the same on each working day and normal on the days away from exposure.

3   If recovery takes longer than 3 days then there will be a progressive decline week by week until a fixed state is reached. Following cessation of exposure recovery may not begin for a week or two and not be complete for as long as 3 months.

4   Rarely in occupational asthma, the deterioration in PEFR may be most pronounced on the first day of exposure and may recover throughout the rest of the week. This type of response is typical of humidifier fever and byssinosis.

Skin prick tests can be elicited in sensitive individuals by a number of soluble allergens including those in wheat and rye flour and rat and mouse urine, alcalase and ammonium hexachloroplatinate. An immediate wheal and flare reaction indicates the presence of a specific IgE antibody to the allergen and provides corroborative evidence for the diagnosis; a negative reaction does not exclude it.

Testing for specific antibodies in serum is not as yet of great help in making a diagnosis although IgE and IgG antibodies have been found against TDI, MDI, trimellitic and phthallic anhydrides and ammonium hexachloroplatinate.

Abnormal bronchial hyperreactivity is present in most subjects with occupational asthma and this can be elicited using methacholine or histamine challenge tests. However, these tests are nonspecific in that they cannot differentiate occupational from idiopathic asthma; moreover many subjects with TDI and colophony asthma do not exhibit an excessive degree of reactivity to these substances.

In a number of well defined circumstances it may be necessary to undertake inhalation bronchial provocation tests; these must be carried out in hospital by a physician experienced in their use. The indications for provocation tests are if the patient's symptoms are so severe that it would be hazardous to allow him or her to return to work to carry out peak flow measurements; if the putative allergen is not one already recognized as causing occupational asthma; if the patient is exposed to more than one agent at work; or if a diagnosis cannot be reached by any other means.

Management and prognosis

If exposure can be entirely discontinued the prognosis is good although in some cases the symptoms may be prolonged and disabling; in these cases there may be cross-reactivity with other allergens. Very often the only way in which exposure can be totally avoided is if the individual is relocated within the place of work or finds another job. Neither may be easy and the individual may prefer to stay in his or her existing job. If this choice is made, then the employee must be offered some form of personal protection which will reduce exposure to the bare minimum—air flow helmets have often been found effective—and prophylactic medication may be necessary.

Pathogenic mechanisms

It was formerly considered that the immediate and delayed responses in occupational asthma were due to type I and type III immunological reactions since immediate symptoms were prevented by sodium cromoglycate and the delayed responses by steroids but not vice versa. As more is learned about occupational asthma, however, it is becoming evident that in many instances there is no identifiable immunological explanation and in many types of the disease neither specific IgE antibodies nor precipitins (IgG or IgM) can be demonstrated.

The evidence which is presently available suggests that the deposition of inhaled agents in the airways leads to a pharmacological reaction resulting in the release of mediators from mast cells and basophils accompanied by an outpouring of eosinophils into the sputum.

There may be different pathological mechanism underlying the type of occupational asthma caused by low molecular weight substances and that caused by those of high molecular weight. Atopic and non-atopic subjects are equally affected by low molecular weight compounds whereas there is a preponderance of atopics amongst those who develop asthma following exposure to compounds of high molecular weight and many also have high serum IgE levels.

Byssinosis

Byssinosis is a disease peculiar to textile workers. It begins with tightness in the chest and breathlessness after a long period of exposure to cotton, flax, hemp or sisal dusts, commonly of the order of several years.

There is some evidence that byssinosis is more common in atopics than non-atopics and it is distinct from the other diseases which may follow exposure to these dusts, mill fever, weavers' cough and mattress makers' fever (q.v.). The

Table 6.2. Clinical grades of byssinosis

Grade	Symptoms
C1/2	Occasional tightness of the chest on the first day of the working week.
C1	Tightness of the chest and/or difficulty in breathing on each first day only of the working week.
C2	Tightness of the chest and/or difficulty in breathing on the first and other days of the working week.
C3	Grade C2 symptoms accompanied by evidence of permanent respiratory disability from reduced ventilatory capacity.

symptoms of byssinosis can be classified into four clinical grades (Table 6.2). Those of grades C½ to C2 behave like those of a late asthma, that is, there is a delay of some hours between the start of exposure and their onset, but the disease can be differentiated from asthma on the grounds that it recovers during the week. The symptoms of grade C3 appear to represent irreversible airways obstruction and the association with smoking is so great that it is difficult to be certain that this grade is an entity which is truly distinct from chronic bronchitis. Recovery from grades C½ to C1 will be complete if exposure is discontinued but slight impairment will probably remain in individuals in C2. Individuals in C3 may go on to develop right heart failure. The asthmatic symptoms are relieved by broncodilators and antihistamines and are probably caused by histamine liberators in the dusts; the extent to which there is also an immunological aetiology is uncertain.

The symptoms first appear on a Monday, usually several hours after the start of exposure, and the worker may be well for the rest of the week. As the disease progresses the symptoms extend further into the week until a state of permanent breathlessness with cough and sputum becomes established. There is no fibrotic change in the lungs and chest X-rays show no distinguishing features although individuals in C3 may have emphysematous changes.

Changes in lung function

The magnitude of the effect on the dust exposure can be determined by measuring the FEV_1 at the start and the end of the shift. For epidemiological purposes the differences between these values can be graded as follows:

F0: No demonstrable acute effect and no evidence of chronic ventilatory impairment;

F½: Slight acute effect; no chronic impairment;

F1: Moderate acute effect;

F2: Evidence of slight to moderate irreversible impairment, and

F3: Moderate to severe irreversible impairment.

Mill fever

This is a mild febrile condition which occurs only on first contact with cotton, flax, hemp or kapok dust. The fever is accompanied by a slight cough and rhinitis. The symptoms are mild and disappear as exposure continues. They are probably caused by endotoxins derived from Gram-negative bacteria in the dusts. It has been suggested that byssinosis does not occur in individuals who have no previous history of mill fever.

Weavers' cough

This was a form of late asthma accompanied by fever and malaise. The symptoms occurred in those handling cotton yarns treated with flour paste or tamarind seed extract and were thought to be caused by contaminating fungi.

Mattress maker's fever

This was probably a form of extrinsic allergic alveolitis occurring in workers handling cotton contaminated by *Aerobacter cloacae*. The symptoms began within 6 hours of exposure and consisted of fever, malaise, nausea and vomiting; asthma did not occur.

Granulomata

Foreign body granulomata may be found in association with talc pneumoconiosis (see below) whilst granulomata resembling those seen in sarcoid are a prominent feature of the acute phase of extrinsic allergic alveolitis and the chronic stage of beryllium poisoning.

Extrinsic allergic alveolitis

This condition is the classic example of a Type III mediated hypersensitivity reaction. The antigen is typically a fungal protein and some of the causes are shown in Table 6.3.

Of the conditions listed in Table 6.3 those most frequently encountered are farmer's lung and bird fancier's lung. The former results from the inhalation of

Table 6.3. Some causes of occupation extrinsic allergic alveolitis

Condition	Origin of dust	Causative agent
Farmer's lung	Mouldy hay	*Micropolyspora faenia* and *Thermoactinomyces vulgaris*
Bird fancier's lung	Bird droppings and feathers	Avian proteins
Bagassosis	Mouldy sugar cane	*T. sacchari*
Mushroom pickers' lung	Mushroom compost	*M. faeni* and *T. vulgaris*
Malt workers' lung	Mouldy malt and barley	*Aspergillus clavatus* and *A. fumigatus*
Wheat weevil lung	Grain and flour dust infected with wheat weevil	*Sitophilus granarius*
Maple bark disease	Mouldy maple bark	*Cryptostroma carticale*
Animal handlers' lung	Dust of dander, hair particles and dried urine	Serum and urinary proteins
Cheese washers' lung	Mould dust	*Penicillium casei*
Fish meal workers' lung	Fish meal dust	Fish proteins
Di-isocyanate alveolitis	TDI and HDI vapour and dust	TDI and HDI
Suberosis	Mouldy cork dust	*P. frequentans*
Pyrethrum alveolitis	Insecticide aerosol	Pyrethrum
Paprika splitters' lung	Mouldy red peppers	*Mucor stolinifer*

spores of *Microspora faeni* and *Thermoactinomyces vulgaris* growing in mouldy hay. The latter is caused by the inhalation of dried serum proteins contained in the faeces of birds. Owners of pigeons and budgerigars are those most often affected.

Bagassosis is a disease of employees inhaling the fibrous residue of sugarcane stalks after the juice has been extracted by crushing. This bagasse is used for a number of purposes, including the manufacture of fibre boards. The hazard arises when the bagasse is dry and mouldy.

Malt workers' lung occurs in distilling and brewery workers handling fungally contaminated grain whilst cheese makers' lung is observed in those engaged in washing moulds off Swiss cheese. Grain workers, animal handlers and those exposed to di-isocyantes may, in addition to asthma, also show the signs and symptoms of allergic alveolitis with basal crepitations and impairment of gas transfer. Fish meal workers' lung was observed in a factory manufacturing animal food in which fish meal was incorporated but allergic alveolitis following exposure to pyrethrum-based insecticides has only been observed following over-exposure in the home. Maple bark stripper's lung occurs in those working in paper mills and has been controlled by spraying the logs during de-barking and by issuing respirators to those at risk. Mushroom workers' lung is an uncommon variety of extrinsic allergic alveolitis and of the remaining types shown in Table 6.3, paprika splitters' lung and suberosis do not occur in this country. Indeed the former is now a historical curiosity. It used to be found amongst the Hungarian women who picked and processed a certain variety of red peppers, but the paprika splitter has been made redundant by advances in horticulture which have produced peppers which need no human processing and with their disappearance has gone the disease. Suberosis is a problem amongst the cork workers in Portugal and arises from the inhalation of mouldy cork dust. Clean cork dust does not cause pulmonary disease.

The symptoms of the disorder are the same irrespective of the external agent although they may vary in severity. After an interval of 4–6 hours, an influenza-like illness develops during which the patient feels unwell, has pains in the limbs and is febrile. The patient also has a dry cough and dyspnoea but no wheeze. The only abnormal sign in the chest is the presence of scattered crepitations heard throughout the lung field. After 2–3 days the symptoms abate.

Repeated acute attacks of extrinsic allergic alveolitis may lead to the development of chronic changes in the lungs. These give rise to progressive respiratory failure and sometimes to airways obstruction. Evidence of cor pulmonale may be found. A few patients have finger clubbing with persistent crepitations.

In acute attacks the chest X-rays show changes which vary from a diffuse haze to widespread nodular shadowing. Chronic changes include shadowing, often most predominant in the upper zones, and honeycombing.

Pathologically the typical feature of the acute phase is the presence of granulomata in the walls of the alveoli and respiratory bronchioles. The granulomata contain multinuclear giant cells and lymphocytes, and plasma cells are common. In chronic cases the normal lung architecture is destroyed producing fibrosis and honeycombing.

In farmers' lung the presence of circulating antibodies is found in asymptomatic farmers as well as in those with symptoms and thus has no diagnostic value. The demonstration of antibodies to pigeon proteins is also of no great diagnostic value since about 40% of symptomless pigeon owners have antibodies. By contrast, the presence of antibodies to budgerigar serum almost always reflects clinical disease. Considerable cross-reactivity occurs from one avian species to another so that an individual sensitive to one bird may develop symptoms when exposed to another species with which he does not normally come into contact.

Patients with bird fanciers' lung have an increased frequency of HLA-B8 antigens, which is interesting in the context of the changes found in the gut since this is also the case with patients who have coeliac disease, and it is tempting to postulate a common aetiological link. However, HLA-B8 is also more common in patients with farmers' lung, in whom gut symptoms have not been noted, so the significance of this observation is not yet clear.

Organic dust toxic syndrome

Exposure to organic dusts may produce an acute febrile illness with respiratory symptoms which closely resembles allergic alveolitis but from which rapid recovery without treatment is the norm and which does not lead to permanent impairment of lung function. This condition has variously been referred to as atypical farmers' lung, precipitin negative farmers' lung and pulmonary mycotoxicosis. Following a symposium held in 1985 it has been decided to call it the organic dust toxic syndrome, a name which could only have been decided upon by committee; the construction is ugly in the extreme and there is no evidence that the condition is toxic in nature.

ODTS is common in farmers who handle mouldy hay; much more common than farmers' lung itself. It also occurs in those who work unloading grain silos or in sewage treatment works. Pyrexia is the most common manifestation of the condition and many individuals experience some degree of shivering with the raised temperature. Difficulties in breathing, with or without a wheeze or a cough, muscular aches and pains, headaches and nausea may also be reported. In the majority of cases the symptoms are sufficiently severe that the patient has to take to his bed; they generally last 2 or 3 days before remitting completely.

Laboratory investigations are helpful only so far as they may exclude other causes of the symptoms. The chest X-ray is normal and the level of circulating antibodies and the results of prick tests do not differ from those in the general population. No treatment is required but efforts should be made to minimize exposure by wearing respiratory protection when undertaking tasks known to precipitate attacks of the disease.

Thesaurosis

Granulomata may develop in the lung following the inhalation of natural or synthetic resins. Thesaurosis is the name given to a sarcoid-like illness which has been reported in a small number of hairdressers and alleged to be due to the inhalation of hair lacquer spray. The patients had complaints of breathlessness and showed radiological changes characteristic of early sarcoid with hilar lymphadenopathy and widespread miliary infiltrates. When exposure to the hair spray was discontinued, the patients made a spontaneous recovery.

Vineyard sprayers' lung

This is a disease found amongst those who are engaged in spraying the French vineyards with Bordeaux solution which contains dilute copper sulphate. After a number of years of exposure, the affected workers develop dyspnoea and their chest X-rays show the presence of nodular and linear shadows. The nodules are granulomata which contain copper.

Humidifier fever

This is a condition which has some of the features of alveolitis, whilst being accompanied by constitutional symptoms like those of metal-fume fever. The characteristic feature of all the case reports is that the patients have been inhaling air contaminated by micro-organisms which have been dispersed from humidifiers of various sorts.

The major complaints are those of malaise, fever, cough, tightness in the chest and myalgia which develop within a few hours of starting work and which usually improve within 24 hours. These symptoms are worse on Monday mornings and may be accompanied by breathlessness and a cough. There are no radiological abnormalities, but physiological studies show impaired gas transfer and reduction in ventilatory capacity.

The micro-organisms responsible for the symptoms grows in the water which is recirculated through the humidifying system and from it, bacteria, protozoa and fungi of many kinds have been cultured. Most of those affected have serum precipitins to the crude water extract and the symptoms can generally be reproduced when the victims cautiously inhale extracts of the contaminated water. The immunological basis of the disease has not yet been worked out and it has been shown that workers without symptoms may also have precipitins in their serum.

The disease can be abolished by using steam humidifiers instead of those which depend upon re-circulating water and steam humidifiers are recommended for all new installations.

A similar disease has been described in workers in sewage disposal plants in which sludge is thermally reduced to powder. It is thought that the symptoms are a response to the protein from the high concentration of Gram-negative bacteria in the environment.

Legionnaires' disease

This is an atypical pneumonia caused by *Legionella pneumophila* of which there are over 20 species with 10 serogroups. The disease is not strictly occupational but since the causative organism is ubiquitous in water it has occurred in those working in large buildings with infected water systems including hotels and hospitals. The disease has no distinguishing clinical or radiological features and diagnosis is based on finding specific antibodies using an indirect fluorescent antibody test. It can be treated effectively with erythromycin or rifampicin and prevented by chlorinating the water to a concentration of 2–4 ppm or by heating it to between 55 and 60°C.

Beryllium disease

Chronic beryllium disease is the other granulomatous disease of major occupational significance and is discussed in Chapter 2.

Chemical pneumonitis

Chemical pneumonitis with pulmonary oedema follows the inhalation of many toxic gases and fumes because of damage to the respiratory epithelium and the alveolar capillaries. The more important are the halogens, nitrous fumes, sulphur dioxide, phosgene and the fumes of cadmium. Further details are to be found in Chapters 2 and 5.

Pneumoconiosis

The term pneumoconiosis is used as a generic name to cover the group of lung disorders which result from the inhalation of dust. Many of these dusts give rise to a fibrotic reaction in the lung with the production of overt clinical symptoms, but there is also a group of dusts of high radiodensity which cause opacities on chest X-rays but no symptoms. These radiographic changes are sometimes referred to as those of benign pneumoconiosis. The opacities are due to the fact that the inhaled dusts contain minerals whose atomic number is high enough to cause significant X-ray absorption. The density of the opacities produced by these dusts is directly proportional to their atomic number.

The International Labour Office (ILO) has issued a standard method for the classification of the radiographic changes seen in pneumoconiosis and an outline of the short classification is shown in Table 6.4. The object of the classification is to enable the radiographic changes seen in pneumoconiosis to be coded in a simple reproducible form. It does not define pathological entities nor enable any assessment to be made of working capacity.

The classification has found worldwide acceptance and it is used in this country by the Pneumoconiosis Medical Panels.

Table 6.4. Outline of the short ILO classification of the radiographic changes seen in pneumoconiosis

Feature	Classification
No pneumoconiosis	0
Pneumoconiosis	
Small opacities	
Rounded	
Profusion	1, 2, 3
Type	p, q(m), r(n)
Extent	—
Irregular	
Profusion	1, 2, 3
Type	s, t, u
Extent	—
Large opacities	
Size	A, B, C
Type	—

Explanation of symbols in Table 6.4

Small opacities	Rounded	Irregular
Type	p = up to 1.5 mm diameter	s = fine, irregular or linear opacities
	*q(m) = >1.5 mm but <3 mm diameter	t = medium opacities
	*r(n) = >3mm but <10 mm diameter	u = coarse opacities
Profusion	0 = opacities absent or less profuse than in Category 1.	0 = opacities absent or less profuse than in Category 1.
	1 = opacities present, few in number.	1 = opacities present, few in number.
	2 = numerous opacities, lung markings visible.	2 = numerous opacities, lung markings partly obscured.
	3 = very numerous opacities, lung markings obscured.	3 = very numerous opacities, lung markings totally obscured.

Large opacities
A = a single opacity with greatest diameter >1 cm but <5 cm or several opacities each >1 cm, the sum of whose greatest diameters <5cm.
B = one or more opacities larger or more numerous than in category A but whose combined area < the area of the right upper zone.
C = as B, but the combined area > area of right upper zone.

*q and r are now used instead of m and n of the previous classification.

Benign pneumoconioses

These are only recognized during life by the presence of small, rounded, dense opacities (ILO categories p or q) on a chest film which are caused by perivascular collections of dust.

Siderosis (iron oxide lung) is the most common of the benign pneumoconioses and results from the inhalation of iron dust (atomic no. 26) as iron oxide fume in iron and steel foundries, in rolling mills, during the mining and crushing of iron ores and during grinding and welding operations. The radiological changes disappear when exposure ceases. The inhalation of iron oxide and silver produces the condition known as argyrosiderosis.

Stannosis, caused by deposits of tin (atomic no. 50) in the lungs, is much rarer than siderosis. The opacities in stannosis are much denser than those seen in siderosis and the hilar lymph nodes often stand out, due to the deposition of tin within them. Exposure to tin dust may occur during the handling of the ore, when it is crushed and during the operations of changing and raking out the refinery furnaces. Tin fume will be encountered during any process which involves the molten metal.

Other causes of benign pneumoconiosis include calcium (atomic no. 20) and, rarely, barium (baritosis, atomic no. 56), antimony (atomic no. 51), chromite (atomic no. 22), zirconium (atomic no. 40), and cerium (atomic no. 58). The shadows seen in baritosis are denser even than those in stannosis, and hilar lymph nodes may be prominent. The deposits in the lungs disappear when exposure is discontinued.

Fibrotic pneumoconiosis

Silicosis

Silicosis is the most important and best known of this group of diseases. In considering the disease care must be taken to differentiate between free silica (SiO_2) and silicates which are the salts formed by the combination of silica and basic materials such as calcium oxide and magnesium oxide. Nonfibrous silicates do not harm the lungs unless they contain free silica.

In nature, free silica occurs in flint and quartz and is extremely dangerous. The dust from newly fractured flint is more dangerous than old dust. Natural noncrystalline silica (diatomaceous earth) is relatively nonfibrogenic although after heating it is converted into highly active forms. The most dangerous forms of silica are those produced by heating. At temperatures of 800–1000°C, tridymite is formed and at 1100–1400°C, cristobalite is produced.

Because of the multitude of uses to which silicaceous rocks have been put, silicosis has acquired a great many colloquial names. For example, the disease has been known at one time or another as dust consumption, grinders' rot, masons' disease, miners' phthisis, potters' rot and stonemasons' disease. Improved methods of dust control and substitution with other materials have resulted in a great decline in the incidence of silicosis although sporadic outbreaks still occur. Substitution has occurred in three principal areas. Artificial abrasives have replaced silica in grinding wheels, calcined alumina replaced ground flint in which pottery was embedded for firing in about 1937 in the pottery industry, and sand has been prohibited for use in blasting operations, being replaced by corundum or silicon carbide.

Signs and symptoms

The principal complaints are of breathlessness and cough but it is important to remember that there may be no symptoms even in those whose chest

X-rays show alarming changes. The cough varies in severity and is unproductive unless a secondary infection supervenes. It tends to occur mainly in the mornings but as the disease progresses there may be distressing paroxysms of coughing which are thought to be caused by the stimulation of nerve endings in the trachea and bronchi by silicotic nodules. Breathlessness is first noted during effort and even in severe cases is not present at rest unless some other lung disease is present.

There are remarkably few clinical signs in uncomplicated cases and finger clubbing is not produced nor is there any evidence of central cyanosis.

The complications of silicosis include pulmonary tuberculosis which tends to occur late in life and after moderate or heavy exposure, and right heart failure. Silicosis is the only pneumoconiosis which predisposes to tuberculosis, the onset of which is usually heralded by loss of weight and haemoptysis. Right heart failure is uncommon in silicosis but in those few cases in which it does occur, death is likely from congestive cardiac failure.

Lung function tests
Alterations in pulmonary function are often less severe than the appearances of the chest X-ray might suggest. There is nothing characteristic about the changes but decreases in total lung capacity, in vital capacity, in residual volume and in compliance may be found; there is no evidene of obstructive airways diseases but occasionally there is a slight reduction in gas transfer.

Pathology
The principal lesion is a nodule composed of connective tissue arranged in a whorled pattern (Fig. 6.1). Between the collagen fibres there are collections of dust particles which are usually doubly refracting so that they may readily be seen through a polarizing microscope. The nodules tend to predominate in the upper zones and may coalesce to form confluent masses. The pleura are often adherent and thickened and the lungs may have a gritty feel. Some degree of bronchiectasis is common but emphysema is not a feature of the disease.

Radiography
Discrete rounded nodules of intermediate density are seen throughout the lung fields (Fig. 6.2). These vary in size from 1 to 3 mm in diameter (p and q in ILO classification). As the disease progresses the opacities increase in size and number (ILO category r) and conglomerations appear which eventually develop into large irregular opacities occupying much of the lung field. Calcification in the periphery of the hilar lymph nodes, so-called eggshell calcification, is a feature in some cases (Fig. 6.3). Marked asymetry in the radiological findings is very rare.

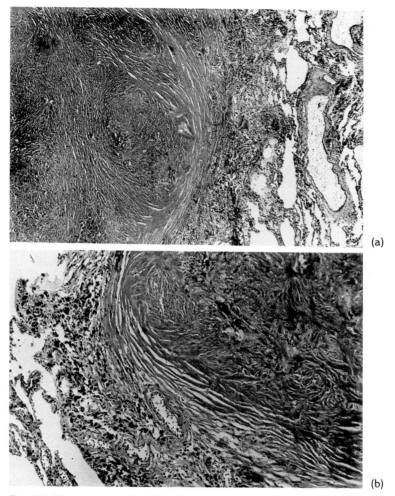

(a)

(b)

Fig. 6.1 Photomicrographs of a silicotic nodule. Sections stained with haematoxylin and eosin, (a) × 39, (b) × 98

Prognosis

Uncomplicated silicosis does not usually cause premature death although in a few individuals the disease progresses and severe respiratory impairment and death follow even if exposure is discontinued. The treatment of silicotuberculosis is generally effective provided that an adequate drug regime is given for a sufficient period. Some cases respond poorly, however, and in them the outlook is poor. The outlook is also poor in those with pulmonary heart disease.

Pathogenesis

There have been a number of theories put forward to explain the fibrogenic effect of free silica. It was at one time thought that minute electrical currents produced by the mechanical deformation of the quartz crystal might damage

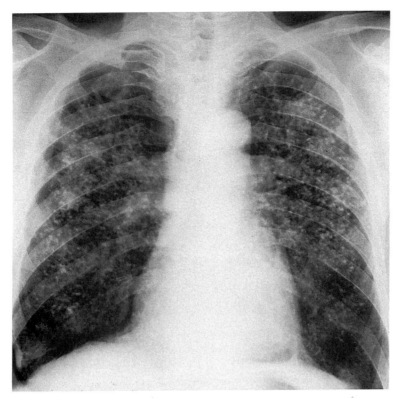

Fig. 6.2 Chest radiograph showing changes of silicosis (category 3.r.) in a flint miller

the fibroblast and initiate fibrosis (the piezoelectric theory) and it has also been considered that crystalline silica might pass into solution in the lung to form silicic acid which would promote fibrosis (the solubility theory). Neither of these theories has many adherents nowadays and most authorities would consider that the initiation of fibrosis results from damage to the alveolar macrophage. Free silica is engulfed by alveolar macrophages and damages the lysosome membrane. The release of proteolytic enzymes into the cytoplasm causes the death of the macrophage and the further release of the enzymes into the lung where a fibrotic reaction is initiated. It is now becoming accepted that the perpetuation of the fibrosis has an immunological basis. It has been suggested that macrophages exposed to quartz release a factor which stimulates the synthesis of collagen against which an antibody is produced and that this anticollagen antibody actually stimulates fibroblasts to produce more collagen.

Acute silicosis

Acute silicosis is a pulmonary fibrosis, typically with considerable pleural thickening, which develops rapidly as the result of a short exposure to dust containing a high concentration of quartz. The alveolar spaces are filled with an

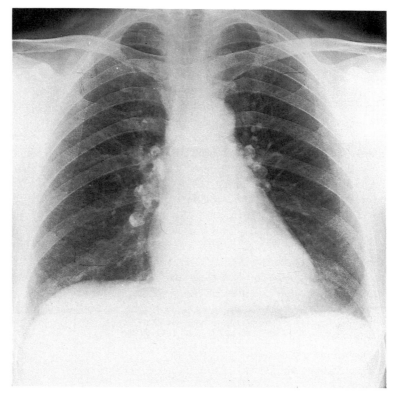

Fig. 6.3 Chest radiograph showing egg-shell calcification in both hilar lymph nodes

albuminous fluid which is PAS positive, and the appearances are like those in alveolar proteinosis. Silicotic nodules are rarely seen and the condition may thus be differentiated from nodular silicosis of rapid onset in which immature nodules are characteristic.

Symptoms develop quickly, often within a few weeks of exposure to the silicaceous dust. The principal symptom is rapidly progressive dyspnoea with malaise, fatigue, loss of weight, productive cough and pleuritic chest pain. Crepitations may be heard throughout the chest and there is often a pleural rub. Depending on the degree of pleural thickening, breath sounds are diminished or of the bronchial type. Finger clubbing may be present.

The disease is usually fatal within a year of the first appearance of symptoms.

Mixed dust fibrosis

This condition results from the inhalation of free silica with substantial amounts of other dusts, most often iron oxides, which reduce its fibrotic activity. The condition occurs in foundry workers, boiler scalers, haematite miners, potters, and in some welders who have worked in foundries.

The lesions produced differ from the classical silicotic nodules in being irregular in shape although they are normally still discrete. The nodules in haematite miners are brick-red in colour, but dark grey in the other groups. In advanced cases, massive fibrosis in the upper zones leads to distortion of the main airways with displacement of the trachea. Tuberculosis is less likely to develop in mixed dust fibrosis than in 'pure' silicosis.

Fibrous silicates

A number of fibrous silicates are used in industry but asbestos is by far the most dangerous. Asbestos is the collective term used to describe some fibrous mineral silicates of which there are two main groups, serpentine and amphibole of differing chemical compositions (Table 6.5).

Asbestos is widely used in industry because of its ability to withstand heat and its excellent insulating properties. Asbestos-cement manufacture consumes the greatest quantity of the fibre and this is followed by the manufacture of floor tiles. An important use is as a component of brake-pads and clutch plates. Of the various forms of asbestos, chrysotile accounts for over 90% of world production. Crocidolite and amosite are next in importance and the remaining forms have a very limited use. In Great Britain the use of crocidolite has been greatly restricted because of its association with malignant mesothelomia but this is not so in other countries of Western Europe, nor in the USA or Japan.

Inhalation of asbestos may give rise to several separate conditions:

1 Asbestosis, by which is meant fibrosis of the lung with or without pleural fibrosis.
2 Benign pleural disease.
3 Bronchial carcinoma.
4 Malignant mesothelioma.

Bronchial carcinoma and mesothelioma are discussed in Chapter 8 and will not be considered here.

Asbestosis

Asbestosis is a form of diffuse interstitial fibrosis and it is most important to understand that it is a dose-related disease. A clear linear relationship between increasing dust exposure and the development of asbestosis has been demonstrated and only those who have been heavily exposed for a long time are in danger of contracting it. The fibrosis which is seen is typically distributed subpleurally over the lower half of the lungs. The pulmonary pleura may be thickened, invariably so when lung fibrosis is advanced, although the degree of

Table 6.5. Classification and chemical composition of asbestos

Serpentine group	
Chrysotile (white asbestos)	$(OH)_6Mg_6Si_4O_{11}.H_2O$
Amphibole group	
Actinolite	$Ca(MgFe)_3(SiO_3)_4.xH_2O$
Amosite (brown asbestos)	$(Fe.Mg)SiO_3.1.5\%H_2O$
Anthophyllite	$(Mg.Fe)_7Si_8O_{22}(OH)_2$
Crocidolite (blue asbestos)	$NaFe(SiO_3)_2FeSiO_3.xH_2O$
Tremolite	$Ca_2Mg_5Si_8O_{22}(OH)_2$

fibrosis in the pleura does not always match that in the lungs. Bronchiectasis is found in a few cases in areas of severe fibrosis but emphysema is uncommon and the hilar lymph nodes are not enlarged. The typical microscopic picture is one of fibrosing alveolitis with gradual obliteration of the air spaces by collagen. Asbestos bodies are seen in the areas of fibrosis and in the sputum (Fig. 6.4).

Asbestos bodies are long structures, up to 80 μm in length, and they consist of asbestos fibres coated with layers of iron-containing protein which imparts a golden-yellow or brown colour to them. The protein coat is usually fragmented so that the asbestos bodies tend to have a beaded appearance. They are readily detected in sections of lung tissue as they stain blue with Perl's reagent.

It is important to realize that whilst the presence of asbestos bodies in the sputum is indicative of past exposure to asbestos it does not signify proof of asbestosis.

Symptoms of asbestosis

The symptoms of asbestosis are insidious and there is a variable latent period between their appearance and first exposure. Dyspnoea is the first symptom to be noted. At first moderate, the breathlessness increases in severity and patients find difficulty in taking a deep breath because of the reduced compliance of the lungs. This is not unique to asbestosis but occurs in any form of interstitial fibrosis. The degree of breathlessness may be out of all proportion to the changes seen on the chest film and may be severe even when there are few physical signs in the chest.

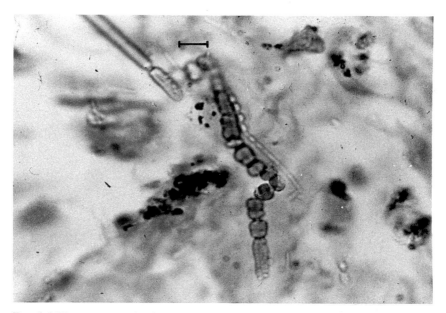

Fig. 6.4 Photomicrograph of an asbestos body in the sputum of a man with asbestosis. Note the characteristic beaded appearance. Bar = 10μ

Cough is absent during the early stages but as the disease advances, becomes much more common. There is usually little sputum. Chest pain is not a feature but most patients with severe disease complain of lassitude.

Physical signs
Signs in the chest are few considering the degree of disability. In advanced cases there is an impairment of chest expansion affecting particularly the lower part of the chest and this is a useful measure by which to screen men at work. Persistent crepitations heard during inspiration are discovered early in the disease, often before there are any changes on X-ray and this is an important sign of pathological change. Finger clubbing is frequently present.

Radiography
Abnormal radiographic signs in asbestosis are more common in the lower zones than elsewhere (Fig. 6.5). This contrasts with the situation in silicosis and coal miners' pneumoconiosis where the changes are more common in the upper zones. The radiological signs are those of diffuse interstitial fibrosis (ILO categories s, t or u) with fine punctate mottling. A cystic or honeycomb appearance may develop but the cystic spaces remain small, usually less than

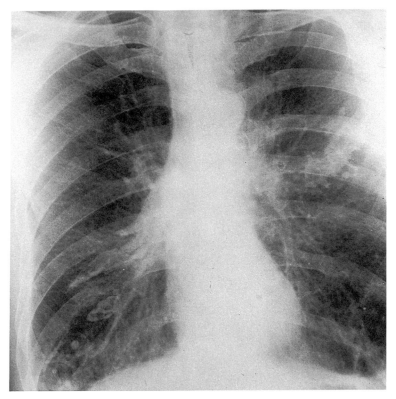

Fig. 6.5 Chest radiograph showing changes due to asbestosis with pleural plaques

5 mm. The costophrenic angles become obliterated and the cardiac outline becomes blurred and there is evidence of pleural thickening.

Pleural plaques are often overlooked unless they are calcified when they are seen as irregular shadows of patchy density. They may be seen in the absence of other evidence of asbestosis and in those with no history of an occupational exposure to asbestos (Fig. 6.6).

Pulmonary function

The earliest abnormality in lung function in cases of asbestosis is decreased compliance and this can be noted before there are any signs or symptoms of the disease. Measuring compliance is difficult under routine conditions and so in the monitoring of asbestos workers the vital capacity (VC) is used. A consistent reduction in VC in the absence of significant airways obstruction or any other chronic chest disease is a good indication that compliance is reduced and is the most sensitive routine test by which to detect the effects of asbestos exposure. Other functional abnormalities which are noted include reduction in total lung capacity and reduction in diffusing capacity for carbon monoxide.

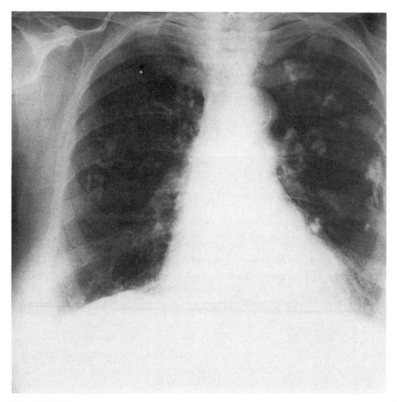

Fig. 6.6 Chest radiograph showing pleural plaques due to asbestos exposure. The patient, a female journalist, had never worked in industry but was brought up near an asbestos mine in Canada

Pathogenesis
The pathogenesis of asbestosis is not fully understood although it is known that asbestos fibres are cytotoxic; this can be demonstrated *in vivo* by their capacity to haemolyze red cells. The fibrogenic property of asbestos fibres is determined by their length, those which are longer than 10–20 μm are fibrogenic whereas shorter fibres are not. Long fibres are incompletely ingested by macrophages and they damage the cell membrane allowing the release of enzymes and other constituents which may initiate the fibrotic process. Long fibres are also poorly cleared from the lung and, since they are not broken down by the macrophages, their potential to harm the cells is increased. As with silicosis, it is probable that immunological responses also have a part to play in the development of the fibrosis. After the ingestion of asbestos fibres the surface of the macrophage shows an increase in the number of receptors for both the C3 component of complement and for IgG antibodies. Asbestos fibres also activate both the classical and the alternative complement pathways. These findings suggest that the activation of complement and the alteration in the antigenic properties of the macrophage may have an important role to play in the development of asbestosis.

The earlier observation that there was an association between HLA antigens and asbestosis has not been confirmed nor have reports that the number of T suppressor cells is diminished. We have not heard the last of the immunology of asbestosis, however.

Treatment
Once established, asbestosis generally progresses to produce some degree of respiratory disability. The time scale is variable, however, and susceptible individuals may become respiratory cripples within 2 or 3 years of developing symptoms whereas others live into their sixties or seventies, finally dying from a cause unconnected with asbestos. Removing workers from contact with asbestos does not materially alter the rate of progress of the disease.

There is no treatment which can be offered except supportive measures as required.

Neighbourhood cases
Cases of asbestosis have been reported in persons living close to asbestos mines or asbestos-using factories even though they themselves have no occupational exposure. There is no doubt that residents living near factories were subjected to a considerable degree of contamination in the past, but modern measures of control have eliminated this hazard in the UK. Another source of hazard to the public was from dust carried out by workers on their clothes, but regulations now forbid the wearing of work clothes outside the factory. Asbestos building materials if not properly sealed may become friable and release dust into the atmosphere and thus constitute a risk. Similarly, the demolition of buildings with asbestos in their fabric may release dust to the atmosphere if the proper precautions are not taken.

Prevention

The Asbestos Regulations which came into force in 1970 controlled the use of asbestos and they have been supplemented by the Asbestos (Licensing) Regulations of 1983. These regulations prohibit anyone carrying out work with asbestos insulation or asbestos coatings unless they hold a licence issued by the Health and Safety Executive. Furthermore all those who are to be engaged on work with asbestos insulations or coatings must be medically examined before they begin the work and at intervals of not more than 2 years thereafter unless their work is of short duration (less than 2 hours in total) or they are engaged solely in the collection of samples or air monitoring.

It is likely that the use of asbestos spraying will be banned in the near future and asbestos is also likely to be banned for most thermal and acoustic insulation purposes. Crocidolite is no longer used and the use of amosite is discouraged. As from 1 August 1984, there are new control limits for asbestos in the air. The concentration of dusts containing crocidolite or amosite must not exceed 0.2 fibres/ml and that of other types of asbestos must not exceed 0.5 fibres/ml when calculated in relation to a 4-hour reference period.

Benign pleural disease

A number of pleural syndromes may be seen in those who have been exposed to asbestos including pleural plaques, pleural thickening and pleural effusion. Pleural plaques are elevated areas which consist of collagen fibres; they tend to become calcified in those parts of the lesion where the collagen has degenerated. They are found on the parietal pleural, and they tend to be more frequent on the posterolateral and basal parts, and on the central tendon of the diaphragm. Their presence indicates exposure to asbestos or to some other mineral fibres; they are not diagnostic of asbestosis. Pleural plaques are common in some parts of eastern Europe and Asia Minor where mineral fibres such as zeolite, but not asbestos, may be present in the environment.

Diffuse thickening of the pleura may be noted with or without pleural plaques. The costophrenic angles may be obliterated and thickening of the parietal pleura in the interlobar fissures may be the only radiological evidence of exposure to asbestos. Thickening of the visceral pleura may on rare occasions produce folding of the lung producing an appearance which mimics that of a tumour.

Pleural effusions are the most troublesome of the benign pleural conditions which may afflict asbestos workers. They may be asymptomatic but they are often accompanied by pleuritic pain and occasionally by dyspnoea. There may also be a slight fever. The effusion is usually small in volume but it is often blood stained, a feature which causes much alarm and fears that a mesothelioma may be present. In some cases diffuse pleural thickening may develop after the fluid has been absorbed and this may cause a restrictive lung defect of such severity that pleurectomy is required.

Other fibrous silicates

Talc

Talc is a hydrated magnesium silicate with the formula $Mg_3Si_4O_{10}(OH)_2$. It also contains calcium, aluminium and iron in variable amounts and may contain other minerals, including asbestos and quartz. Three clinical syndromes which have been reported to follow the inhalation of talc are:

1   An irregular nodular fibrosis.
2   Interstitial fibrosis with talc bodies similar to asbestos bodies.
3   Foreign body granulomata.

The inhalation of pure talc gives rise to the formation of granulomata, but the first lesions are probably due to the inhalation of contaminating minerals such as quartz or asbestos whose action is modified by the talc. Any or all of the three lesions may be present in an exposed population. The radiological changes, which are confined mainly to the lower and midzones, are similar to those found in asbestosis. Thus fibrotic change is the major feature, and calcified pleural plaques may also be present, usually bilateral in distribution. In addition, there may be signs of pleural adhesions and enlargement of the hilar shadow. There are no nodules, such as might be found in silicosis.

Symptoms develop gradually after prolonged exposure. Fifteen or twenty years is the usual time scale. Dyspnoea and cough are most frequently noted. The disease usually progresses slowly and does not significantly alter life expectancy except in those cases who develop massive fibrosis or diffuse interstitial fibrosis. There is no predisposition to tuberculosis or mesothelioma. There has been some suggestion that the incidence of bronchial carcinoma may be higher than expected in talc workers but this is not a generally accepted view.

Sillimanite minerals

The sillimanite minerals, andalusite, kyanite and sillimanite are all forms of aluminium silicate ($AL_2O_3SiO_2$). They have the properties of being extremely resistant to acids and alkalis and of being able to withstand very high temperatures. They are used mainly to make laboratory porcelain, spark plug casings and refractory bricks.

At most, these minerals cause only mild fibrosis and few reported cases of pneumoconiosis have been convincingly shown to be due to their sole action.

Man-made mineral fibres

Man-made mineral fibres are used increasingly to replace asbestos for thermal and acoustic insulation. There are three main groups, slag wools, rock wools and glass wools and filaments; all are amorphous silicates. The mineral wools are made from melts of natural limestone rock or smelter slags sometimes with the addition of wollastonite or kaolinite. Glass fibres are made either from borosilicate or calcioalumina silicate glass. The fibres are commonly coated with a binder which is a biologically inert resin but may be mineral oil. Unlike asbestos fibres which tend to split longitudinally into particles with a smaller diameter than the parent fibre, man-made fibres split transversely to produce short fragments with the same diameter.

There are no convincing reports of respiratory effects following exposure to man-made mineral fibres nor have any radiographic changes been consistently noted. There is some concern that these fibres may cause bronchial carcinoma; they are not thought to cause mesothelioma. The results of a recent large scale epidemiological study in Europe do suggest that there was a slightly increased risk in the past but with present very low levels of exposure, the risk has probably disappeared.

Non-fibrous silicates

This group includes mica, kaolin and other clays, fullers' earth and bentonite.

Mica

The family of mica minerals comprises muscovite (potassium aluminium silicate), biotite (a complex silicate containing magnesium aluminium, potassium and iron) and vermiculite (magnesium-aluminium silicates derived from biotite).

There is little in the way of firm evidence to show that any of these minerals causes pulmonary fibrosis although a few workers exposed to mica dust have been found to have minor changes on X-ray consistent with pneumoconiosis.

Kaolin (china clay)

China clays are predominantly composed of hydrous aluminium silicate ($2H_2O.Al_2O_3.2SiO_2$), also known as kaolinite. Other than as the main ingredient of china clay, it is used as a filler in rubber, paints, plastics and papers, and high purity kaolin is used medicinally.

Pneumoconiosis affects only a small minority of those exposed and then only after a prolonged period, and it is by no means certain whether the symptoms are due entirely to kaolin or to contaminants such as quartz. The lesions reported include nodular fibrosis, sometimes massive fibrosis and mild diffuse interstitial fibrosis, whilst reported symptoms include breathlessness with cough and sputum.

Non-kaolin clays

These clays contain a higher proportion of quartz than china clays, hence pneumoconiosis is rather more frequent and of the silicotic, nodular type.

Fullers' earth and bentonite

Fullers' earth is a clay so named because of its one-time use to remove grease from wool and cloth, a process known as fulling. It is a fine-grained, absorbent clay composed mainly of calcium montmorillonite. Quartz is found in some deposits and this may produce silicotic lesions in those working or mining it. Other radiographic changes which have been found include small, discrete opacities of low density, especially in the upper zones, which occasionally coalesce. This form of pneumoconiosis is essentially benign and does not

shorten life expectancy. Bentonite clays contain 85% or more of montmorillonite and are harmless unless they contain quartz.

Coal miners' pneumoconiosis

This disease occurs in miners exposed to coal dust whether at the coal face or
elsewhere. The pathological lesions which develop are caused by the inhalation
of carbon, and similar lesions may develop in workers exposed to other forms
of carbon. The development of the disease is dependent upon the amount of
dust inhaled and the duration of exposure. It is distinct from silicosis although
mixed dust fibrosis is found in coal miners who have also been exposed to silica.

Simple pneumoconiosis

The early lesions are small discrete macules of dust found mainly in the upper
zones. They are found to be concentrated around the respiratory bronchioles
and are enmeshed in reticulin fibres. Collagen is found in early lesions but later
fibrotic changes ensue to produce black fibrous nodules. Pseudo-asbestos bodies
are sometimes found in the dust-containing lesions. They consist of spicules of
coal or carbon and a covering of iron-containing protein which gives a positive
Prussian blue reaction.

Progressive massive fibrosis (PMF)

Large black fibrotic masses consisting of coal dust and bundles of collagen occur
in some cases. These lesions tend to concentrate in the upper and midzones but
there are many exceptions to the rule. When near the periphery, the overlying
pleura is involved and may become fibrotic and adherent to the parietal layer.
A lesion is defined as PMF when its diameter is greater then 3 cm. Necrosis and
cavitation of the lesions are well known complications.

Caplan's syndrome

Caplan's syndrome is a modified form of pneumoconiosis found in association
with rheumatoid arthritis. The majority of cases occur in coal miners, but the
disease may be found in workers in a wide variety of dusty trades. The nodules
in the lung are scattered irregularly through the lung and are up to 2 cm in
diameter. They have a characteristic concentric appearance with alternating
laminae of coal-dust and necrotic collagen. Cavitation is common and sometimes the nodules aggregate to form structures which closely resemble a
collection of silicotic nodules. Coal-dust macules are typically absent but where
they are in evidence, they are the same as in nonrheumatoid miners.

Symptoms

Simple pneumoconiosis is asymptomatic. In PMF symptoms may be trivial or
such as to cause severe disability. There is little correlation between radiological
findings and the severity of symptoms. In most miners cough and sputum are
more related to the development of bronchitis which seems to be due to coal
dust exposure, aided in many instances by smoking. In some cases of PMF a
severe unproductive cough brought on by effort is a distressing feature of the

disease. If a massive fibrotic lesion ruptures into a bronchus large amounts of jet-black sputum are brought up and this may continue for several days.

Signs
Coal pneumoconiosis has no characteristic signs although wheezes and rhonchi may be heard throughout the lung field. In patients with PMF the trachea may be displaced by lesions in the upper zones. Large PMF may be accompanied by signs of right heart failure. Finger clubbing is extremely rare.

In patients with Caplan's syndrome, signs of pleural effusion may indicate the onset, or the exacerbation, of the symptoms of rheumatoid arthritis.

Radiology
The earlier radiological signs to appear are a few small, ill-defined opacities in the mid and upper zones. Opacities of different size may be present in one film but most come into the q category. As simple pneumoconiosis progresses the opacities come to be found more or less equally distributed throughout the lung fields (Fig. 6.7).

PMF opacities (Fig. 6.8) are also usually seen in the upper zones and may be unilateral or bilateral, symmetrical or asymmetrical. These appearances are usually set on a ground of simple pneumoconiosis but this is not invariable. The

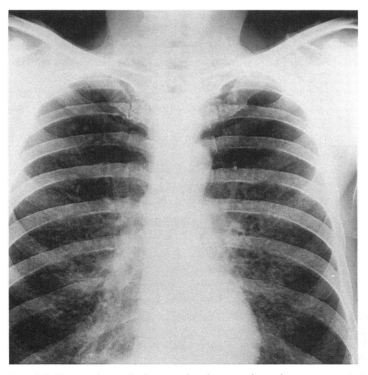

Fig. 6.7 Chest radiograph showing the changes of simple pneumoconiosis in a coal miner who had worked 26 years underground. Changes are in categories 2.q. and 2.s.

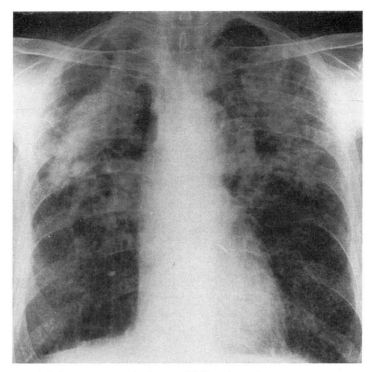

Fig. 6.8 Chest radiograph showing PMF and simple pneumoconiosis in a miner who had worked underground for 30 years. Changes are in category 3.q./C.

shape of the opacities in PMF varies considerably and cavitation is indicated by an area of translucency within an opacity.

In a few cases 'eggshell' calcification of the hilar lymph nodes is seen, similar to that which is seen in silicosis. It happens more frequently in conjunction with PMF than with simple pneumoconiosis.

The dense, round opacities in Caplan's syndrome are irregularly scattered throughout the lung fields and are usually few in number. There are normally no signs of simple pneumoconiosis.

Exposure to coal dust and emphysema

For some years there has been a debate as to whether exposure to coal dust predisposes to the development of emphysema. The most recent information shows that there is a clear relationship between measured exposure to respirable coal dust and both FEV_1 and decline in FEV_1 over time. Postmortem studies have also shown that miners have a higher prevalence of emphysema than controls and that the more coal dust present in the lung, the greater the likelihood that the lung will show centriacinar emphysema.

Respiratory function in occupational lung diseases

Respiratory function tests are being used increasingly to monitor workers exposed to dust and other materials known to affect the lungs. The tests most often used for routine screening purposes are the measurement of forced expiratory volume (FEV), usually the volume expelled in 1 second (FEV_1), the forced vital capacity (FVC) and the vital capacity (VC). These are all measurements which can be made using a simple, portable respirometer and are thus most suitable for use in industry.

Three broad categories of impairment in lung function can be recognized.

Airways obstruction

Asthma, bronchitis and emphysema produce some narrowing of the airways with a resultant obstruction to air flow, predominantly during expiration. In asthma this is usually reversible but only rarely so in bronchitis and emphysema. As a result FEV_1 values are low but VC is larger than FVC because forced expiration increases the degree of narrowing in the airways.

Reduced compliance

A reduction in compliance is found in those diseases which produce diffuse interstitial fibrosis. The lungs are unable to expand fully and there is a resultant decrease in VC and FVC. Asbestosis is the most important occupational disease in this class and the VC is an excellent screening test for lung damage in asbestos workers.

Impairment of gas exchange

Gas exchange is impaired whenever ventilation is reduced relative to blood flow, either locally or generally, or vice versa. It is also impaired by diseases which affect the architecture of the alveoli such as diffuse interstitial fibrosis and granulomatous lung disorders.

Table 6.6. Patterns of change in lung function tests in occupational lung diseases

	VC	FVC	FEV_1	Gas exchange
Silicosis	↓↓ (in advanced cases)			↓
Acute silicosis	↓↓	↓↓		↓↓↓
Coal pneumoconiosis				
Simple	↓	↓		↓
PMF	↓↓			↓↓
Asbestosis	↓↓	↓↓	↓↓	↓↓
		(FEV$_1$: FVC greater than normal)		
Chronic beryllium disease	↓	↓	↓	↓↓
Extrinsic allergic alveolitis	↓↓			↓↓
Byssinosis			↓↓ (progressive fall during working day)	
Asthma	↓	↓↓	↓↓	

↓ Slightly reduced; ↓↓ reduced; ↓↓↓ greatly reduced.

Tests of gas exchange need to be conducted in a laboratory and on this account are not suitable to be used for screening purposes.

A summary of the changes in respiratory function seen in the occupational lung diseases is shown in Table 6.6.

Chapter 7
Diseases of the Skin

Occupational dermatitis

The prevalence of occupational dermatitis is high in all industrialized countries. In Great Britain more days are lost as a result of skin disease than from all the other prescribed diseases put together. In men, approximately 650 000 working days a year are lost, and for women, approximately 200 000 days a year are lost. These figures are some indication of the cost to the community, but they give no indication of the amount of misery and discomfort experienced by the patients, much of which could be avoided by proper precautionary measures.

The agents which cause skin lesions are many and varied but can be divided into five classes as follows:
1 Mechanical factors, such as friction, pressure and trauma,
2 Physical factors including heat, cold, electricity, sunlight and radiation,
3 Chemical agents, both organic and inorganic,
4 Plants and their products, resins and lacquers, and
5 Other biological agents such as infective organisms, insects and mites.

The relative importance of each of these naturally depends on the occupation being considered, but in general, chemical agents are by far the greatest cause of occupational skin disorders.

Mechanical factors

Mechanical factors give rise to cuts and abrasions which may become secondarily infected. Repeated trauma produces callosities, the sites of which are determined by the particular occupation and will often identify a man's job to the knowledgeable observer.

Callosities may develop at specific points of pressure between the skin and any tool or instrument which is being used constantly. Workers in whom one might expect to find them thus include carpenters, painters, cobblers, dressmakers, floor sweepers and so on. In other workers, the callosities develop on the whole palmar surface of the hand in response to general trauma. The callosities are of no pathological significance but rather, they have a function to protect underlying tissues.

Physical factors

Heat may affect the skin by causing excessive perspiration which softens the protective horny layers. When combined with frictional stress, it can produce intertrigo, the so-called heat rashes of furnace men, stokers and others who work under hot conditions.

Cold injuries to the skin include chilblains, and if associated with damp or wet conditions may produce trench foot in extreme cases. In our climate, extremes of temperature are unusual so that frost bite is not a condition which is likely to be encountered.

Burns resulting from accidents at work are a real hazard in industry, although they rarely result from electrical accidents. They may occur from an overenthusiastic exposure to the sun on the part of those whose work takes them outdoors. Prolonged exposure to sunlight can undoubtedly be a factor in the production of skin cancer. Exposure to ionizing radiation also has the dual effect of burning and inducing malignant change, but adequate safety measures should ensure that neither is seen nowadays.

Chemical agents

These are responsible for the great bulk of occupational skin disease and they act either as primary irritants or sensitizers (or both).

Primary irritants

Primary irritants are agents which produce lesions by direct action at the site of contact. Their speed of action depends on their concentration and the length of time for which they are in contact with the skin. Their effects are caused by chemical reactions with the skin; by degreasing or dehydrating, by denaturing proteins in the skin, or by disturbing the osmotic pressure of the cells in the skin. Alkali seems to cause most skin trouble, but the list of primary irritants is enormous and constantly on the increase as the number of chemicals in use rises steadily year by year. Some of the more important primary irritants are listed in Table 7.1 but it must be emphasized that this list is far from being complete.

Sensitizers

Many chemicals do not have a primary irritant effect. Instead, contact with them results in a type of cell-mediated hypersensitivity reaction. The resultant lesion is referred to as contact dermatitis. The sensitizing chemical passes through the epidermal barrier and reacts with a protein to produce a hapten against which antibodies are formed. Once the antibodies are produced, the skin reaction will occur whenever the hapten is formed.

The list of sensitizers is again formidable and some primary irritants such as the bichromates, the phenols, and formaldehyde are also sensitizers. Table 7.2 shows some of the more important sensitizers. These chemicals have in common a great affinity for keratin with which they form haptens.

Clinical picture

Whether the skin lesion is produced by primary irritants or by sensitizers, the changes are essentially the same, although it should be noted that sensitivity rashes may occur away from the area in contact with the sensitizer. The first change to be noted is erythema often accompanied by irritation. Following this, vesicles are formed, which burst to produce a red weeping lesion. Healing is associated with crusting and the damping down of the inflammatory reaction.

Table 7.1. Principal primary skin irritants in industry

Alkalis

Inorganic
  Alkaline sulphides
  Sodium hydrate, carbonate, silicate
    and metasilicate
  Potassium hydrate and carbonate
  Ammonium hydrate and carbonate
  Barium hydrate and carbonate
  Calcium oxide, hydrate carbonate and
    cyanamide
  Trisodium phosphate

Organic
  Ethanolamines
  Methylamine

Acids

Inorganic
  Arsenious
  Chloroplatinic
  Chlorosulphonic
  Chromic
  Hydriotic
  Hydrobromic
  Hydrochloric
  Hydrofluoric
  Hydrofluosilic
  Nitric
  Perchloric
  Silver nitrate
  Phosphoric
  Sulphuric

Organic
  Acetic
  Carbolic
  Cresylic
  Formic
  Lactic
  Maleic
  Metanilic
  Oxalic
  Salicylic

Elements and their salts

  Antimony and salts
  Arsenic and salts
  Chromium and
    alkaline chromates
  Copper sulphate
  Copper cyanide
  Mercuric salts
  Nickel salts
  Zinc chloride

Solvents

  Petroleum solvents
  Coal tar solvents
  Chlorinated hydrocarbons
  Esters
  Ketones
  Turpentine
  Terpenes
  Carbon bisulphide
  Alcohols

Acne producers

  Petroleum oils
  Cutting oils
  Pitch
  Tar
  Paraffin
  Chloronaphthalenes
  Chlorodiphenyls
  Chlorodiphenyloxides
  Solid chlorobenzols
  Solid chlorophenols

From Schwartz L., Tulipan L. & Birmingham D.J., *Occupational Diseases of the Skin*, Kingston, London, 1957.

Table 7.2. Principal skin sensitizers in industry

Dye intermediates

Aniline and compounds	Naphthalene and compounds
Chloro compounds	Benzidine and compounds
Nitro compounds	Benzanthrone and compounds
Acridine and compounds	Naphthylamines

Dyes

Paraphenylendiamine	Metanil yellow
Aniline black	Brilliant indigo, 4 G.
Paramido phenol	Erio black
Chrysoidine	Hydron blue
Bismarck brown	Indanthrene violet, R. R.
Nigrosine	Ionamine, A. S.
Amido-azo-toluene	Pyrogene violet brown
Amido-azo-benzene	Orange Y
Crystal and methyl violet	Safranine
Malachite green	Sulphanthrene pink
Auramine	Rosaniline

Photographic developers

Paraphenylendiamine	Pyrogallol
Hydroquinone	Bichromates
Para-amido-phenol	Paraformaldehyde
Metol	

Rubber accelerators and anti-oxidants

Hexamethylene tetramine	Para toluidine
Guanidines	Ortho toluidine
Mercapto benzo thiazole	Triethyl tri-methyl triamine
Tetromethyl thiuram monosulphide and disulphide	

Insecticides

Creosote	*Arsenic compounds
Nicotine	*Fluorides
Tar	*Lime
Pyrethrum	Rotenone
*Mercury compounds	Thiocyanates
*Phenol compounds	Organic phosphates
*Petroleum distillates	

Oils

Cutting oils (the inhibitor or antiseptic they contain)	Coconut oil
Coning oils (cellosolves, eugenols)	*Cashew nut oil
Sulphonated oils	Tung oil
Linseed oil	Essential oils of plants and flowers
*Mustard oil	

Natural resins

Pine rosin	Japanese lacquer
Wood rosin	Dammar
Burgundy pitch	Copal

Table 7.2. Principal skin sensitizers in industry (*Continued*)

Synthetic resins

Alkyd	Chlorobenzols
Vinyl	Chlorodiphenyls
Acrylic	Chlorophenols
Phenol formaldehyde	Cumaron
Urea formaldehyde	Epoxies
Melamine formaldehyde	Polyesters
Sulphonamide formaldehyde	Urethane
Chloro-naphthalenes	

Coal tar and its direct derivatives

Acridine	Fluorene
Anthracene	Naphthalene
Phenanthrene	*Phenol
Carbazole	*Cresol
Pyridine	

Explosives

Trinitrotoluene	Lead styphnate
Trinitromethylnitramine (Tetryl)	Ammonium nitrate
Fulminate of mercury	Sodium nitrate
Hexanitrodiphenylamine	Potassium nitrate
Dinitrophenol	Picric acid and picrates
Dinitrotoluol	Sensol

Plasticizers

Propylene stearate	Methyl cellosolve oleate
Butyl cellosolve stearate	Methyl phthalylethylglycol
Diamyl naphthalene	Phenylsalicylate
Dibutyl tin laurate	Stearic acid
Dioctylphthalate	Triblycol di (2, ethyl butyrate)

Others

Enzymes derived from *B. subtilis*

*Compounds which also act as primary irritants. From Schwartz L., Tulipan L. & Birmingham D.J., *Occupational Diseases of the Skin*. Kingston, London, 1957.

The organic arsenic and mercury compounds are powerful vesicants and other chemicals such as chrome, alkalis, washing soda, brine and lime cause ulceration. The ulcers are often sufficiently characteristic to be identified with a fair degree of precision. Mercury fulminate causes small necrotic lesions known as powder holes and a more generalized, pruritic, papular lesion called fulminate itch.

The site of the lesion will depend upon which parts of the skin have been in contact with the pathogenic chemical and this alone may give the clue to its identity. Often the easiest forms to recognize are those which occur on the fingers or hands due to the wearing of rubber gloves. It is not always so easy to identify the substances which are responsible, however, if only because many workers will not know the chemicals with which they have been in contact, or know them only by trade names. Again, the employee's description of the job may often give no clue to the chemicals, mineral oil, epoxy resins, and so on. It is always helpful to ask whether any other employees have had skin trouble, since the diagnosis of occupational skin disease is made much more certain if fellow workers have experienced similar troubles.

Once the field has been narrowed down the responsible agent (or agents) can be sought through patch testing. Patch testing is not infallible and indeed may sometimes be misleading. It may sometimes exacerbate the condition and should only be done by experts. Despite the drawbacks of the technique it should always be attempted, since if the cause for the dermatitis can be identified, then the patient can be protected from it.

Occupational acne

This common form of occupational dermatitis is caused by oils, pitch and tar, and some chlorinated hydrocarbons. The chloronaphthalenes are the most potent acne producers but the greatest number of cases are caused by exposure to mineral oil.

The chemicals which cause acne have a dual action, plugging the pores of the skin whilst at the same time promoting the production of keratin. The result is the formation of comedones and cysts, which in the case of exposure to oils is almost always preceded by folliculitis. Inflammatory reactions are the rule when considering acne due to cutting oils; they are the exception in acne due to tar or chlorinated hydrocarbons.

Plants and their products

Plants and their products cause dermatitis by virtue of the chemical compounds which they contain. The list of those plants which are harmful is of majestic length. Fortunately the family of plants which is most effective in causing skin lesions, the Anacardiaceae, does not grow in this country. Those which do sometimes give trouble are predominantly members of the Liliaceae and the Primulaceae. Those affected are farmers, gardeners, nurserymen and florists as would be expected.

Tulip finger is a condition found amongst farmers handling bulbs from which the juice is oozing. The lesion is confined around and under the nails although the nail itself is not affected. Painful lesions of the same sort may also occur amongst those picking tulips, daffodils or narcissi and it is thought that lime salts in the sap are here acting as primary irritants, though, of course, almost any plant is liable to produce an idiosyncratic skin reaction in a susceptible individual. In some cases there is an itching, desquamating rash accompanied by fissuring and this is known as lily rash. The incidence of both types of dermatitis shows a marked seasonal variation as would be anticipated, and on occasion has been severe enough to disrupt the flower industry in Cornwall and the Scilly Isles.

The Primulaceae secrete a toxin in the form of a sticky yellowy-green liquid and gardeners and florists are frequently affected by it. The rash typically consist of numerous close-packed shiny red punctiform papules which may coalesce to form small vesicles or large blisters. There is much smarting and itching as an accompaniment. The toxin may be conveyed by other agencies to the affected individual. For example, cow men have been affected by touching the udders of cows which have passed over cowslips picking up the toxin as they do so.

Of all the species, the hot house *Primula obconica* is the most irritant and affects something like half of those coming into contact with it.

Toxic woods

Dermatitis from woods is frequent amongst carpenters, wood machinists, workers in wood yards, cabinet makers, shipbuilders and furniture makers. The culpable substances can be the saw dust, the sap and the polishings, or the oil of the wood. It is usually imported woods, or woods not handled before which cause trouble. Some wood dusts can produce respiratory symptoms in susceptible individuals (see Chapter 6).

Woods usually produce a sensitivity reaction so that the worker becomes affected several days after beginning to work with a new wood. Most of those affected become desensitized, but there is a minority of men who remain highly sensitized. The reactions occur when the wood is in a certain stage of drying out and so outbreaks of dermatitis occur when consignments in the appropriate condition are used. Once the consignments are finished, the outbreak ceases.

Most cases have minimal symptoms with a papulovesicular rash on the hands and arms which clears quickly with treatment. In some cases, however, more severe symptoms may be produced. *Gonioma kamassi*, known more often as Kamassi boxwood, will cause systemic effects in susceptible individuals due to the liberation of an alkaloid which has curare-like effects. The myocardium is affected and a marked bradycardia is produced. Those affected become subject to a marked languor with mental dullness in addition. There may be repeated episodes of an influenza-like illness. This wood was at one time widely used in the manufacture of shuttles for the cotton industry. It had to be discontinued from this use, however, because of the epidemic lethargy induced in the men who made the shuttles. Iroko wood, which is used as a substitute for teak, has also been known to produce symptoms resembling influenza, particularly if the wood is badly seasoned. Asthmatic symptoms may also occur. This skin rash is intensely irritant and is accompanied by facial oedema, conjunctivitis and blepharospasm in some cases.

Many other woods will produce dermatitis but good preventive measures will minimize the hazard. These include exhaust ventilation to remove dust, and the provision of protective clothing and respirators where appropriate.

Other biological agents

Grain itch, barley itch, copra itch and grocers' itch are all varieties of dermatitis caused by mites. Grain itch and barley itch occur in men handling cargoes of grain infested with *Pediculoides ventricosus*, a mite which normally feeds on the grain moth. The skin lesion develops after a period of 12–16 hours and consists of papules, vesicles, pustules and urticarial wheals on the face, neck, arms and trunk. Copra itch is found to occur in dock workers handling copra infested with *Tryoglyphus longior* which causes intensely irritant papules to develop after an incubation period of 1 day. The cheese mite is of the same family and it causes skin eruptions in grocers amongst others, hence the eponym. Another of the family lives in raw vanilla and attacks those coming into contact with it. Decomposing figs harbour a mite, *Carpoglyphus passularum*, which causes a pruritic rash in handling this fruit. The mite is also found in other fruits such as prunes and dates.

Outbreaks of scabies are well known to occur in camps occupied by soldiers and other groups such as miners and lumberjacks and in any group of people working in closely crowded, unhygienic conditions. It is the lack of hygiene rather than the occupation which predisposes to the infestation. Certain forms of animal scabies, on the other hand, may be found in humans by reason of their work. Thus veterinary practitioners can become infected with the mites that give rise to sarcoptic mange in horses, dogs and cats. Rarely, dairymen are infected by cattle mange and the condition is then known as dairyman's itch. The rash produced is intensely pruritic. In horse mange, which was very common in the days when the horse was the main form of transport, the itching is accompanied by red papules about the size of pin head. The mite does not propagate in human skin so that the lesions are transitory and the burrows which are typical of the human variant are not found.

Colour changes in the skin

Colour changes in the skin are specific to several occupations. Workers handling dyes and other chemicals are especially prone, the colour change being dependent upon the dye or dyes in use. Those handling chromates develop yellow stains on their hands, so do those employed in the manufacture of TNT and DNB. Picric acid imparts a light yellow colour to the skin whilst tetryl gives it an apricot tint. Those who handle silver nitrate have darkened skin; the photographer's fingers and nails are brown from metol and men handling pitch and tar have black skins. People who worked for several years in contact with arsenic are often found to have a fine, mottled brown pigmentation, the so-called raindrop pigmentation. It occurred predominantly on the face and neck but in severe cases, there was an intense bronze colour on the chest, abdomen and back. The argyria of silver workers has already been mentioned in Chapter 2. Most coal miners carry pigmented scars on their bodies due to the impregnation of small cuts and abrasions with coal dust and the same is true of other miners, the ultimate colour of the scar depending on the material being worked. Men chiselling steel are also liable to show the same phenomenon as small chips of metal enter the skin and become oxidized.

Vitiligo

Vitiligo occurs amongst workers handling *p*-tert-butylphenol (PTBP) which is used in the production of resins which go to make adhesives used in the car industry. The depigmentation has been noted in those manufacturing the raw product and in car workers using the adhesives prepared from it.

The condition is morphologically indistinguishable from true vitiligo but there is no evidence of an autoimmune disorder as in the true condition; those affected do not have an unusual incidence of thyroid antibodies, for example. On the other hand, there may be minor abnormalities in liver function tests and other signs of liver damage which are not found in true vitiligo. The main histological features seen on liver biopsy include moderate or severe focal fatty change, fibrosis and hepatocellular necrosis. The liver function tests return to normal when exposure to PTBP is discontinued.

Workers exposed to PTBP should be regularly screened with a Wood's lamp to detect those with early vitiligo, and in addition, tests of liver function should be undertaken at periodic intervals.

Prevention

The aim in reducing occupational skin disease is to prevent dangerous substances from coming into contact with the skin. As a preliminary it is necessary to identify those substances which are dangerous and then, wherever possible, enclose the processes in which they are used. When this cannot be done, operators should be given protective clothing, the nature of which will depend on the process and the substance under consideration. Masks and goggles will form part of the protective outfit if appropriate.

Personnel exposed to substances which are liable to produce skin diseases should be told of the potential dangers and informed of the ways in which they can protect themselves. Personal cleanliness is essential and the management should indicate this by seeing to it that standards of factory hygiene are of a high order and by providing good washing facilities and plentiful protective clothing. A factory-based laundry service can sometimes encourage the employees to change their overalls more often than they otherwise would.

The use of barrier creams is often advocated. Barrier creams are of three types, (1) simple vanishing creams which fill the pores of the skin with soap thus preventing the entrance of irritants and facilitating their removal by washing, (2) water-repellent creams which prevent water soluble irritants, such as acids and alkalis from coming into contact with the skin, and (3) oil and solvent repellents.

Creams such as these are best provided in dispensers in washrooms since it is essential that they are applied to clean skin otherwise irritants may be trapped under them. It goes without saying that the barrier creams must be nonirritant and this rule ought also to apply to the many proprietary brands of skin cleansers which are available. Unfortunately, this is not always the case, and there are many instances in which dermatitis is caused by skin cleansers. Excessive use of cleansers can lead to drying of the skin and this is so particularly when detergent cleansers are used, the injury often being compounded by virtue of their defatting properties. Of the detergent cleansers, the cationics are more likely to produce skin reactions than the anionics, whilst the nonionics are the least harmful of the three types available.

The use of solvents to remove materials on the skin must be actively discouraged. Many employees working in machine shops are often tempted to remove oil from their skin by this means, and whilst there is no doubt that they achieve this objective, they do so at the risk of causing the skin disease they are trying to avoid. Solvents used in this way are probably the most important cause of dermatitis in machine room workers, they being tempted into the habit by the unwelcome prospect of the walk to the washroom.

Chapter 8
Occupational Cancer

The first recognized association between occupation and malignant disease was made in 1775 by Percivall Pott, a surgeon at St Bartholomew's Hospital, when he described the occurrence of scrotal cancer in chimney sweeps. Although more tumours of occupational origin have been recognized since Pott's day, both the number of sites at which they occur and the number of undisputed occupational carcinogens is relatively small; there are a great many chemicals which are suspected to be carcinogens on the basis of *in vitro* mutagenicity tests. Some attempts have been made to estimate the proportion of all malignant disease which might be of occupational origin. The results show an extreme variation (from less than 1% to more than 50%), and are based as much on political or economic considerations as on epidemiology; the true proportion lies towards the lower end of the range and probably does not exceed 5%. Tumours of occupational origin have no pathological features to distinguish them from those which appear to arise spontaneously, nor does their symptomatology differ, but they all share the same characteristics.

1 They tend to appear at an earlier age than tumours which arise in the same sites simultaneously. Because of this, death also occurs at a younger age.

2 They arise as a result of repeated exposure to the putative carcinogen, although the exposure need not be continuous.

3 There is usually a long latent interval between the time of first exposure and the appearance of the tumour. This latent interval is commonly of the order of 20 years or more.

These features, particularly the earlier age of onset, ought to alert doctors to the possibility of an occupational origin for a tumour, but they are of no help in preventing its occurrence. The long latent interval is such that the carcinogenicity of a new material will go unnoticed until many years after its introduction into industrial use unless experiments with animals raise the possibilities of its dangers, or its chemical structure is similar to that of a known carcinogen.

Chemical carcinogens

Experiments which began in the period between the two world wars helped to establish that at least two processes are involved in chemical carcinogenesis, initiation and promotion. Initiation is seen as a process whereby an irreversible potential for malignancy is induced in a target cell; this malignant potential becomes manifest only when the cell is further acted upon by a promotor. Some chemicals act as both initiators and promotors and are referred to as complete carcinogens.

The underlying mechanisms of initiation and promotion are not fully understood, but it is generally considered that the most common event is the induction, by initiators, of mutations in somatic cells. Since not all chemical carcinogens are mutations, it is clear that some epigenetic phenomena are also involved. For example, chemical carcinogens may affect DNA repair mechanisms leading to an increased proneness to produce faulty genetic material; they may also interact with cellular mediators of genetic expression, alter the cellular response to normal growth by nongenetic effects or perhaps reduce the efficacy of the immune system.

The majority of initiators are mutagens, however, and initiation, unlike promotion, is not dose-dependent. A mutagen changes the structure of the DNA molecule, frequently by changing the sequence of purine or pyrimidine bases in the molecule. The simplest way by which this is achieved is base pair transformation in which one base is replaced by another. This may be accomplished by chemical modification as, for example, when adenine or cytosine are deaminated to form hypoxanthine or uracil respectively. Alternatively, mutation may be accomplished by the incorporation of an abnormal base analogue into the DNA molecule during replication; the mutagen 5-bromouracil, for example, is an analogue of thymine and will replace it during replication. One or more bases may also be added or deleted from the DNA molecule to produce what is known as a frame-shift mutation. Whatever the mechanism, however, a change in the sequence of bases alters the triplet code and will result in errors in the amino acid sequence of formed proteins.

Mutagens may also affect whole chromosomes by causing breaks or faulty repair; these effects are similar to the base pair changes but on a grander scale.

Cancer of the skin

Cancer of the scrotum was the first instance of an occupational malignancy to be recognized and Pott's description of the clinical course of the disease has no equal.

> It is a disease which always makes its first attack on, and its first appearance in, the inferior part of the scrotum; where it produces a superficial, painful, ragged, ill-looking sore, with hard and rising edges: the trade call it the sootwart. I never saw it under the age of puberty, which is, I suppose one reason why it is generally taken, both by patient and surgeon, for venereal; and being treated with mercurials, is thereby soon and much exasperated. In no great length of time, it pervades the skin, dartos, and membranes of the scrotum, and seizes the testicle, which it enlarges, hardens, and renders truly and thoroughly distempered; from whence it makes its way up the spermatic process into the abdomen, most frequently indurating and spoiling the inguinal glands: when arrived within the abdomen, it affects some of the viscera, and then very soon becomes painfully destructive.

Since Pott's day occupational skin cancer has been noted to occur at other sites, most usually on exposed skin surfaces. The disease has been recorded in men working with pitch and tar, with arsenic, and in those exposed to mineral oils. In the 1920s and 1930s there was a virtual epidemic in the Lancashire cotton industry which necessitated the introduction of new safety measures and the introduction of oils of low carcinogenicity. More recently workers exposed to cutting oils in the engineering industry have been found to be at risk. Agricultural workers are another high risk group since their outdoor work exposes them to ultraviolet light from the sun. This is not as substantial a hazard in England as in some other more favoured countries. In the early days of radiography, many radiologists unwittingly exposed themselves to high doses of X-rays which produced malignant changes in their skin.

New cases of epitheliomatous ulceration of the skin have to be notified to the Health and Safety Executive and most cases are still due to exposure to pitch and tar, although mineral oil exposure is becoming of increasing importance. Many cases go unnotified, however, because an adequate occupational history is not obtained from the patient.

Men exposed to pitch and tar frequently develop hyperkeratotic lesions which they refer to as warts, on exposed skin. These sometimes fall off, or the men treat themselves with applications of caustic solutions. In the same way, a proportion of workers exposed to mineral oils develop folliculitis and hyperkeratotic lesions which in the majority of cases do not become malignant. When malignant change does supervene, the lesion (or lesions) becomes ulcerated, bleeds and enlarges. Local spread to lymph nodes may be apparent by the time the patient seeks medical advice.

Prevention

Protective clothing and the provision of good washing facilities are essential for those coming into contact with pitch, tar and mineral oil. Unfortunately, most protective clothing is uncomfortable to wear since it is not only impervious to pitch and oil but also to water vapour, so that the worker tends to sweat whilst wearing it. Those at risk should be made aware of the dangers of the substances with which they are working and encouraged to examine their skin regularly and report any suspicious lesions to their own doctor or their works doctor, if there is one. Regular medical inspections may help by detecting growths at an early stage, but these are not yet required by law, except for mule spinners and patent fuel workers, and so the onus is on the works doctor and the employees to co-operate in voluntary schemes. Machines on which cutting oils are used are nowadays guarded to prevent splashing and only oils of low carcinogenicity should be used.

Carcinogens in pitch, tar and oil

These are considered to be polycyclic aromatic hydrocarbons, largely concentrated in the fractions with the highest boiling points. A great deal of work has gone into defining mineral oils which have low carcinogenicity. Much of the early work was done in Manchester in the wake of the outbreak of skin cancer amongst the mule spinners in the late 1920s. It was then found that the carcinogenic potency of oil could be related to a number of physical properties, the most important of which were the refractive index and the density. More recently, solvent extraction has been used to reduce the carcinogenicity of mineral oils and since the mid-1960s, so-called solvent refined oils have come into general use.

Carcinoma of the bladder

The first cases of occupational bladder cancer were reported in Germany in 1895 as occurring in workers employed in the manufacture of aniline dyes. Thereafter it became common practice to refer to such tumours as aniline tumours although, in fact, aniline was not responsible for their production. Compounds which are responsible for causing bladder tumours are certain aromatic amines used as intermediates in the manufacture of dyes and pharmaceuticals, as antioxidants and accelerators in the rubber industry, and as curing agents for polymerized elastomers in the plastics industry. Some of the more important of these aromatic amines are shown in Figure 8.1.

β-naphthylamine has probably contributed most to the production of bladder cancer in industry and it was withdrawn from use in this country in 1949. The fumes inside gas retort houses may contain β-naphthylamine and this probably accounts for the excess of bladder tumours found in gas workers.

α-naphthylamine in the pure state is usually considered noncarcinogenic but it is difficult to prepare the pure compound for industrial use and it usually contains up to 4% of β-naphthylamine as a contaminant. The difference in activity between the two compounds relates to the position of the NH_2 radical and as a general rule, compounds with a free position para to the NH_2 are noncarcinogenic.

Benzidine was widely used as a laboratory reagent for the detection of occult blood in faeces. Since 1962, however, it has not been used for this purpose in the UK but in the USA this use continues. Benzidine is an essential intermediate in the dyestuffs industry. It is not manufactured in this country, however, and can only be imported in the form of its hydrochlorides provided a licence has been obtained and that the compounds contain a minimum of one-third water.

Dimethylbenzidine (o-tolidine) was once used in medical laboratories for occult blood testing but it should now no longer be used as it is carcinogenic in animals and probably in humans also.

Dichlorobenzidine, another analogue of benzidine, is a potent experimental carcinogen but is still used in the dyestuffs industry and for curing polyurethane elastomers. Xenylamine (4-amino diphenyl) is a highly potent carcinogen and is not used in this country.

MOCA (3,3'-dichlor, 4,4'-diamino diphenyl methane)* is used as a hardener for some types of urethane foam rubber. It has been shown to produce lung and liver tumours in experimental animals and to cause haemorrhagic cystitis in workers exposed to it. For these reasons its use in industry is kept under close supervision and most manufacturers in this country prefer not to

---

*This compound is also known as MbOCA from its alternative chemical name, methylene-bis-o-chloraniline.

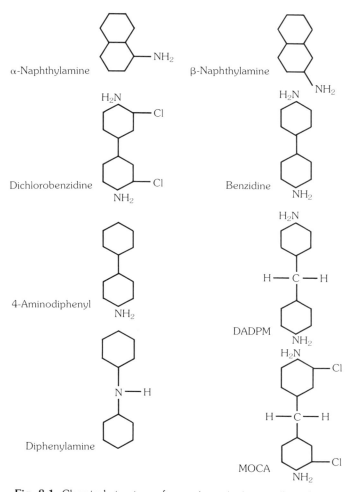

Fig. 8.1. Chemical structure of some important aromatic amines

use it. The closely related compound DADPM (4,4'-diamino diphenyl methane) causes liver tumours in rats but it has not been shown to cause bladder cancer. This compound was responsible for what was become known as the Epping jaundice. A total of 84 people presented with abdominal pain and jaundice and an influenza-like illness due to eating bread which had become contaminated with DADPM. The lorry in which the sack of flour was transported from the mill to the bakery had previously carried a solution of DADPM, some of which had been split on the floor of the lorry. The lorry was not thoroughly cleaned between trips and so the sack containing the flour became impregnated by the residual fluid.

Diphenylamine is used as an intermediary in the dyestuffs industry and in the manufacture of rubber antioxidants. There is no evidence that it is carcinogenic in humans or animals but it has been found to contain 4-amino diphenyl as an impurity and its use must be closely monitored.

Prevention

The manufacture of compounds which are essential intermediates in the production of important materials and for which no substitute can be found is controlled by a Code of Practice drawn up by the British Association of Chemical Manufacturers. The importation of β-naphthylamine, benzidine, 4-amino diphenyl, 4-nitro diphenyl and their salts, and substances containing them has been prohibited since 1967 except where they are present as a chemical by-product in a concentration not exceeding 1%.

The manufacturing processes in which potentially carcinogenic compounds are used, and the workers employed in these processes must obviously be meticulously supervised. The clinical course of the disease is no different from that of the spontaneously occurring variant and early diagnosis affords the best hope of a cure. All those exposed must be warned of the possible dangers in order that they co-operate with monitoring schemes.

Cytological examination of urinary sediment has become an established part of screening procedures for those at risk and should be undertaken at least twice a year, supplemented by cystoscopy when necessary. Malignant cells may be found in the absence of haematuria but the latter sign is always an indication for further investigation.

Other tumours of the renal tract

Tumours of the renal pelvis, the ureter and the urethra have been reported in workers exposed to aromatic amines, usually in those who have already had a bladder tumour. The incidence of these tumours is said to be increasing, and relates to the improved survival rate in those with tumours of the bladder. Adenocarcinoma of the kidney is not found to have an increased incidence in workers exposed to aromatic amines. Experimentally these tumours have been induced in rats by lead salts administered either orally or subcutaneously, but no excess of kidney tumours has been shown in industrial lead workers.

Tumours of the liver

Tumours of the liver are occasionally noted in workers exposed to benzidene and they have also been reported in those exposed to arsenical insecticide sprays but these men also had hepatic cirrhosis which has a well-known association with hepatic tumours.

Experimentally, a number of azo dyes and solvents produce liver tumours in animals, but no undue risks appear to be associated with industrial exposure.

Angiosarcoma of the liver has been found in men exposed to VCM. To date less than 30 cases have been reported in the world and the tumour has occurred only in those who have been exposed to very high concentrations, usually those cleaning the reaction vessels. In view of the long latent period it is likely that more cases will appear and a control limit for VCM has recently been introduced.

Cancer of the bronchus

Tumours of the lung were noted to occur amongst the miners of Schneeburg in the Erzgebirge. Later the uranium miners in Joachimstal, on the other side of the Erzgebirge, were also found to be subject to a high risk of developing bronchial tumours. The mines were worked successively for silver, nickel, and uranium and provided the ore from which the Curies isolated radium. There was a very high level of radioactivity in both mines and many years later, when the ventilation had been substantially improved, the average concentration of radon in the air was 3×10^{-9} curies/litre. Radon decays to form a series of daughter products with the emission of α-particles. There is no doubt that the α-particles are the carcinogenic agent and they produce an undifferentiated carcinoma which arises from the bronchial epithelium. It has been suggested that when conditions were at their worst, the miners in the Schneeburg and Joachimstal mines were receiving doses of 100 000 rads of α-particles to the lungs.

The increased risk of lung cancer experienced by uranium miners in other areas of the world is also due to exposure to radon.

Uranium miners, however, are by no means alone in their occupational exposure to radon since the gas is found in almost all metaliferrous mines, sometimes in concentrations which are in excess of the limits laid down by the atomic energy industry for their own workers.

Nickel

Tumours of the lung were a risk to those employed to refine nickel from its ores by the Mond process, but this risk now seems to have disappeared, although it is still experienced by those refining nickel by electrolytic processes. Men who ran the greatest risk in the Mond process were those engaged in calcining the ore or in extracting the ore with sulphuric acid which contained large amounts of arsenic. In 1920–24 an acid which was virtually free of arsenic was substituted and thereafter the risk declined. This has led to speculation that the arsenic was responsible for the disease, but not all authorities agree. Nickel in powdered form has been shown to be carcinogenic to animals and the reduction in airborne dust due to improvements in the process is a more likely reason for the decline.

Carcinoma of the nasal passages has also been attributed to exposure to nickel, but as with lung cancer, the risk appears to have diminished in recent years. Adenocarcinoma of the nose and air sinuses, however, is still a risk for workers in the furniture industry exposed to wood dust and to a lesser extent, for those using leather in the shoemaking industry.

Chromates

Workers manufacturing chromates from chrome ores have been shown to have a higher than expected incidence of lung tumours, monochromate ores seeming to represent the greatest hazard. Exposure to dichromates frequently gives rise to ulcers of the skin and the nasal septum but these do not undergo malignant change.

Asbestos

There is no doubt that prolonged exposure to asbestos may lead to the development of bronchial carcinoma and about half of those who develop asbestosis die from lung cancer; it is debatable whether lung cancer develops in an asbestos worker in the absence of asbestosis. Not only the degree of exposure but also the type of exposure is important, however. Thus, the risk of developing lung cancer is much greater in those who have been engaged in the manufacture of asbestos products than in those who have worked in mining or milling processes. This difference is probably due to the fact that a higher proportion of submicroscopic fibres is produced during textile manufacture than during mining and milling. Cigarette smoking considerably enhances the risk of lung cancer in those exposed to asbestos.

Gas-workers

Employees who have worked in retort houses in gas works experience a higher risk than normal of developing cancer of the bronchus. The tarry material which is produced during the process of distillation of coal to make coal gas contains a large number of polycyclic aromatic hydrocarbons which are found also in the generated fumes. This fume contains benzo (a) pyrene and in the horizontal retort houses very high concentrations (>200 μg^3) were recorded above the retorts. Apart from this special case, there are no differences in the concentrations of benzo (a) pyrene in horizontal retort houses and vertical retort houses, although there is an increased risk of lung cancer in the horizontal as opposed to the vertical retort houses. It is not clear how far this difference can be accounted for in terms of the experience of those who worked in the most polluted areas.

Haematite

The iron ore miners in West Cumberland who work underground experience an occupational risk of lung cancer about 70% greater than normal. Miners working on the surface do not have the same risk. Also in France, iron ore miners have been found to have a similar lung cancer risk. As mentioned earlier, the risk arises because of exposure to radon. In the Cumberland mines, the average radon concentration in the air is 100 Ci/l.

Mesothelioma

This rare tumour affecting principally the pleura, but also the peritoneum, is particularly a hazard of exposure to crocidolite but other forms of asbestos will, with the exception of antophyllite, produce the disease. Crocidolite from the north-west Cape Province is far more dangerous in this respect than crocidolite from the Transvaal. The exposure need not be prolonged and nonoccupational cases are known in persons living in the neighbourhood of asbestos factories or mines.

The main symptom is dyspnoea which rapidly increases in severity and may be accompanied by cough, haemoptysis and chest pain. A chest X-ray will demonstrate massive thickening of the pleura with pleural effusion and perhaps signs of lung collapse. Straw coloured pleural fluid, often bloodstained, can be aspirated from the chest and malignant cells will be found on cytological examination. Abdominal tumours give rise to ascites with a bloody exudate containing malignant cells.

The tumour is a dense white growth which may spread to the whole of the lung and cause collapse. Ultimately the whole pleural cavity becomes obliterated. The pericardium may become affected and the mediastium becomes progressively widened by tumour growth. Peritoneal tumours sometimes involve all the abdominal organs but more usually the growth is unevenly distributed. Metastatic spread is not common but in some cases there is a generalized lymphadenopathy and subcutaneous nodules may be found over the neck and chest. Rarely nodules are found on the tongue. The diagnoses should be confirmed by pleural biopsy but no treatment is sufficient to prevent the fatal outcome of the disease and this takes months rather than years.

Leukaemia

Ionizing radiation

Ionizing radiation is well known to produce leukaemia in experimental animals and in humans. The evidence for the latter association has come from the increased rates which were formerly shown in radiologists and others working in diagnostic X-ray units, in patients irradiated for ankylosing spondylitis and in survivors of the atomic bomb explosions in Hiroshima and Nagasaki. The relationship between the mean dose of radiation to the spinal marrow and the age-standardized incidence of leukaemia in patients with ankylosing spondylitis is shown in Table 8.1. It should be noted that the doses to which these patients were exposed are much higher than those which could be encountered by patients undergoing diagnostic radiology or by persons who are exposed to radiation either in hospitals or in industry during the course of their occupation. Nevertheless, ionizing radiation is becoming increasingly used in both situations and there is no room for anything but the most stringent control (*see* Chapter 9).

Benzene

Exposure to benzene has occasionally been found to result in the production of leukaemia, frequently superimposed as a terminal event on aplastic anaemia.

Table 8.1. Standardized incidence rates for leukaemia in men with ankylosing spondylitis after different doses of irradiation to the spinal marrow

	Mean dose (rads)					
	0	250	750	1250	1750	2500
Standardized incidence rate/ 10 000 men/year	0.49	1.98	4.66	7.21	13.44	72.16

From Court-Brown W.M. & Doll R. *Medical Research Council Special Report* Series No. 295, HMSO, 1957.

The myeloid types are the most common, but all other varieties have been recorded from time to time.

Other volatile solvents such as toluene and xylene have sometimes been incriminated in causing leukaemia, but as used industrially they often contain large amounts of benzene as an impurity. There is no evidence that in the pure state they are capable of inducing malignant changes in the marrow.

Osteosarcoma

Radium salts were first used in industry in the manufacture of luminous paint which was then applied to watch and clock faces with brushes. The women employed in this work kept the point on their brushes by licking them, and in this way they swallowed considerable quantities of the radioactive paint. A high proportion of the women subsequently developed anaemia and necrosis of the jaw, but in addition some also developed osteosarcomata. This process now takes place under carefully controlled conditions.

Testing chemicals for carcinogenicity

In many countries manufacturers are not permitted to introduce new chemicals into use unless they have undergone carcinogenicity tests. The testing schedules are laid down by the regulating authorities in the countries concerned and vary one from another. In general, however, the schedule requires both *in vitro* and *in vivo* tests.

In vitro tests: Because they are relatively quick and cheap, there has been a great deal of effort in recent years to develop reliable *in vitro* tests of carcinogenicity. Many are available but the one which is still in most common use is the Ames' test which actually determines the ability of chemicals to induce a specific mutation in bacteria. Another frequently used test, technically more difficult than the Ames' test, measures the ability of chemical compounds to induce transformations in cell cultures. It is also a test of mutagenicity but this is accepted as satisfactory since the majority of chemical carcinogens are also mutagens. There is no absolute certainty, however, that the converse is true, that is, that all mutagens are also carcinogens. Nevertheless, short term tests may be used to screen chemicals in the first instance and *in vivo* tests are usually required only if at least two *in vitro* tests give positive results.

The Ames' test relies on the ability of chemicals to induce a mutation in a histidine requiring strain of *Salmonella typhimurium*. To conduct the test, the chemical is mixed with the bacteria and an enzyme rich rat liver fraction. It is invariably the case that the active carcinogens (or mutagens) are metabolites of the parent compound and the liver fraction is thus essential to ensure that this transformation takes place. The mixture is then plated out onto nutrient agar which lacks histidine and incubated for 3 days. After this, the number of revertant colonies, that is those which have derived from a mutant not requiring histidine, is counted. The background reversion rate is low, of the order of 10 or less colonies whereas in the presence of a mutagen the count may be as high as 10^4 per plate.

In vivo tests: With *in vivo* tests, a compound may be tested for carcinogenicity rather than for mutagenicity. Various protocols exist for carrying out these tests, but all are time consuming and expensive. One which is commonly used is that proposed by the National Cancer Institutes of America. The dose to be used in the study is determined by a preliminary subacute study carried out on rats and mice of both sexes. The animals are tested in groups of 5 and six dose levels are administered for 42 weeks followed by a 2-week observation period. From these experiments the maximum tolerated dose (MTD) is determined and for the main study, animals are given a high (MTD) or a low (0.5 MTD) oral dose of the chemical for 5 days a week for 78 weeks. This period is followed by further observation, the extent of which is variable but may be until 80% of the animals have died. The animals which have survived until the end of the experiment are then sacrificed and a full pathological examination is carried out and a histological examination is made of any tumours present; those animals which have died before the end of the experiment will already have been treated likewise. The prevalence of tumours in the experimental animals and in control animals is then determined.

Chemicals which are shown unequivocally to be carcinogenic or mutagenic must clearly be treated with the utmost caution and not introduced into use unless there are overriding reaons for doing so and there is no suitable alternative. Positive results in *in vivo* or *in vitro* tests, however, must not necessarily lead to the conclusion that the chemicals in question are human carcinogens. With a number of chemicals the dose which is needed to produce tumours in animals is far in excess of that which would be encountered in industrial use and the mode of administration is often different; in many test schedules an oral dose is given whereas in industry the major route of entry is by inhalation or, to a lesser degree, through the skin. Thus, trichloroethylene has been found to induce hepatic tumours in mice when given in massive oral doses but there is no evidence that it is carcinogenic in humans. It should also be remembered that chemical carcinogens do not produce the same effects in all species. For example, tar has little carcinogenic effect on the skin of rats or dogs whereas in mice and rabbits tumours are produced with ease. Conversely, mice and rabbits are relatively unresponsive to β-naphthylamine which produces bladder tumours in dogs. A recent report that exposure to formaldehyde produced tumours of the nasal sinuses in rats set in train a series of human epidemiological studies, none of which produced positive results. The cause of this particular discrepancy seems to lie in the anatomy of the rat's nose; it has extremely large ethmoids with a large surface area for absorption and it is thus prone to the effects of substances which are mucosal irritants.

Despite these caveats it is obviously prudent to treat mutagenic substances with circumspection taking care to tread the narrow line between alarmism and indifference. Moreover, it must also be remembered that materials which are not animal carcinogens may nevertheless be carcinogenic to humans and only long usage will give a definite answer.

Non-specific cancer

Some occupations involve exposure to specific carcinogenic hazards and the site of the disease is characteristic for the occupation; bladder in rubber workers, mesothelioma in asbestos workers, skin in oil workers and so on. Certain other occupations, however, appear to have an excess risk of developing tumours in various sites, even though in most cases there is no well-recognized specific hazard.

In Table 8.2 a list of these occupations and the tumour sites is shown. The data have been taken from the Occupational Mortality Tables of the Registrar General and to avoid the social class bias discussed in Chapter 1, only those occupations in which there is an excess in the husbands but not their wives (as indicated by a significant t-value) are shown.

Table 8.2. Malignant causes of death, by occupation, with high t-values in husbands but not their wives

Site of cancer	Occupation
Mouth	Textile workers
Oesophagus	Food, drink and tobacco workers
Stomach	Gas, coke and chemical workers
	Furnace, forge, foundry, rolling mill workers
	Painters and decorators
Rectum	Furnace, forge, foundry, rolling mill workers
Pancreas	Clothing workers
Larynx, lung, bronchus and trachea	Food, drink and tobacco workers
	Glass and ceramic workers
	Furnace, forge, foundry, rolling mill workers
	Electrical and electronic workers
	Construction workers
	Painters and decorators
	Warehousemen, storekeepers, packers, bottlers
Kidney	Electrical and electronic workers
Bladder and other urinary organs	Gas, coke and chemical makers
	Transport and communication workers
Bone	Furnace, forge, foundry, rolling mill workers

From the Registrar General's *Occupational Mortality Tables*, HMSO, 1971.

There is only one case in which it is possible to suggest a specific carcinogenic hazard and that is for the excess of bladder carcinoma in gas, coke and chemical workers where exposure to aromatic amines is the probable carcinogenic risk. Otherwise it is difficult to see the connection between the occupation and the apparent enhanced risk of malignancy. In all probability, however, there are many carcinogens, or groups of carcinogens acting in concert, which have not been identified, and this is a fertile region for epidemiological exploration.

Chapter 9
Physical Hazards

Decompression sickness

This syndrome can occur in three groups of persons.

1 Those working in compressed air who are too rapidly decompressed.

2 Divers who surface too rapidly from depths greater than about 33 feet (10 m).

3 Crew or paratroopers in aircraft who ascend too rapidly from sea level to heights of greater than 18,000 feet (5487 m).

In the first category the syndrome is sometimes called caisson disease, after the apparatus which is used when underwater excavation is being carried out during the course of constructing piers, bridges, etc. The caisson is an iron or concrete tube open at the bottom, which is weighted and driven into the mud or sand below water. The men working in the caisson descend through a series of airtight chambers in which the atmospheric pressure is successively raised. it is the high atmospheric pressure in the final working chamber which prevents it from being flooded. The usual maximum working pressures in compressed air work in building or in civil engineering is 4.5 kg/cm^3 (441.2 x 10^3 Pa) and generally much less. When the worker ascends back to the surface, the air pressure is reduced to atmospheric as successive chambers are passed through.

The manifestations of decompression sickness are due to the formation of nitrogen bubbles in the body fluids and in the tissues. Bubbles of nitrogen large enough to cause symptoms form when the partial pressure of nitrogen in the tissues rapidly becomes twice as great as its partial pressure in the atmosphere.

The symptoms produced depend upon the site in which the bubbles are formed whilst the size and rate of growth of the bubbles determines the severity of the symptoms.

Symptoms

The acute symptoms of decompression sickness are usually divided into two types (see Table 9.1); some chronic symptoms also occur.

Type I: The main symptom is acute pain in the limbs usually in the joints, sometimes preceded by numbness; the pain may come on at any time during the 12 hours following decompression. The affected part is often held in a semiflexed position from which it is difficult to move, hence this condition is known amongst divers as the bends. Skin mottling and itching may occur with or without joint pain.

Type II: Type II symptoms are much more serious than Type I but are seen much more rarely. The most striking are paralysis of one or more limbs which

Table 9.1. Symptoms in different types of decompression sickness

Type I	Mild or severe limb pain
	Skin mottling or skin irritation
Type II	Paralysis or weakness of the limbs
	Tingling or numbness in the limbs
	Vertigo
	Headache
	Dyspnoea
	Fits or convulsions
	Chest pain
	Hypotension
	Coma
Chronic	Aseptic necrosis of the bones
	Neurological or psychological symptoms

may be accompanied by vertigo, nausea or vomiting. If nitrogen bubbles occur in the pulmonary vasculature the worker experiences a sensation of burning retrosternal distress with a cough. This may be at first relieved by shallow breathing but after a while the coughing becomes paroxysmal and uncontrollable. These symptoms are referred to as the chokes. In the most serious cases the patient may pass into a coma and die unless immediate treatment is given. Post-decompression shock with haemoconcentration is another serious complication.

Aseptic necrosis

Aseptic necrosis of bone is thought to result from infarcts brought about by nitrogen emboli lodging in the nutrient arteries (Fig. 9.1). The changes are often symmetrical but the condition is only serious or disabling if the articular surfaces of the humerus or femur are affected. About a quarter of all compressed air workers have aseptic necrosis but only 3% are disabled. By contrast, aseptic necrosis is seen in only about 5% of deep sea divers and only about 0.2% are disabled.

Prevention and treatment

In most cases decompression work is carried out in accordance with a statutory set of tables many of which have been based on the 1958 British tables which owed much to the work of Haldane. In the UK these tables have now been superseded by the Blackpool Decompression Tables which are published in the Medical Code of Practice for Work in Compressed Air.

Those who are to work at reduced atmospheres should be carefully selected, weeding out the fat, the alcoholic and those with pre-existing cardiovascular or pulmonary disease. People over 35 years of age are also best not newly recruited. A radiographic examination of the chest and the major joints should be carried out and the major joints should be X-rayed every 2 years. Anyone who has had Type II symptoms must not be allowed to work in decompressed conditions again unless there are the most overwhelming reasons for him or her to do so.

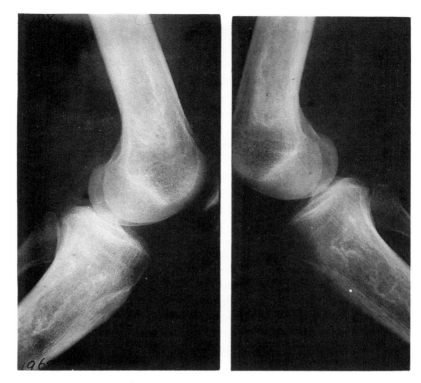

Fig. 9.1 Radiographs showing aseptic necrosis in the bones around both knee joints in a naval diver.

The symptoms of decompression sickness are relieved by recompressing the patient and reducing the pressure in accordance with a protocol laid down in a set of tables; the one contained in the US Navy Diving Manual is frequently used.

Other effects of diving or increased atmospheric pressure

Divers are at risk from several other hazards which may or may not be due to increased atmospheric pressure. The risk of drowning is everpresent and this is far and away the most common cause of death in divers. At great depths there is the danger from cold and some provision must be made to maintain the normal body temperature. Anyone who dives into water—whether using breathing apparatus or not—may develop a spontaneous pneumothorax if he or she surfaces too rapidly; there is also the risk of being attacked by other creatures in the sea.

When the pressure on a diver exceeds 4 atmospheres (equal to about 100 feet or 30 m of water) a diver breathing air may suffer from nitrogen narcosis. Judgement, thought and movement all become impaired and if the diver does not surface, he or she may become unconscious. The symptoms rapidly clear when the diver returns to normal pressure. Substituting helium for nitrogen in a breathing apparatus prevents the onset of symptoms.

Adverse effects are also noted from exposure to high partial pressures of oxygen. Divers breathing pure oxygen are at risk in depths greater than 25 feet (7.5 m) and those breathing helium/oxygen mixtures are at some risk at very great depths (greater than 500 feet or 150 m) and a vague feeling of discomfort may precede more serious symptoms, but convulsions and coma can occur with little warning.

All divers using oxygen apparatus should be able to recognize the symptoms of oxygen narcosis and come to the surface as soon as they notice them. The only treatment required is to breathe fresh air.

Patients in hyperbaric chambers and their attendants should also be on their guard against oxygen poisoning.

Heat

So-called heat cramps may be a symptom amongst forge and foundry workers, metal casters, iron and glass workers, and miners, as well as those who work out of doors in hot climates. They may also occur as the result of heat generated by microwave radiation. The incidence of the disease shows seasonal variations, well over three-quarters of the cases occurring during the summer months.

The symptoms usually occur during the second half of the shift and those affected are generally of poor physique. Sometimes there are prodromal symptoms such as headache and dizziness, but characteristically there is a sudden onset of severe cramping pain in the muscles being used at the time. Most often the attack begins in the calves and spreads to the muscles of the upper limbs and abdomen. The pains are of an intermittent nature, occurring with increasing severity every few minutes. Albuminuria is frequently found but there are no other abnormal signs.

The condition is, in effect, a form of water intoxication, brought about because the workman drinks a lot of water in response to the sweating experienced in the hot environment, which, in turn, leads to a decrease in the plasma osmolality. Treatment with a drink containing sodium chloride is all that is required to prevent this. In factories where it is impossible to eliminate the heat hazard entirely, a stock of tablets from which such drinks can be made should be kept for use by the employees. If they drink this salt solution regularly, the symptoms do not appear.

Those who work regularly in a hot environment gradually become acclimatized and it is found that they conserve sodium and chloride so that the concentration of these ions in the sweat falls. This phenomenon explains why heat cramps are not more common.

Heat exhaustion and heat stroke

Heat exhaustion is associated with a depletion of both salt and water. The concentration of the body fluids is not altered greatly but there is a dimunition in blood volume which accounts for the symptoms. Over a period of a few days the patient complains of weakness, fatigue and headache, with perhaps anorexia and vomiting. If the vomiting is persistent, circulatory collapse may follow. Generally the patient is incapacitated before this stage is reached and the disease is rarely fatal.

When seen by the doctor, the patient will have signs of peripheral circulatory failure with pallor, hypotension and profuse sweating. There is generally little elevation of the body temperature.

Treatment consists of removing the patient to a cool place, rest in bed and replacement of salt and water, which can be achieved in the majority of cases by the oral route. If the patient is severely ill, recourse to intravenous replacement will be necessary.

In heat stroke, the symptoms are due to a defect in thermoregulation producing a positive heat balance. The onset is abrupt. The patient falls unconscious and is found to have a temperature of at least 40.6°C. Management consists of rapid cooling by whatever means possible and the aim must be to reduce the temperature to 40°C within 1 hour, thus minimizing the danger of damage to the central nervous system.

Treatment may be required for as long as a week before sweating returns and temperature can be regulated unaided.

Neither of these conditions is likely to be encountered with any frequency in this country.

Occupational cataracts

Most cases of occupational cataracts are the late result of penetrating injuries to the eye, although in the past heat-induced cataracts were the most common variety. Cataracts may also be a sequelae of exposure to ionizing radiation and may follow an electric shock.

Traumatic cataracts

These follow penetrating injuries to the eye in which the lens capsule is ruptured, although they do sometimes form following a simple contusion to the eye with no penetration.

The hazard is particularly great where workers are using explosives or working on lathes and presses, where small pieces of metal may fly into the eye. Protective goggles should be worn by all those at risk but this ideal is seldom achieved.

Heat cataracts

In the early part of the century this form of cataract was common amongst glass blowers and it was subsequently reported in other workers exposed to radiant energy, most notably chain makers and furnacemen. The cataract was often unilateral, forming in the eye closest to the source of the heat. It has since become established that X-irradiation of the eye can produce a cataract, the minimum dose for this effect being about 500 rad. Fast neutrons are particularly hazardous in cataract production.

In all cases of radiation cataract the lens changes began in the posterior pole of the lens immediately under the posterior capsule. The opacity was often disc-shaped and had a golden colour when viewed through a slit lamp. In time the opacity spread to involve the remainder of the posterior cortex. The anterior cortex also became involved in the disease process and ultimately the cataract became indistinguishable from the ordinary senile form. The pathognomonic change of a radiation-induced cataract was said to be the exfoliation of the zonula lamella of the anterior capsule. This lamella peeled off in sheets and it was said that in the absence of this change it was difficult to blame an occupational exposure for the production of the posterior cataract.

Heat cataract is seldom met with nowadays. Bottles are usually made mechanically so that one of the most potent sources of hazard has been removed through an advance in technology. Where exposure to heat is unavoidable, workers are protected by wearing goggles made from glass containing metallic oxides which cut off heat radiation but transmit light. Standards for such goggles are laid down by the British Standards Institute.

Electric shock

Rarely, cataract formation has been noted following electric shock. The cataract may be present only on the side on which electrical contact was made or it may be bilateral. There is usually a delay of a year or so before it begins to form, but thereafter it often matures rapidly. Spontaneous regression sometimes occurs within a few weeks of the onset of the lens changes.

Microwave radiation

There have been some reports of cataract formation in workers exposed to relatively high intensity microwave radiation, usually above 100 mW/cm^2, but the association is controversial. It is less readily accepted as proven in the countries of western Europe than in the east principally because, in none of the published reports, has it been possible unequivocally to rule out other causes for the cataracts.

Treatment
The treatment of cataract is the same regardless of the means of formation. The affected lens is removed and the sight defect corrected by suitable spectacles.

Miner's nystagmus

This condition is thought to result from poor lighting conditions underground. The relative absence of rods at the macula causes a defect in fixation which is often symptomless. Where there are symptoms they are, in addition to nystagmus, those of vertigo, photophobia, headache, insomnia and blepharospasm. The vertigo may be so severe as to be disabling but in cases where this is so, there appears to be a considerable functional overlay. Defective vision is sometimes reported, but there is no retinal lesion to account for it.

Improvements in lighting underground, including the provision of reflecting surfaces have done much to minimize the condition. Patients who develop symptoms should be reassured that there will be no permanent loss of vision but it may be necessary, nevertheless, to find alternative work for those who are severely affected.

Ionizing radiation

The number of radiation sources has increased spectacularly during the last two or three decades as they find ever wider application both in industry and in hospital practice.

Ionizing radiation can be divided into two main groups; electromagnetic radiations, such as X-rays and γ-rays and corpuscular radiations such as α-particles, β-particles (electrons), protons and neutrons. Unlike the first three particles, neutrons carry no electric charge.

When X-rays or γ-rays are absorbed, high-energy electrons are produced in the irradiated tissue and it is these β-particles which are the effective ionizing agents, being capable of breaking chemical bonds to release positively and negatively charged ions. The radioactive particles are capable of ionization with no intermediary, but for all practical purposes there is no distinction between the biological effects of the different groups.

Definitions

Different units are used to define absorption, dose equivalence and radioactivity.

Absorption is measured in grays (Gy); 1 Gy is defined as an energy absorption of 1 joule per kilogram. It can be applied to all sources of radiation but since not all sources produce equivalent effects in the tissues it is customary to introduce a modifying factory which allows for this variation. The value of the modifying factor, which is sometimes known as the Relative Biological Effectiveness (RBE) is 1 for gamma rays, X-rays and β-particles whereas for α-particles, fast neutrons and protons it is 10. The product of the RBE and the absorbed dose provides the dose equivalent in sieverts (Sv).

The dose equivalent provides an index of the risk of harm following exposure to radiation. Not all the tissues are equally at risk from radiation, however, and to account for this, a series of risk weighting factors has been recommended as shown in Table 9.2.

If a single tissue is irradiated the dose can be converted to a dose equivalent for the whole body by applying the appropriate weighting factor. If, as is more common, several tissues are involved, then the weighting factors can be applied to each and the sum of the products is the dose equivalent to the whole body

Table 9.2. Risk weighting factors for ionizing radiation

Tissue or organ	Factor
Gonads	0.25
Breast	0.15
Red bone marrow	0.12
Lung	0.12
Thyroid	0.03
Bone surfaces	0.03
Remainder	0.03

which would yield the same overall risk. The sum of the weighted dose equivalents is known as the effective dose equivalent and is also expressed in sieverts.

Radioactivity is measured in becquerels (Bq), 1 Bq being equivalent to the quantity of radioactive material in which there is one disintegration per second.

Effects of radiation

Acute radiation syndrome

Doses of whole body irradiation of the order of 5–20 Gy delivered over a short period of time result in severe tissue destruction and death within a week. With lower doses, say about 1–5 Gy the patient will survive long enough to develop the acute radiation syndrome, although this will seldom be of much comfort to him. In the typical case, four more or less distinct stages can be distinguished. There is first a short latent period of a few hours during which no ill effects are observed. The second stage is heralded in by nausea and vomiting which passes off within about 24 hours to be followed by a period of minor symptoms including malaise, anorexia, diarrhoea, thirst and lassitude. These persist for a few days and then the patient enters the third stage of comparative well-being although anorexia and malaise may persist and there may be a low grade fever. After about 3 weeks the patient enters the final stage. If the dose has exceeded 2 Gy a sudden loss of hair may sometimes precede the other symptoms by a few days. Total loss of body hair is a bad prognostic sign since this generally indicates a whole body exposure of at least 5 Gy. Symptoms of this final stage include increasing malaise with pains in the throat and mouth, both of which become inflamed, oedematous and ulcerated. Blood examination at this time reveals profound thrombocytopaenia and leucopaenia which give rise to purpuric haemorrhages, epistaxis and bloody diarrhoea. The bleeding, or an overwhelming infection, is likely to kill the patient, and even if it does not, then the severe damage sustained by the gastro-intestinal tract will produce chronic diarrhoea and a more gradual demise.

The time scale described above may, in very severe cases, be considerably shortened or it may be considerably delayed. If part of the body is shielded from the radiation, then recovery is greatly assisted, generally by a much greater amount than would be expected.

If the patient is to recover, he or she must survive long enough to allow the cells of the bone marrow and gastric and intestinal mucosa to recover and repair the damage. During this time, blood transfusions, platelet transfusions, intravenous feeding and prompt antibiotic therapy will be required.

Chronic effects of radiation

Conditions which produce the acute radiation syndrome are, fortunately, very rare, although minor accidents are not uncommon. In industry, serious radiation hazards are likely to be encountered only in critical accidents in establishments handling fissile materials. Chronic effects from radiation of which carcinogenesis, leukaemogenesis and genetic disturbance are the most important, are potentially a greater hazard. Cataract formation is discussed elsewhere (p. 149).

Carcinogenesis

Many different types of tumour have been found to have increased frequency in irradiated populations. These include tumours of the skin in those radiologists who were working when X-rays had just been introduced into medical practice, carcinoma of the lung in miners in Schneeburg and Joachimstal, thyroid carcinoma in patients given irradiation to the neck in childhood for thymic enlargement, tumours of the reticuloendothelial system in patients given Thorotrast* and osteosarcomas in the women painting luminous watches with radium and other radioactive elements. The survivors of the two nuclear bomb explosions in Japan have developed a number of different types of tumour in addition to having shown an earlier increased incidence of leukaemia. Patients who had received irradiation therapy for ankylosing spondylitis were also found to be more at risk from leukaemia.

An attempt has been made to quantify the increased risk of cancer on the basis of a linear dose–response relationship. The International Commission on Radiological Protection has estimated the number of cases of cancer likely to occur in a population of a million persons each exposed to 0.01 Gy (Table 9.3). Their

Table 9.3. Estimated risk of cancer from exposure to 0.01 Gy*

Type of cancer	Estimated no. of cases per 10^6 persons exposed[†]
Fatal neoplasms	
Leukaemia[‡]	20
Others	20
Thyroid carcinoma[§]	10–20

*A linear dose–response relationship is assumed. Since the evidence is based on irradiation by X-rays or γ-rays, the absorbed dose is approximately equal to 1 mSv.
[†]Effects would be experienced over 10–20 years.
[‡]Risk may be enhanced by a factor of 2–10 if the fetus is exposed.
[§]Estimated refers to exposure in childhood. Unlike other types of cancer for which estimates are given, incidence is not equivalent to mortality.
Based on data from International Commission on Radiological Protection *The Evaluation of Risks from Radiation*, Pergamon Press, 1966.

estimates should not be taken to be precise, however, but rather as showing a trend. The increased incidence of leukaemia found to result from irradiation given for the treatment of ankylosing spondylitis is shown in Table 8.1)

Genetic effects

It is generally assumed that irradiation during pregnancy carries a risk to the developing fetus and may cause childhood leukaemia. Diagnostic X-rays to the abdomen are discouraged in pregnant women and in other women should be restricted to the 10 days following the onset of menstruation.

Radiation protection

The philosophy underlying all schemes of radiation protection is that exposure to any amount of ionizing radiation carries some risk of harm. Therefore no exposure is permissible unless there is a benefit associated with the exposure. The benefit may not necessarily be received by the person exposed, but may be a benefit to society as a whole. The dose which an exposed person, or society as a whole, receives must therefore be kept as low as possible taking into account all the social and economic costs. There are recommended maximum dose limits for both the general public and for radiation workers (see Table 9.4); in practice in the UK, received doses are much lower than those shown in the Table 9.4; the average annual effective dose for radiation workers is 4 mSv whilst for the general public the average effective dose from occupational sources is 9 μSv per year and approximately 530 μSv per year from all sources.

Recently there has been some concern about the permitted levels of exposure to ionizing radiation since it seems that some of the premises on which these have been calculated were in error. Thus HSE says that levels should be reduced to as low as is reasonably practicable and is likely to reduce the limits of acceptable exposure in 1990. The National Radiological Protection Board has already advised that individual exposures should be reduced to a level of 15 mSv and so the figures in Table 9.4 will almost certainly be shortly out of date.

The doses which radiation workers in the UK receive are routinely monitored by the National Radiation Protection Board and a national register of such workers has been established in which lifetime dose and cause of death are recorded. As the data accumulate, it should be possible to determine whether the causes of death differ as between radiation workers and a comparable group not exposed to radiation, and between groups of radiation workers with different lifetime dose levels.

Table 9.4. Dose limits (mSv per year) for radiation workers and members of the general public

	Worker	General public
Effective dose equivalent	50	5
Dose equivalent to single organ or tissue	500	50
Dose equivalent to the eye	300	30

Radioactive elements

A large number of radioactive elements are used in industry, in universities and other research establishments and in hospitals for diagnostic purposes. The principles governing the use of radionuclides are the same as for the use of any other source of ionizing radiation; when being administered to volunteers (and patients count as volunteers) it is now a legal requirement throughout the countries of the European Community that prior authorization must be obtained. This authorization must take into account the training and experience of the practitioner, the facilities which are available and the types and amount of radionuclides to be used. Radionuclides are classified according to their toxicity per unit activity and use of the most toxic is very restricted. It goes without saying, that patients and volunteers should be properly advised of the procedure and the degree of risk attached to the procedure so that their consent is truly informed.

When using radionuclides, precautions must be taken not only to avoid exposure to the radiation but also to prevent the unsealed sources from coming into contact with the skin or being taken into the body accidentally. Great care must be given to the design of units in which radionuclides are to be handled, and to the disposal of all waste materials. Sealed sources generally present no problems and they can safely be stored until they have decayed to a low activity or are collected by an approved disposal service. The doses used in experiments are low and most waste will be only minimally contaminated and items such as swabs or paper towels can generally be disposed of normally or held for a time until they have decayed to safe levels. Some items may require special laundering. The urine from patients receiving radio-iodine therapy for thyroid carcinoma may be sufficiently radioactive to require retainment with appropriate shielding until the activity has decayed to safe levels, but otherwise, the excreta from subjects who have been administered radionuclides do not present a hazard. Gaseous wastes may arise from radium stores or fume cupboards or from incinerator stacks. Any point of release must be sited so that the gas is rapidly diluted and unable to re-enter the building from which it was emitted.

The activity of radionuclides used for experimental or industrial work is usually so low that it presents no serious hazard provided that normal work practices are adhered to. The supervision of the use of radionuclides should be in the hands of an expert Radiation Protection Officer who would be an ex officio member of any works safety committee. Hospital workers should be carefully instructed in the safe way to handle excreta or vomit from patients treated with radionuclides; there is no danger from implanted sources. Because the degree of exposure is low, it is not necessary to undertake any form of routine monitoring of workers handling radioactive elements; some special investigations may be required if they suffer accidental contamination.

Nonionizing radiation

Electromagnetic radiations with a wavelength greater than 10 nm are incapable of ionizing biological important atoms or molecules because their energy (10 eV) is not sufficiently great and so it is conventionally referred to as nonionizing.

The following categories of nonionizing radiation are of importance in occupational health practice, ultraviolet (UV), infrared (IR) and microwave and radiofrequency (MW/RF); lasers will also be considered here.

Ultraviolet radiation

It is usual to categorize UV radiation into two types on the basis of their harmful potential. UVA occurs in the wavelength 315–400 nm and has relatively little biological effect beyond causing mild erythema and pigmentation. UVB, wavelength 280–315 nm, produces much more serious effects on the skin and on the eyes. It causes marked erythema with a peak effect at 297 nm and, with prolonged exposure, it produces chronic effects such as loss of elasticity and carcinoma.

If the eyes are irradiated by UVB photokeratitis may develop after a variable interval depending on the degree of exposure but usually within 6–12 hours. The condition is known as arc eye because it is seen most frequently in those who look at arc welding without protective goggles—rarely the welder. Arc eye is marked by a painful conjunctivitis and blepharospasm which disappears within 24–48 hours. In the most severe cases the patient may be photophobic for a few days after the incident. The eyes do not develop a tolerance to repeated UV exposure so they must always be protected. Intense UV irradiation may induce the formation of cataracts and there is a suggestion that the cataracts found in furnacemen and others exposed to red heat may be caused by UV rather than infrared radiation. Exposure to solar UV radiation may be responsible for a gradual yellowing of the lens and for the production of senile cataracts.

Exposure standards

Maximum permissible exposures for UVA are expressed in units of Joules per square metre (J/m^2) or in irradiation units of watts per square metre. The limits for the eye and skin for periods of exposure exceeding 10^3 seconds are 10^4 J/m^2 or 10 W/m^2. For UVB, the limits vary according to wavelength. If exposure is to a broad band of UV—as is usually the case—the maximum permitted exposure is calculated from the sum of the relative irradiance from each spectral component, each being weighted by a factor known as the relative spectral effectiveness which is taken as 1.0 for a wavelength of 270 nm. The effective irradiance, E_{eff}, is expressed in W/cm^2. Permissible exposure times per day vary from 8 hours when E_{eff} is 10^{-3} to 10 minutes at 5×10^{-2} and 0.01 seconds when E_{eff} is 3×10^2.

Infrared radiation

IR radiation has a wavelength in the range 700 nm to 1 mm. Its biological effects lie not only in its capacity to heat the tissues by which it is absorbed (the skin and the eye), but also because it can excite vibration in large molecules which releases emissions of UV; hence those exposed to red heat receive both UV and IR radiation.

Radiation in the range 400–1400 nm is transmitted through the eye and focused on the retina. Since it is difficult to look at a bright light for more than a few milliseconds, the eye is protected from the effects of IR. If this aversion reflex is overcome, however, severe retinal burns may be produced and since the radiant energy is focused on the most sensitive part of the retina, the injury can have a catastrophic effect. IR radiation with a wavelength greater than 1400 nm can burn the corneal epithelium; the iris is susceptible to radiation with a wavelength of 1300 nm and the lens is sensitive to two bands, 1400–1600 and 1800–2000 nm. Long-term exposure to IR can produce cataracts because of the increase in temperature in the tissues of the eye which results from absorption. Skin burns may occur at all wavelengths but most people remove themselves from exposure when the skin becomes uncomfortably hot, before any serious damage occurs.

Microwave and radiofrequency radiation

This is defined as radiation having a wavelength in the range 1 mm to 30 km (or a frequency in the range 0.3–300 000 MHz). The main use of MW/RF radiation is in providing a source of heat (as in microwave cookers or heat sealing operations) and in communications. It is the thermal properties of MW/RF radiation which provide the principal risk to health; cataract formation is discussed elsewhere. Local irradiation may cause burns whilst whole body irradiation can induce thermal stress which, if sufficiently severe, may cause death. Such deaths have been produced in animals which have been experimentally exposed to continuous-wave whole body irradiation but no undisputed human case has been reported.

In the countries of eastern Europe it is widely held that low levels of MW/RF radiation can cause a variety of nonthermal effects including changes in behaviour. None of these effects has been recognized in the west where the exposure limit of 10 mW/cm^2 is several orders of magnitude higher than that in the eastern bloc countries.

Lasers

A laser is a device which is used to generate high-intensity beams of electromagnetic energy; the word laser is an acronym for light amplification by stimulated emission of radiation. The device is used to generate a high energy beam of coherent radiomagnetic energy and has three basic components, the active medium, an energy source and a resonant optical cavity. The active (laser) medium contains a population of atoms of molecules which can be raised to a high energy level from the normal ground energy level; in this so-called inverted state, the atoms or molecules can be stimulated to emit photons of the same energy and all in phase. To raise the electrons to high energy levels in a laser, a pumping system is necessary. The pumping system supplies energy to the laser medium until population inversion occurs. There are many pumping systems available including optical, electron collision and chemical reaction. In optical pumping systems, a strong light source is used such as a xenon flashtube or another laser such as a nitrogen or an argon laser. Electron collision pumping is achieved by passing an electric current through a laser medium which may be a gas (as in the case of the helium–neon laser) or a semiconductor junction (as in the gallium arsenide laser). Alternatively, electrons may be accelerated in an electron gun to impact on the laser material. Chemical pumping is based on the energy released during the making or breaking of chemical bonds; some hydrogen fluoride and deuterium fluoride lasers are pumped in this way.

The optical cavity is formed by placing mirrors at each end of the laser medium so that the beam of radiation is passed through the medium several times in order to amplify the number of protons in the medium. One of the mirrors is only partially reflecting so that part of the beam is permitted to escape from the cavity; the geometry of the mirrors determines the shape of the emitted laser beam.

Lasers are generally known by the type of medium which is employed. Thus, they may be solid-state (in which a glass or crystalline medium is used), gas, semiconductor or liquid (in which an organic dye is used). Lasers may operate continuously, in which case they are termed continuous wave lasers and the beam irradiance is constant with time; alternatively they may operate in pulses, delivering repetitive pulses of energy, the duration of which vary from a few milliseconds to fractions of a microsecond.

Laser may emit radiation in the ultraviolet, visible light of infrared spectra and the hazard which is presented by a particular type of laser is dependant upon which is emitted; as expected, however, the target organs are the skin and the eye. Great care must be taken when using lasers that appropriate control is exercised; if the radiation emitted is outside the visible spectrum an aiming beam should be incorporated so that the position of the laser beam can be inferred. Locks must be included in the design of the laser so that the instrument cannot be switched on accidentally and the device should be used only by authorized personnel. All workers involved with lasers should be issued with and wear the appropriate safety goggles and when used for surgery, the patient must be protected. For CO_2 lasers (which emit IR) cotton wool pads soaked in saline can protect the patient's eyes and saline soaked clothing may also be required. It should be noted that CO_2 lasers can set dry cotton or paper drapes on fire and this must be taken into account when using them in the operating theatre. For all uses, a local code of practice must be established and a laser safety officer should be appointed.

Maximum permissible exposure limits (MPELs) have been recommended for both direct exposures and for exposure from a diffuse reflection of a laser beam. The MPELs are expressed in terms of the radiance (in watts or J/cm^2) falling on the cornea. On the basis of the type and energy of their emissions, it is possible to put lasers into four classes:

Class 1: These are the lowest powered lasers and are not considered hazardous if they are incapable of damaging the eye or burning the skin.

Class 2: Only lasers which emit visible light (within the spectrum 400–700 nm) fall within this class and they are considered to be low risk because damage to the eye will occur only if the normal aversion response to bright light is overcome. Since there will always be a few people who will force themselves to stare fixedly into an intensely bright light for a minute or two, lasers in this class should bear a label to warn of the dangers of this practice.

Class 3: Lasers in this class are moderate risk because they can cause damage to the retina within the natural aversion response time (about 0.25 seconds). They do not cause serious skin damage and their diffuse reflections are not dangerous under normal use. The safety precautions which must be taken in their use, however, are often considerable.

Class 4: These are the lasers of highest power and most risk. They may cause serious injury to the skin by direct exposure and their diffuse reflections may cause damage to the eye. In addition, class 4 lasers present a serious fire risk.

Noise

There are many occupations in which the daily exposure to noise may impair hearing or reduce efficiency, or both. The intensity of sound is expressed in terms of the square of the sound pressure. By convention the units are in steps or ratios of tenfold intensity, each unit known as a bel. For practical purposes units of one-tenth of a bel, the decibel (dB) are used.

On instruments used to measure sound the zero point on the scale is taken as being equal to a sound pressure of 0.0002 microbars, the weakest sound pressure which can be detected by a child under very quiet conditions. With any given sound pressure, however, the response varies with the frequency of the sound, maximum sensitivity occurring between 1000 and 4000 cycles per second or Hertz (Hz). The auditory field lies between 20 and 20 000 Hz but the threshold of differentiation between two sounds varies with frequency, each frequency having specific maximum and minimum audibility thresholds. Between 1000 and 4000 Hz the differential threshold varies very little and this is the zone of maximum sensitivity to sound intensity. The threshold of audibility is at its minimum at 4000 Hz and at this frequency is located the zone of impairment of high pitched tones that occur in the very early stages of hearing loss.

When measuring sound, allowance is made for the variation in response to sound of different frequencies. Sound level meters incorporate electrical circuits, known as weighting networks, which provide for variation in sensitivity to sound of different frequencies, the objective being to simulate the character-istics of the ear. A number of scales are in use, but the A weighting is the one generally used for descriptive purposes and sound levels are reported in dB(A). Some typical sound levels are shown in Table 9.5.

Acoustic reflex

The ear is protected to some extent from noise by the acoustic reflex. In response to loud sounds, the stapedius and tensor tympani muscles contract, with the result that less energy is transmitted to the sound receptors of the inner

Table 9.5. Sound levels of some sources of noise

Source	level dBA	
Conversation	60	Quiet
Light traffic at 30 m	66	Moderately loud
Dishwasher	76	
Key-punch machine	82	
Milling machine	90	Very loud
Bench lathe	95	
Newspaper press	101	
Textile loom	112	Uncomfortably loud
Pneumatic drill	122	
Aircraft carrier jet deck	140	Painfully loud

ear. The protection afforded is limited by muscle fatigue and by the delay in response so that it is impossible to cope with sudden, unexpected sounds.

Auditory fatigue and masking

Auditory fatigue and masking are physiological effects noted on exposure to noise. Auditory fatigue causes a temporary shift in threshold with a consequent decrease in hearing. As the intensity of the sound increases, auditory fatigue becomes more marked and may be associated with tinnitus. It is greatest at 4000 Hz.

Recovery may take several hours, especially if the threshold has risen by more than 50 dB. Pure tones have more effect than broadband noise, and intermittent sounds more than continuous sound. In individuals with a high susceptibility towards a temporary threshold shift there appears to be an association with occupational hearing loss.

Masking refers to the process whereby the threshold of hearing of one sound is raised by the presence of another. The effect becomes more noticeable as the frequencies of the two sounds approach each other. Masking can interfere with the understanding of speech and this can have important repercussions in industry, limiting communication or threatening safety.

Hearing loss

Occupational hearing loss represents the transition from a temporary threshold shift to one which is permanent and it usually has a gradual and often unsuspected onset; it should not be forgotten, however, that severe acoustic trauma such as that experienced in an explosion, may cause immediate deafness by rupturing the ear drum, disrupting the ossicles and damaging the inner ear. The first sign of occupational hearing loss is usually a slight impairment of hearing, detected by audiometry in the 4000 Hz range, spreading at a later stage to the 3000–6000 Hz range (Fig. 9.2). This characteristic pattern allows occupational hearing loss to be differentiated from other forms of deafness. The patient may be completely unaware of any defect in hearing until the speech

(a)

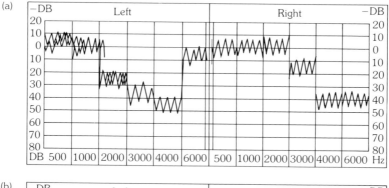

(b)

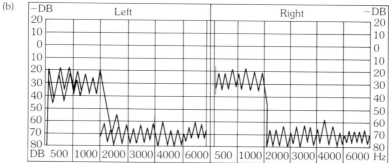

Fig. 9.2 Audiograms showing mild (a) and more extensive (b) hearing loss of occupational origin

frequencies are affected. The speech frequencies lie between 500 and 2000 Hz and may be subdivided into vowel (500–1000 Hz) and consonant frequencies (1000–2000 Hz).

When hearing loss occurs in these frequencies, speech becomes increasingly difficult to understand, and the patient suffers from some degree of social handicap. It may take years for deafness of this severity to develop but there is no possibility of its reversal since it implies permanent damage to the organ of Corti.

Impulse noise is the most dangerous form, gunfire being notorious for damaging the hearing of those behind the rifles. The intermittent noise of drop-forging is another source which can lead to a rapid deterioration in hearing.

Aetiology of occupational deafness

The ultimate site of the damage induced by noise is the sensory hair cells on the basilar membrane of the cochlea but why the damage is restricted to a relatively small region of the basilar membrane (that which responds most sensitively to 4000 Hz) is not clear. It has been suggested that noise may induce strong mechanical forces along the organ of Corti which physically shake the cells of the membrane and that the 4000 Hz area on the membrane is most susceptible to physical damage. Other authorities have noted that intense noise stimulation induces vasoconstriction in the capillaries in the cochlea which reduces the supply of oxygen and nutrients to the hair cells; under this theory, the cells at 4000 Hz would be inherently more sensitive to this deprivation than cells in other areas.

Nonauditory effects of noise

Noise has been shown to produce effects on the body in addition to causing hearing loss. The heart rate is modified in response to noise, being either increased or decreased depending on the type of noise, and the respiratory rate often increases. Cardiac output is generally decreased and peripheral vasoconstriction may cause blanching of the skin in some people.

All these changes reflect a response on the part of the adrenal gland or the autonomic nervous sytem to the noise stimulus analogous to those demonstrated by someone who is frightened, and it is unlikely that they are specifically caused by the noise but rather by the individual's reaction to it. None of these changes is permanent and the suggestion than those exposed to noise are more likely than average to develop hypertension has not been confirmed.

Psychological effects

Noise can affect the performance of psychomotor tasks either adversely or beneficially depending upon its intensity, frequency, duration and intermittence. Sudden, unexpected noise always interferes with the performance of a task, whether mental or physical. Canned music is often introduced into works and other situations with the notion that it engenders a sense of well-being and improves efficiency. Some studies appear to bear out this assumption. Many individuals, however, find that such intrusions are annoying and that they interfere with their performance. The attitude to noise at work seems largely determined by the significance which the individual attaches to it.

Noise and mental illness

There is little reliable evidence that there is any connection between noise and neurotic illness although some categories of neurotic patients show responses to noise which are markedly different from those of normal subjects. For example, hysterical patients fail to habituate noise whilst anxious patients will show a much greater than normal adrenal response.

Deafness is associated with significantly higher rates of mental illness in the community and in hospital populations. In the elderly, deafness is likely to be associated with paranoid states, whereas in young patients, affective disorders are more common. Deafness acquired during late childhood or early adult life causes a profound change in life style and leads to an increased feeling of isolation. The deaf are treated with much less sympathy by their fellows than the blind, and this may help foster the sense of isolation.

Since noise may induce deafness, it can thus be said to have a secondary effect on mental illness.

Hearing conservation

There are many components to a hearing conservation programme, including the reduction of noise at source, limiting exposure with or without ear protectors, and routine monitoring of the workplace and of the work population exposed.

Reducing noise at source can be achieved by enclosing noisy areas with sound insulating partitions, by silencing exhaust systems, and by enclosing noisy machines, or by enclosing the operator of a noisy machine in an insulated box. When choosing new machinery or deciding which of a number of different processes to use, the industrialist should take noise control into account as an important factor in making the decision.

Under the Noise at Work Regulations which came into force on 1 January 1990, employers must make noise assessments where workers are likely to be exposed to levels of 85 dB(A) or more. Employees should be given some indication of the risks which they run with this degree of exposure and ear muffs must be made available to them. When exposure levels reach 90 dB(A), employers must do all that is reasonably practicable to reduce the need for people to work in these areas but where this cannot be avoided, hearing protection must be worn; it should be noted that employees are *required* to wear hearing protection when noise levels are 90 dB(A) and above.

Ear protectors are of several forms and they vary considerably in their ability to cut out noise. The simplest forms are ear-plugs, either reusable rubber or plastic plugs which come in several sizes, or disposable plugs fashioned from 'acoustic wool'. For the re-usable plugs to be effective, they must be of a correct size and make a good seal in the auditory canal. Care must be taken to keep them clean by regular washing. Acoustic wool is extremely fine glass fibre which can be formed to make a plug for insertion into the ear. It is discarded after use. The wool comes in dispensers which automatically supply the correct amount to make a plug. It is cheap and effective but some people develop an eczematous reaction to the glass fibre which may require them to discontinue its use. Cotton wool is an extremely poor protector and should not be used.

The most effective form of protection is the earmuff of which there are two varieties, those with a liquid seal and those with a seal of soft plastic foam. The degree of protection they afford is tested by audiometry and their efficiency varies according to the frequency of the sound (Table 9.6). Their main

Table 9.6. Typical performance of fluid seal ear muffs*

Frequency (Hz)	125	250	500	1000	2000	4000	8000
Mean attenuation (dB)	13	20	33	35	38	47	41
Standard deviation (dB)	6	6	6	6	7	8	8
Assumed protection (dB)	7	14	27	29	31	39	33

*The assumed protection is the sound reduction given to the majority of users, and is obtained by subtracting the standard deviation from the mean attenuation. From Department of Employment *Code of Practice for Reducing the Exposure of Employed Persons to Noise*, HMSO, 1972.

disadvantage is that they are uncomfortable because they are sweat-traps and workers cannot always be persuaded to continue with them, preferring the less effective ear-plugs.

Routine audiometry is often used to monitor hearing loss in individuals exposed to noise, the results being compared with those of a test performed before the worker was exposed. It would be clearly unwise for an individual who already has some hearing deficit to be employed in a job which entails some risk of further deterioration. Many firms now use audiometry programmes on their employees and apparatus is available which enables the employees under test to administer it themselves.

Ultrasonic and infrasonic noise

Ultrasonic waves are those generated at frequencies above the limit of human hearing. They occur in the range from about 16 kHz up to about 10 MHz. Ultrasound has a number of industrial applications including cleaning and welding plastics, drying fine powders, emulsification and detecting flaws in materials. It is also becoming increasingly used in medicine, mainly in the fields of obstetrics, cardiology, neurology and ophthalmology.

It has been suspected that ultrasonic waves may lead to the local generation of heat in biological materials. Experimental studies have shown that tissue damage can result from ultrasound but follow-up studies of mothers and fetuses have not revealed this to be a hazard in obstetric use.

Hearing loss and vasoconstriction have been reported concomitants of its industrial use, but some effects attributed to ultrasound have been blamed on sound in the high frequency audible range.

Infrasound, such as is generated by diesel engines, generators and turbo-jet and rocket engines has been shown to produce dramatic effects in exposed subjects. Vertigo and nausea are caused by the excitation of the semicircular canals and the vibrations may produce resonance in the internal organs producing a sensation of discomfort. Vibrations in the chest wall may induce changes in respiration. Subjective symptoms such as headache and fatigue have been recorded.

Careful experimentation using human volunteers has indicated that men wearing ear protectors can tolerate noise in the 1–100 Hz range for short duration even when the sound pressure levels are as high as 150 dB. For the frequency range above 40 Hz, however, such exposure approaches the limits of tolerance.

Vibration

Vibrating tools may give rise to injury to the soft tissue of the hands and cause pains in the joints of the arms, most commonly the elbows and wrists. Workers using pneumatic tools and chain saws are commonly found to have small cysts and vacuoles and osteoporotic changes in the bones of the wrist on X-ray examination. These are usually symptomless and do not give rise to any complaint. The other common disorder, however, is vibration induced white finger. This condition occurs in a variety of occupations and all those who use pneumatic tools or rotating tools for grinding and other purposes are potentially at risk. Chain saw operators are a high risk group who have been intensively studied in recent years.

Vibration induced white finger (VWF) takes several years to develop as a rule and is commonly preceded by tingling and numbness in the fingers. Blanching is first noticed in 1 or 2 fingers in the winter but as the condition progresses, all the fingers become involved and episodes of blanching occur in both winter and summer. The condition can be arbitrarily divided into a number of stages for descriptive purposes (Table 9.7).

Table 9.7. Stages of vibration induced white finger

Stage	Condition of digits	Work and social interference
O	No blanching of digits	No complaints
O$_T$	Intermittent tingling	No interference with activities
O$_N$	Intermittent numbness	
1	Blanching of one or more fingertips with or without tingling and numbness	No interference with activities
2	Blanching of one or more complete fingers with numbness usually confined to winter	Slight interference with home and with social activities. Restriction of hobbies
3	Extensive blanching usually all fingers bilateral. Frequent episodes summer as well as winter	Definite interference at work, at home and with social activities. Restriction of hobbies
4	Extensive blanching. All fingers; frequent episodes summer and winter	Occupation changed to avoid further vibration exposure because of severity of signs and symptoms

The mechanism by which the changes found in VWF are induced is not clearly understood. Arteriograms of affected patients show that the proximal segments of the digital arteries may be occluded but the occlusion is related to attacks of finger blanching only to the extent that the degree of occlusion affects the blood flow through the finger. Thus, reducing the blood flow will make the finger more susceptible to the effect of cold, but this, in itself, does not produce the blanching effect.

Histologically, the occluded arteries show marked medial hypertrophy and fibrosis with extreme intimal thickening and elastosis. These changes reduce the size of the lumen but the final obliteration often results from thrombosis and the organization of the thrombus.

There is no doubt that during an attack of white finger the circulation of the finger has ceased but, as already mentioned, arterial occlusion does not cause blanching of the skin, rather it is due to the loss of blood from the subpapillary venous plexuses. Fingertip blood flow is diminished in response to cold in users of vibrating tools, whether or not they have VWF, but in contrast to normal subjects, there is no subsequent phase of cold dilatation. Various hypotheses have been put forward to explain this phenomenon, including failure of local biochemical regulations due to damage to the vessel wall or nerve endings in the fingers. The fact that the condition frequently progresses even when the man changes his work, suggests that the damage sustained is permanent. The more popular hypothesis is that the damage sustained by nerve endings is the most significant, but an alternative point of view holds that the formation of callus in the finger pads eliminates the reservoir of blood which is normally present in the small blood vessels and which is necessary to accommodate sudden changes in blood volume.

The question as to whether VWF progresses to produce the clinical features associated with Raynaud's phenomenon is still a matter for some dispute. Most authorities, however, incline to the view that Raynaud's phenomenon of occupational origin is a definite entity and patients have been described with severe trophic changes in the hand, including gangrene, apparently as the result of their work. Despite this, the Industrial Injuries Advisory Council has declined to recognize this disease as qualifying for industrial compensation.

Prevention

A number of countries, including the USSR, Czechoslovakia and Japan have regulations governing the use of vibrating tools. In Great Britain, the British Standards Institute has produced draft recommendations but as yet there are no regulations. The British Standards Institute recommendations are based on the acceleration produced in m/s^2 in a wide range of frequencies and on the time and type of exposure. For a 5-hour period of continuous exposure, or an 8-hour period of interrupted exposure the maximum acceleration allowed is shown in Table 9.8.

For exposure of shorter duration, greater accelerations may be permitted. Where this is less than 30 minutes continuous exposure, then the values in Table 9.8 may be increased by a factor of 10.

Whole body vibration

Mechanical vibration between 5 and 11 Hz will cause the body to resonate. Exposure to vibration of this frequency occurs in bus, truck and tractor drivers and in helicopter and aeroplane pilots. Whole body vibration is thought to predispose to back pain and changes in the lumbar and thoracic vertebrae have been recorded. In the USA, prostatitis seems to be a particular hazard amongst army drivers who refer to the condition as jeep drivers' disease.

Table 9.8. Maximum accelerations recommended in each frequency range in vibrating tools

Frequency	Up to 16	31.5	63	125	250	500	1000	2000
Maximum acceleration m/s^2	1	2	4	8	16	32	64	128

BSI Draft Recommendations.

Sick building syndrome

This is an inaccurate and inelegant term which is applied to the symptoms which may be experienced by those who work in new, or newly renovated, buildings. It is characteristic that the building is entirely artificially lit and air conditioned so that it is impossible for the worker to open a window, alter the temperature or change the lighting. The symptoms invariably occur in epidemics and those most commonly complained of include headaches, irritation of the eyes, nose and throat, pains in the joints or muscles, fatigue, and tightness in the chest. The symptoms are generally thought by the patients to be caused by some contaminant in the environment, perhaps coming from the air conditioning system. They may begin after urea-formaldehyde insulating foam has been installed. In many cases the most extensive surveying of the environment reveals no abnormality other than low humidity and the symptoms may remit when the humidity is increased; sometimes altering the lighting also has a beneficial effect. This condition can be clearly distinguished from humidifier fever and the air conditioning is generally blameless if it is not sending round air which is too dry. If urea-formaldehyde foam is installed badly there may be a leakage of formaldehyde from cracks in the walls or around window frames or central heating pipes and the concentration of gas may be sufficient to produce conjunctivitis and irritation of the upper respiratory tract. The concentration of formaldehyde rapidly falls as the foam hardens, however, but symptoms noted after the event may be considered to have been caused by the gas. In a small number of cases, patients appear to have become sensitized to formaldehyde or to dust from the foam and they develop asthma.

In the majority of cases no external agent can be found to account for the symptoms and it is most probable that workers are somatizing their dislike for an environment over which they have no control. There is obviously an overlap between this syndrome and mass hysteria and it can be a most difficult condition with which to cope.

Chapter 10
Infectious Diseases

Dirt in one form or another is an inevitable accompaniment of many forms of work and thus sepsis following accidental cuts at work is common. For this reason employees in many factories are encouraged to have courses of immunization against tetanus.

In some occupations there is a considerable risk from general infections, medical and veterinary practice being outstanding examples. Workers in laboratories in which micro-organisms are handled for diagnostic or experimental purposes are also at risk and in an attempt to contain this risk, a strict code of practice must be adhered to. Pathogens can be classified according to the risk they present and the precautions taken when handling them vary accordingly. Four risk categories have been proposed, as follows:

Group 1: A biological agent that is most unlikely to cause human disease;

Group 2: A biological agent that may cause human disease and which might be a hazard to laboratory workers but which is unlikely to spread in the community at large. Laboratory exposure rarely produces infection and effective prophylaxis or treatment are available;

Group 3: A biological agent that may cause severe human disease and present a serious hazard to laboratory workers. It may also present a risk of spread within the community but effective prophylaxis or treatment are usually available; and

Group 4: A biological agent which has all the properties of Group 3 organisms but for which there is usually no effective prophylaxis or treatment.

The majority of pathogenic bacteria fall into Group 2 whilst all the *Rickettsiacae* are put into Group 3. Most fungi are Group 2 organisms as are most parasites. All viruses are classified as at least Group 2; the hepatitis B virus is a Group 3 pathogen whilst the viruses which cause haemorrhagic fever are in Group 4.

Specific infectious disease of occupational origin are relatively few in number; those which are most serious or which occur most commonly are discussed below.

Hepatitis B

Amongst the various forms of viral hepatitis, A and B (formerly known as non-A and non-B), only hepatitis B presents a serious occupational risk at present, particularly to hospital staff and others whose work brings them into contact with blood and blood products. The risk from hepatitis B was highlighted during the rapid introduction of renal dialysis units when there were several cases in the staff of the units, some of them fatal. In due time, a code of practice was evolved which has considerably diminished the risk to staff in renal units.

Contact with the virus is most often brought about by inoculation injuries or when blood comes into contact with mucous membranes, following a splash of blood in the eyes, for example. The incubation period varies between 30 and 150 days and the symptoms of the disease include malaise, myalgia, headache, nausea, vomiting, anorexia, abdominal pain and pruritus. The patient becomes jaundiced, passing dark urine and pale stools, and the liver may be tender and enlarged. Liver function tests will be wildly abnormal; the diagnosis is confirmed by demonstrating the presence of surface antigen (HBsAg). The normal course of events is that the patient will show a brisk antibody response and recover completely. At the end of the illness, the patient will retain a relatively high antibody (HBAB) titre but will be antigen negative. A proportion of patients will become carriers, however, and some may develop chronic hepatitis.

Prevention

All staff who work in renal units should be screened for the presence of HbsAg and those who are found to be positive should be employed elsewhere. Patients who are known to be antigen positive should be dialysed away from the main unit; donor blood is screened for surface antigen and not used if it is found to be positive.

Hepatitis B vaccination

Hepatitis B vaccination is offered as a prophylactic measure to hospital staff; sometimes to all and sundry and sometimes only to those considered to be at risk of contracting the disease. The first vaccine to come onto the market was plasma derived but this fell out of favour because of fears that it might be contaminated with HIV although there was never a reasonable foundation for this fear. The vaccine which is now used is derived from yeast through genetic engineering and consequently does not suffer from the stigma attached to its predecessor. Those to be vaccinated receive three injections each of 1 ml of vaccine. The vaccine should be given into the deltoid muscle and not into the buttock as conversion rates are higher with the former route. The first and second injections are separated by 4 weeks and the second and third by a further 20 weeks. There is no need to screen potential vaccinees for the presence of antibodies prior to vaccination since their prevalence in the community is too low to make this a cost-effective procedure. Three months or so after finishing the course it is customary to check the antibody response; those whose antibody titre is greater than 10 m-international units/ml are considered to have produced a satisfactory response. In practice, the great majority of individuals have a much greater response than this and about 95% of those vaccinated have a satisfactory response and can be considered immune. Individuals who are negative after three injections of the vaccine can be offered a fourth dose after which their antibody levels should be checked again a month later; many will be found to have an adequate response following the fourth dose. There are no absolute guidelines as to the action which should be taken for individuals who persist in refusing to produce antibodies to a fourth dose but it seems reasonable to offer another booster. Some individuals may not convert because they are carrying the hepatitis B antigen, and so it is worth considering testing persistent nonresponders to see if they have antibodies to the hepatitis B core antigen which indicates past infection and then go on to test for antigen status in those who are HBcAB positive.

It must be emphasized to those who are at risk from contracting hepatitis B at work that vaccination is no substitute for safe working practices and indeed, it may even be more cost effective to employ sufficient occupational health personnel to ensure that there are appropriate codes of practice and that these are adhered to, rather than continue with wholesale vaccination.

High risk injuries

In all establishments where contact with hepatitis B is possible there should be provision for dealing with those who have had an inoculation or other high risk injury. No matter how seemingly trivial, any such injury should be reported to the occupational health department as soon as possible. There are two people involved in a high risk accident, the person who has had the accident and the patient whose blood was inoculated or who may otherwise have placed the member of staff at risk. Action needs to be taken on both. If the patient can be identified, then his or her antigen status should be determined. If they are antigen negative no further action need be taken. If they are positive, or if they are considered to be at high risk of being positive in the absence of being able to determine their antigen status in the laboratory, then the antibody status of the member of staff must be checked, assuming that they have had a course of vaccination. Those with a satisfactory response within the last 2 years need no further action; where more than 2 years has elapsed since the determination of the antibody levels, a further booster dose of vaccine is advisable.

Those who have not had a course of vaccination or who have not produced a satisfactory antibody response should be given immediate passive protection through an injection of specific immunoglobulin and a course of vaccination started at the same time to encourage the development of active immunity.

Although medical and nursing staff may be at risk from contracting the disease from their patients, there have been few instances in which it has been shown that antigen positive doctors or nurses have infected their patients. A few outbreaks of hepatitis have been traced to dentists but this risk can be minimized if the dentist wears gloves when working, since infection usually results from the leakage of serum from small lacerations on the hand into the patient's mouth. In a very few cases, hepatitis B has been transmitted from surgeons to their patients as a result of blood from the surgeon getting into the wound following a laceration on a scalpel or needle. Scrupulous attention to technique and wearing an additional pair of gloves have been found to eliminate the risk. There is at present a misconception amongst medical and surgical staff that if they were found to be antigen positive this would lead to their sudden and premature retirement. This is not so and shows a curious, not to say complacent frame of mind. An antigen positive surgeon does not pose less of a risk to his patients because he does not know he is antigen positive; indeed, by knowing, he is much more likely to be safer since he will then take greater care when operating.

One other preventive method which can be employed is to screen all high risk patients when they are admitted to hospital; if any are found to be antigen positive when the hospital staff can be forewarned to take extra care when taking blood or giving any form of treatment which necessitates the use of knife or needle.

Aids

When patients with AIDS were first admitted to hospitals and clinics there was great alarm amongst the staff that they might be greatly at risk of contracting the disease themselves. The risks are similar to those of contracting hepatitis B, that is, following inoculation injuries or other incidents which result in intimate contact with blood or other body fluids. In fact, AIDS appears to be very much less infective than hepatitis B and the number of health workers who have become HIV positive following such an incident is extremely small. There is very little to be done after a high risk accident except to save serum to serve as a base line in case the individual develops symptoms at some time in the future. Clearly the risk of becoming HIV positive applies only if the patient involved in the incident is positive themselves. If it is possible to determine that this is in fact the case, then the member of staff must be counselled by someone with the necessary skills and experience and must be followed up and their HIV status determined—with their consent and after proper counselling—at an appropriate interval which should certainly not be less than 3 months. The prophylactic use of zidovudine (Retrovir) does not seem to be indicated in our current state of knowledge.

Anthrax

Anthrax is the result of infection with the *Bacillus anthracis*, a Gram-positive, spore-forming organism. The spores are extremely resistant and can survive for long periods in the soil and in animal remains. Cattle are the main reservoir of infection, but these days, imported foodstuffs such as bone and fish meal account for most cases. All those handling infected meat, hides and skin, wool or other animal products are potentially at risk. Workers in bone meal factories are probably the group with the highest exposure and cases have occurred in gardeners handling infected bone meal. Hides and skins, wool and hair imported from the Far and Middle East are notorious for their potential to transmit the infection.

Three varieties of the disease occur, cutaneous, pulmonary and gastro-intestinal, the last two being rare in this country, the g-i form very rare.

Cutaneous anthrax

This form of the disease usually occurs on an exposed part of the body and is caused by spores from infected material gaining entry through cuts or abrasions on the skin. The condition is sometimes referred to as malignant pustule, but this is an inaccurate description since the lesion is rarely malignant and never pustular. In three-quarters of all cases the lesions occur on the face, head and neck.

After an incubation time of 1–4 days a small, irritant red papule develops which rapidly becomes vesicular and necrotic in the centre forming a characteristic black eschar. This lesion may be surrounded by a ring of secondary vesicles from which B. anthracis can be cultured. Pain is not common, but itching is. Widespread nonpitting oedema often surrounds the lesion but lymph node involvement is rare. Constitutional symptoms and fever are usually absent unless the skin infection is severe or the infection becomes disseminated, when pyrexia, collapse and death are all possible events. In cases where the lesion is on the face or neck, the intense oedema may threaten life.

The disease can usually be diagnosed on clinical grounds and by the culture of fluid obtained from the vesicles or from under the eschar. Blood cultures should also be made. Serological tests are available if necessary, the best known being Ascoli's test, and fluorescent antibody techniques can also be used for the identification of bacteria in cultures or tissue sections.

Pulmonary anthrax

Pulmonary anthrax was once relatively common amongst workers in the woollen industry and was referred to as 'wool-sorters' disease'. Nowadays, only a very small percentage of cases are of this sort. There is no external lesion and this makes diagnosis difficult. The illness begins abruptly and there are severe toxaemic symptoms. Haemorrhagic mediastinitis with widening of the mediastinal shadow on X-rays and haemorrhagic meningitis may occur. There is widespread pulmonary congestion and oedema with frothy bloodstained sputum. Death is very common in this form of anthrax and the disease may run its complete course in just a few days.

Treatment

Penicillin and tetracycline are both effective, penicillin being the drug of choice. In cutaneous cases recovery is the rule and there is usually no scarring. The pulmonary disease may progress so rapidly that death results even with appropriate treatment.

Prevention of the disease depends upon its eradication in animals. In Great Britain anthrax in cattle is rare and when it does occur the animal is destroyed and the carcase deeply buried or cremated without autopsy, and the rest of the herd is vaccinated. Disease control in other countries is often ineffective and thus it is difficult to prevent the importation of potentially infective material. Regulations exist governing the importation and disinfection of wool and hair but other animal products are exempt. Bone meal is almost impossible to sterilize and those handling it should be protected by wearing gloves and by the downwards ventilation of working surfaces.

Immunization against anthrax is now freely available to those for whom the disease may be an occupational hazard. Three intramuscular injections of vaccine are given at intervals of 3 weeks, followed by a booster dose 6 months after the third injection. An annual booster is recommended for those who continue at risk. Reactions to the vaccine are rare and when they do occur, are usually mild. Cases of anthrax have not occurred in those who have completed the course of immunization.

Glanders

Glanders, or farcy, is a disease of horses, mules and donkeys, although most warm-blooded animals, except the ox, pig and the white mouse, may become infected. The infecting organism is a Gram-negative bacillus variously called *Pfeiferella mallei* or *Bacillus mallei*. Infection in humans is now very rare and is the result of contact with an infected animal. Horsehair is also said to be a potential source of infection. The disease occurs in both an acute and a chronic form.

Acute glanders

There is an incubation period of 2–3 days before the patient experiences symptoms of general malaise, headache, anorexia and joint pains. The site of infection becomes ulcerated and there is a marked lymphangitis. Nodular abscesses form along the lymphatics and these break down to form painful ulcers. There is a marked pyrexia, highest between the sixth and twelfth days after which time a characteristic eruption appears on the face and on the nasal, palatal and pharyngeal mucosae. The lesions begin as erythematous patches which rapidly become papular and then pustular. The pustules ulcerate with the destruction of bone and cartilage to produce a thick, bloodstained purulent discharge. A destructive arthritis may also occur with abscess formation in the muscles.

Diagnosis is difficult, but can be established by a history of contact with horses, by agglutination and/or complement fixation tests, by skin tests and by isolation of the organism.

Chronic glanders

This is rarer than the acute form of the disease and is characterized by the formation of abscesses, which break down to form destructive, painful ulcers. The lungs may be involved with the production of pneumonia, pleural effusion, lung abscesses and emphysema. The disease runs a long course and an acute phase may supervene at any time.

Treatment

There are reports of successful treatment with sulphonamides. Streptomycin, tetracycline and chloramphenicol may all be useful but there is, as yet, little clinical experience of the use of antibiotics in the disease. Treatment should be rigorous since the disease carries a 90% mortality rate.

The disease has ceased to be a public health problem with the identification and destruction of infected animals.

Leptospirosis

Infection with pathogenic leptospires produces a wide variety of clinical signs and symptoms. The disease is transmitted to humans from the many animals which act as reservoir hosts, including dogs, cats, cattle and pigs. Seven separate sero-groups of pathogenic organisms are known in Great Britain, *Australis, Autumnalis, Ballum, Canicola, Hebdomadis, Ictero-haemorrhagiae* and *Javanica*. They are not all equally virulent, but the clinical manifestations and the pathological lesions produced by each and their modes of transmission are similar enough to justify considering them all together.

Transmission may occur by direct contact with the blood, tissues or organs of infected animals, the kidneys being the most likely to be infective. More commonly, however, infection occurs from indirect contact with urine. The leptospires have a tendency to persist in the convoluted tubules and to multiply on the epithelium. From this site they are shed in the urine to contaminate the soil, water, or vegetation on which the urine chances to fall.

The occupations which are thought of as being traditionally most at risk, sewer workers, miners and workers in slaughterhouses and fish markets are now seldom affected, and most cases occur in farmers, usually due to *Hebdomadis* infections.

Leptospires can easily pass through intact skin to reach the blood stream. The infection consists of two overlapping phases, leptospiraemia, during which antibodies are produced, and leptospiruria. Symptoms occur mainly in the leptospiraemic phase.

There are no local signs of infection and there is a latent interval of about 7–12 days before the patient develops a fever. At this time the leptospires multiply in the blood and may be carried to and affect any organ.

There are no pathognomonic signs or symptoms and so clinical diagnosis tends to be unreliable. In addition to fever, the patient may complain of malaise, myalgia, arthralgia, sore throat, conjunctivitis, abdominal pain and tenderness often localized to the right hypochondrium, headache, neck stiffness and photophobia. Conjunctival haemorrhages may also be noted, together with a macular rash often accompanied by petaechial haemorrhages. Lymphadenopathy and hepatomegaly may be found on clinical examination. Epistaxis, haemoptysis and haematuria when they occur are generally slight, but may be severe enough to require transfusion.

Albuminuria with cells and granular casts are common in the early stages of the disease and are usually transient phenomena but in some cases severe urinary symptoms develop, the blood urea rises and anuria may follow.

There is often mild hepatocellular damage with a moderate increase in transaminase levels, and jaundice may be noted 2–5 days after the onset of fever.

The ESR is invariably raised and there is often an elevation in the white cell count, with a preponderance of polymorphs.

There is usually a steady clinical improvement during the second week of the illness and mild cases recover completely without specific treatment; fatalities are rare unless renal damage is severe.

The diagnosis rests on serological testing; leptospirosis is distinguished in the first place from other causes of fever or jaundice by a complement fixing test using a compound screening antigen. If this is positive, further agglutination tests will identify the serogroup to which the organism belongs.

Pencillin is the treatment of choice, although most other antibiotics are effective, the principal exception being chloramphenicol. Large doses should be used, and treatment begun as early in the course of the disease as possible and continued for 7 days. There are usually no long term sequelae of the disease.

Erysipeloid of Rosenbach

This disease is caused by a Gram-positive organism *Erysipelothrix rhusiopathiae*. It occurs following contact with infected animals or animal products, especially pig, fish and game, but it may also develop in those who handle root vegetables grown in contaminated soil. Those who follow high risk occupations are veterinary surgeons and workers in slaughterhouses and fish or meat markets.

Generally it is a trivial condition, the site most often affected being the finger. Infection occurs through an abrasion on the skin and is signalled by pain and swelling in the affected part. The lesion is red or purple in colour with a sharply defined margin. It may spread up the finger to the web and descend from there into the next finger. Commonly it spreads onto the dorsum but not the palm of the hand and it seldom extends above the wrist. The pain may be severe but most often is not and there is no throbbing as in pyogenic infection. Lymphgangitis is uncommon. Constitutional symptoms are rare and the lesion rapidly resolves leaving no disability. The lesion is usually sufficiently distinctive to enable a diagnosis to be made without resort to the laboratory.

The disease may in rare cases become generalized and give rise to toxaemic symptoms. In these cases widespread erythema is followed by severe urticaria presenting in the form of rhomboid-shaped lesions, 1–2 cm in size. A bacteraemia form is also known which may be complicated by bacterial endocarditis.

Treatment with penicillin will shorten the duration of the disease but those who contract it know its self-limiting nature and seldom seek treatment. All those who handle material likely to be infected should wear protective gloves, but seldom do.

Ankylostomiasis

This disease is due to the presence of nematode worms in the gut. Man is the natural host for two species of nematode, *Ankylostoma duodenale,* and *Necator americanis.* There is no intermediate host and the ova are excreted in the faeces and hatch in warm moist conditions. The larvae gain entrance to the new host through abraded skin.

Ankylostomiasis is common in the tropics, in southern Europe and in Asia. As an occupational disease it is now an historical curiosity although still one of the prescribed occupational diseases. It was once prevalent in the Cornish tin miners where the hot, moist and insanitary conditions favoured the hatching of the ova (the ovum requires a temperature in excess of 75°C to hatch).

Brucellosis

Brucellosis in humans is caused by contact with infected animals. The organism is Gram-negative and three species account for most human disease. These species show an affinity for particular animal hosts so that *Br. abortus* is found in cattle, *Br. melitensis* in sheep and goats and *Br. suis* in pigs.

The disease may occur in employees working in slaughterhouses or in those handling meat and meat products. Veterinary surgeons are an outstandingly high risk group. The routes of infection include ingestion, inhalation and direct contact with infected material. Of these, direct contact is the most important and in cases where vets contract the disease, it is usually through handling the placenta or fetal parts during the delivery of a calf. The organism may gain access to the body through abraded skin or through the mucous membranes, including the conjuctiva. Members of the general public are infected from time to time by drinking raw milk from infected animals, usually when on holiday in the country.

Having entered the body by whatever means, the organisms spread through the lymphatics and lodge in the regional lymph nodes. Entrance to the thoracic duct allows widespread dissemination to take place through the bloodstream.

The disease is characterized by the formation of granulomata which occasionally caseate and form abscesses. This happens particularly in infections with *Br. suis*. The organisms are found within monocytes in which situation they are protected to some extent from the action of bacteriocidal antibodies.

Acute brucellosis

The incubation period is variable, from a few days to a few weeks. Onset may be gradual with nonspecific signs and symptoms such as fever, headache, joint pains, insomnia and low back pain, or it may be abrupt with fever, rigors and prostration. The temperature is in the range of 38–40°C but occasional spikes of fever greater than this are found. There are few abnormal clinical findings apart from generalized lymphadenopathy and a palpable spleen. The peripheral blood count shows a leucopenia with a reduction in the number of polymorphs.

Usually the disease subsides within 2 weeks and the patient makes a complete recovery. Some patients, however, enter a subacute stage and continue to have intermittent bouts of fever, back pain, a feeling of lethargy and depression which may last several months.

Positive blood (or bone marrow) cultures provide the definitive diagnosis but repeated cultures may be necessary as the organism is notoriously difficult to isolate. In most patients, levels of IgM and IgG are raised and both agglutination and complement fixation tests are positive. If a rise in antibody titres can be demonstrated this is good confirmatory evidence for diagnosis. Some patients with positive cultures, however, never develop a positive agglutination or complement fixation test. Conversely, some patients with no evidence of an acute attack of brucellosis nevertheless have persistently raised antibody titres.

Chronic brucellosis

The diagnosis of this condition presents many problems. The main symptoms are like those of the subacute stage, that is, lassitude, headaches, malaise, joint pains and depression of many months duration. Unlike the subacute illness, however, there is by no means always a history of an acute attack. Some patients have serological evidence suggestive of past infection, but serology is unhelpful in making the diagnosis; there is no elevation of IgM or IgG levels as in the acute attack. In many cases the occupation is the only clue which there may be to the diagnosis.

Complications of chronic brucellosis include endocarditis, principally affecting the aortic valve, and spondylitis. The radiological picture in the latter condition may mimic tuberculosis, but can usually be distinguished by the rapid growth of osteophytes from the affected vertebrae which meet to form bridges of lamellar bone. In some patients, chronic, suppurative lesions of the liver and spleen have been described. The lesions usually calcify and the appearance of areas of calcification on an abdominal X-ray may suggest the diagnosis.

Allergy to Br. abortus

Patients with an allergy to *Br. abortus* develop skin rashes or a transient febrile illness with arthralgia following exposure to infected animals or animal products. These patients have a high IgE titre and a strongly positive reaction to the brucellin skin test. They become asymptomatic when removed from contact with infected animals.

Treatment

Tetracycline is the treatment of choice in both acute and chronic brucellosis. It is difficult to achieve a complete cure in chronic brucellosis, however, and long courses of antibiotic therapy are often required. Co-trimaxazole is also effective in both conditions. Streptomycin has no therapeutic value used alone, but may be useful in combination with tetracycline.

The ultimate eradication of the disease depends upon eliminating it in the animal reservoirs and maintaining herds of animals free from the disease.

Q fever

Q fever is a rickettsial infection caused by *Rickettsia burneti*. The infection is seen most frequently in farmworkers who usually contract the disease from sheep and cows by the inhalation of infected dust or by the ingestion of raw milk. Veterinary surgeons and abattoir workers constitute other high risk groups.

The symptoms of the illness are like those of influenza and many cases of Q fever are given this diagnosis. The mistake can be corrected in retrospect when the patient is found to have a raised antibody titre.

Typically the illness begins with the sudden onset of fever accompanied by shivering, sweating and backache. The throat is often inflamed and the conjunctiva are suffused. The patient may complain of photophobia and muscular pain. About half the patients have an unproductive cough. An erythematous rash appears in a few patients.

Patients with a cough often have signs of patchy consolidation and chest X-rays frequently show the presence of single or multiple soft shadows, usually in the lower zones. The consolidation of the chest takes 2–3 weeks to resolve and may be complicated by pleural effusions.

In severe cases headaches and neck stiffness may suggest a diagnosis of meningitis but the cerebrospinal fluid is invariably normal. Lymphadenopathy is sometimes found and pericarditis is a rare complication. Occasionally patients develop signs and symptoms similar to those of subacute bacterial endocarditis months, or even years after an acute attack. The organism attacks only valves previously diseased, the aortic valve being most commonly involved.

The diagnosis is suggested by the knowledge that the patient is in a high risk occupation and confirmation depends upon the presence of a raised antibody titre. Treatment with tetracycline or co-trimoxazole singly or in combination, will produce good results in the acute illness. The results of treatment in cases of endocarditis are poor and the best hope for a cure is with surgical replacement of the damaged valve.

Prophylaxis is difficult because although vaccines are available, animals carrying the organism do not manifest any symptoms so that there is little or no incentive for farmers to maintain *Coxiella*-free herds.

Orf

Orf is a viral infection of sheep and goats which is occasionally transmitted to those who look after the animals or who handle the meat or its products.

The disease in humans, commonly known as contagious pustular dermatitis, takes the form of a mild exanthematous lesion, usually single, occurring at the site of infection. Clinical signs appear 4–12 days after infection, with the development of a red macule or papule. This enlarges until it becomes about 1–4 cm in diameter. It then becomes umbilical and vesicular, containing firstly clear fluid and then pus. There may be some local tenderness and lymphadenitis and the lesion is sometimes painful or itchy. Healing is complete within 4–6 weeks with little or no scarring.

Treatment is symptomatic and the main objective is to secure healing without secondary bacterial infection. The incidence of orf has declined since the introduction of an effective cheap vaccine.

Milkers' nodes

This is a disease of dairy cattle handlers, the infective agent being a virus closely related to the orf virus. It is transmitted from the mouths of calves or from the handling of teats of lactating cows.

The lesion is clinically indistinguishable from orf except that it is not painful, nor does it itch.

Ovine encephalomyelitis

This is a viral disease of sheep which produces a form of cerebral ataxia in affected animals. It is commoner in Scotland and the north of England then elsewhere in Britain. In Scotland it is commonly known as the louping-ill because of the characteristic leaping movements which the diseased animals make. It has been found to occur in shepherds, in farmers, in those engaged in sheep-dipping and in men working in slaughterhouses. The tick, *Ixodus vicinus*, which spreads the animal disease is also responsible for cases in humans with the exception of some laboratory workers who have become infected from cultured material.

The disease has two phases, the first of which lasts about a week, during which time the patient has an influenza-like illness with fever, headache and malaise. Leucopenia is common. This is the viraemic phase and the clinical improvement which follows it lasts for up to a week when the neurotropic phase has its onset. The patient then has fever and meningism with headache, photophobia and neck stiffness. He may vomit, and in severe cases pass into a coma. Physical examination may show signs of ataxia, nystagmus and strabismus due to paralysis of the external rectus muscle. The intracranial pressure may be raised with the cerebrospinal fluid showing a lymphocytosis and a varied protein level.

The disease is usually self-limiting and complete recovery within 3–4 weeks is to be expected.

The diagnosis is usually made in the knowledge of the patient's likely exposure to sheep ticks and these may even be found upon him at the time of examination. Protection from the disease depends upon ridding sheep of the ticks. There is no specific treatment although work is in progress to produce a vaccine with which those at risk could be immunized.

Ornithosis

Ornithosis is a specific infection of birds caused by *Chlamydia psittaci*. Although the disease may occur in all birds, humans usually contract it from those in the order Psittaciformes, and so the disease is frequently called psittacosis regardless of the species of the culprit bird.

The disease is usually transmitted to humans through the inhalation of dried, infected droppings, more rarely through contact with the feathers or tissues of infected birds and least often through the bite of an infected bird. It is most usually caught from parrots, parakeets or budgerigars and those at risk include veterinary surgeons, pet shop keepers and pet owners; outbreaks may also occur in poultry workers.

There is a variable incubation period of 7–15 days, and occasionally much longer. The illness is ushered in by slow rise of temperature over the first week. There is a severe headache and malaise with anorexia, myalgia and asthralgia. There is usually a pronounced cough, but it may not appear until the end of the first week. The cough is associated with small amounts of sputum, occasionally streaked with blood. In severe cases, the patient may become delirious and stuporous with signs of extensive pulmonary involvement. Cyanosis will be evident in these cases. Pleuritic signs are rare as are neurological signs. Nausea and vomiting, on the other hand, are common. A macular rash similar to that seen in typhoid has been described, but the spots are smaller. In severe cases jaundice and azotaemia have been reported.

Physical examination reveals relatively few signs. The respiratory rate is rapid and fine crepitations may be heard in the lungs. Changes due to consolidation are only rarely heard. The liver is often slightly enlarged and so also is the spleen. The pulse rate remains low.

Radiographs of the chest may show the presence of areas of patchy infiltration radiating from the hilum, more prominent in the lower zones.

In mild cases the illness lasts only for about a week. In more severe cases it may be up to 3 weeks before recovery is complete and relapses are common.

The diagnosis is usually made on the basis of a rising antibody titre or by the isolation of the organism in specialized laboratories.

Tetracycline is the treatment of choice and early diagnosis and prompt initiation of treatment may be life-saving. Chloramphenicol and penicillin are less effective.

Those who own or sell birds should be warned that sick birds may transmit this disease. If they suspect that either they or their birds have the disease, they should promptly seek advice.

Streptococcus suis

Streptococcus suis type 2 infections are common in pigs giving rise to septicaemia, meningitis, arthritis and endocarditis. Those who work with pigs or pig meat are at risk of contracting the organism which probably gains access through cuts and abrasions in the skin. Meningitis is the most common manifestation of the infection and this may be followed by deafness in a high proportion of cases. Other complications of the infection include arthritis, vestibular disturbances, uveitis and, rarely, myocarditis; endocarditis has not been reported in human infections.

The diagnosis of *S. suis* infection should always be considered in patients with meningitis in whom there is a history of exposure to pigs or pig meat and in whom nongroupable or group D streptococci are isolated. The organism is usually susceptible to penicillin but one resistant strain has been reported.

Chapter 11
Accidents and Trauma

Accidents

Accidents at work are an important cause of personal and national loss, both in terms of loss of lives and loss of working time. In Great Britain there are between 400 000 and 500 000 accidents at work each year. Whilst only a small percentage of these are fatal, this nevertheless represents an annual loss of life which is usual in excess of 1000 (Table 11.1).

Something of the order of 20 million working days a year are lost as the result of accidents at work but, as one might expect, the accident rate shows considerable fluctuations between different industries. This is illustrated in Table 11.2 where the number of days lost each year per thousand employees at risk is shown. It can be seen from this table that the nonmanufacturing industries have by far the highest accident rate and this again is what would be anticipated when one considers that it includes such occupations as coal-mining and fishing, both of which are of such a nature as to render them particularly hazardous. Each of the subgroups in the nonmanufacturing category has a high accident rate as shown in Table 11.3.

The overall economic cost of industrial accidents is difficult to compute with any accuracy since it is the sum of at least four separate costs, none of which is capable of precise quantification. The four divisions of the main cost are: those met by the employee; those met by the employer; those met by the community at large; and those met by the state. As a rough estimate, accidents probably cost the victims or their families a total of not less than £100 000 000 per year (1989), whilst other costs, including lost production, the award of damages, and the provision of hospital and ambulance services, probably accounts for a sum in excess £200 000 000.

The causation of accidents

A number of theories have been elaborated to account for accidents at work, the most influential of which has been that of accident-proneness. This theory states that some people are more liable to have accidents than others because of some innate physical or psychological characteristics. Another theory which enjoyed a considerable vogue was that all the members of a population at risk had an equal risk, that is to say, the occurrence of accidents was due to pure chance. Yet another accepted that the first accident was due to chance, but that having sustained one accident, the probability of having a second increased or decreased. These are all difficult theories to test by epidemiological means, however, because the basic hypothesis requires that all those in the sample population shall be exposed to the same risk. Research has tended to

Table 11.1. Accidents at work in Great Britain, 1961–1970*

	1961	1962	1963	1964	1965	1966	1967	1968	1969	1970
Factories	161 655 (368)	157 600 (351)	168 106 (332)	217 950 (344)	239 158 (358)	241 051 (372)	247 058 (342)	254 454 (359)	266 857 (357)	255 907 (325)
Docks and warehouses	7506 (37)	7220 (36)	7815 (36)	10 207 (40)	10 178 (39)	9952 (41)	10 483 (25)	11 407 (28)	10 963 (27)	8865 (28)
Construction	23 356 (264)	25 338 (281)	28 348 (242)	40 491 (271)	44 381 (230)	45 607 (288)	46 475 (197)	46 569 (238)	44 570 (265)	39 823 (203)
Mines and quarries	191 208 (284)	201 389 (288)	206 234 (295)	201 364 (244)	209 935 (256)	188 909 (191)	169 763 (181)	144 046 (158)	121 402 (126)	93 983 (124)
Agriculture	12 846 (80)	13 553 (71)	14 548 (65)	13 276 (64)	11 839 (49)	10 680 (73)	10 069 (58)	8722 (63)	8783 (70)	7366 (41)
Offices, shops and railway premises	18 000 (28)	18 000 (28)	18 000 (28)	18 000 (28)	17 225 (34)	18 533 (29)	19 903 (16)	19 075 (39)	19 018 (20)	16 871 (32)
Railways	14 233 (167)	12 139 (118)	11 846 (116)	11 064 (96)	9838 (103)	8236 (72)	8003 (78)	6912 (62)	7335 (69)	7625 (68)
Road transport	16 200 (57)	16 400 (55)	16 600 (65)	18 700 (70)	22 700 (86)	22 900 (78)	25 300 (82)	26 700 (90)	26 300 (81)	33 800 (80)
Civil Aviation	30 (24)	27 (17)	25 (12)	17 (12)	22 (13)	35 (27)	28 (19)	14 (8)	6 (3)	15 (13)
Seamen	8817 (154)	8783 (131)	8805 (70)	9090 (90)	8672 (91)	8769 (118)	8361 (94)	8177 (98)	8421 (52)	8491 (71)
Total	453 851 (1463)	460 449 (1376)	480 327 (1261)	540 159 (1259)	573 948 (1259)	554 672 (1289)	545 443 (1092)	526 076 (1143)	513 655 (1070)	472 746 (985)

*Fatal cases are shown in brackets. From *Report of the Roben's Committee*, HMSO, 1972.

Table 11.2. Accident rates in different industries

Industry	Days lost each year through accidents/10^3 men at risk*
Non-manufacturing	6000
Construction	1800
Transport	1700
Manufacturing	1200
Distributive	800
Service	700
Professions	200

*Means for 5 years, 1968–72.
From *Digest of Statistics Analysing
Certificates of Incapacity*, HMSO 1974.

concentrate, therefore, on assessing the relative risks associated with such factors as age, experience, medical condition and so on.

Age is one of the most frequently investigated factors in accident research and there seems little doubt that there is an increased incidence in the 'teens and early twenties. In the third and fourth decades the number of accidents declines, thereafter rising again slightly until retirement is reached. The high accident rate in the young seems to be due to their lack of experience in the job, although after a year or two, length of service is not related to the accident rate, whereas age is, indicating that some other factors are also at work.

The state of health might well be expected to be at the root of some accidents and in some cases this does seem to be true. Accidents due to the onset of hypoglycaemia in diabetes or to myocardial infarction in men with coronary artery disease are obvious examples of acute medical states which might cause an accident, but ill health is a much less common precipitant of accidents than is generally supposed. Similarly, although defects in vision or in hearing do sometimes cause accidents, this happens only rarely and the defect is job-specific, that is to say, only jobs where good vision is essential will show a relationship between the accident rate and poor sight; the same is true so far as hearing is concerned. Some personality traits, including extraversion, neuroticism, aggression and anxiety have been suggested as being related in some way to an excess accident rate, but the evidence is a long way from being

Table 11.3. Accident rates in different non-manufacturing industries

Industry	Days lost each year through accidents/10^3 men at risk*
Coal mining	10 700
Agriculture	1100
Fishing	3500

*Means for 5 years, 1968–72.
From *Digest of Statistics Analysing
Certificates of Incapacity*, HMSO 1974.

conclusive or of being of help in accident prevention schemes. Intelligence does not correlate with accident rates.

Some characteristics of the work pattern have been shown to be determinants in accident causation. Accidents occur at a peak when the work rate is fastest and when the rate of productivity is greatest. There are more accidents when the length of a shift is increased, but generally there are fewer accidents on the night shift and at the end of the working week. Factories in which there is a good working relationship between the employees seem to enjoy a lower accident rate than those bedevilled by internal strife, probably because communications are better where there is a good *esprit de corps*.

The effect of environmental factors such as extremes of temperature, poor lighting and noise have all been studied but with inconclusive results and the possible interactions between these variables has not been studied at all.

Accident prevention

The high social and economic cost of accidents requires that all those involved with occupational health work strenuously towards their prevention. It must be realized that the burden of implementing a safety prevention programme has to be shared equally and is not the prerogative of one particular section of the working population.

There are broadly four means by which accidents can be prevented although not all are of equal importance. The most important measure is to inculcate an attitude of mind in those at risk which makes them aware of the necessity to comply with safety measures, including the wearing of safety clothing.

This attitude will only be fostered if the management recognize that the safety of their work force is their responsibility and thus accept the need to support vigorous safety campaigns. Each factory should have a team of safety engineers whose task it is to see to it that due attention is given to all aspects of safety and that safety regulations are complied with. In order that there should be no misunderstanding on the part of men and management, safety rules and safety instructions ought to be set down for each job where some hazard exists. These must be as comprehensive as possible and amended as required in the light of new knowledge. It will fall to the safety engineers to ensure that these rules are implemented and to do so often requires considerable tact and diplomacy if they are not to be seen as acting in some way as an unofficial 'police force', constantly on the watch for malpractice.

Safety regulations and good habits of work are encouraged by propaganda of one kind or another, one of the most popular being the safety poster. To be effective, posters should be placed in areas where their message has some relevance to the work in progress and they should be changed at frequent intervals so that their message does not become so familiar that it is ignored. They should instruct, and emphasize the positive benefits of working safely. Some firms operate incentive schemes whereby areas of the factory compete with each other in a 'safety league' but the utility of such schemes remains to be assessed.

One of the greatest challenges in a safety programme is to ensure the use of safety clothing since it is well known that its mere provision is no guarantee of its use. As mentioned in other parts of this book, safety clothing is often cumbersome and uncomfortable to wear and this is an area which would benefit from a well directed research effort. Some simple considerations, however, often tend to be overlooked. For example, the appearance of the clothing should not be such that the wearer feels embarrassed or ill at ease in it. This is particularly so when considering safety clothing for women at work. For example, the provision of safety glasses with fashionable frames instead of the standard, rather unattractive ones, may be critical in encouraging their use.

Safety clothing must also be designed so that it does not hinder normal activities. The provision of safety boots which are too heavy to allow comfortable walking is not calculated to gain many users. Because those who design and provide safety equipment are not often called upon to use it under working conditions, elementary considerations such as these may be over-looked, although this happens less often when the workers are consulted during the design stage.

Two other points about safety clothing remain to be noted; firstly, no one should consider him or herself exempt from wearing safety equipment in a designated area. If management does not set a good example in this respect then it follows that safety rules will be given less than enthusiastic support. Secondly, workers must not be out of pocket if they comply with safety regulations. This means that protective clothing should be provided free, or, as in the case of safety shoes, for example, at subsidized rates.

Trauma

The eye

Injuries to the eye are unfortunately commonplace in industry. The most frequent injuries are those caused by foreign bodies, usually splinters or metal. Every time metal strikes metal there is a hazard from flying splinters; this seems so obvious that it is surprising that men disregard the hazard, risking serious injury, or blindness by not wearing goggles, or by using them to protect their foreheads. Grinding and polishing and all forms of metal entail some risk from eye injuries. Burns caused by splashes of acid or alkali or by molten glass or metal are common events.

Prompt treatment at hospital is required to salvage a burnt eye. Superficial foreign bodies can often be removed in the works surgery (where there is one). Where the foreign body has penetrated the globe its position will have to be located radiographically (always assuming it is radio-opaque) and then removed surgically.

Physical trauma to the eye

The damage sustained by the eye depends upon the direction in which the force of a blow is transmitted. If directed along the axis of the eye, then the lens may be dislocated, partially or completely, with a resultant distortion of vision. If the lens is completely dislocated backwards, it falls into the vitreous leaving the iris unsupported and tremulous (a condition referred to as an iridodonesis). Frontal dislocation results in the lens falling into the anterior chamber and if this happens it may produce secondary glaucoma by interfering with aqueous drainage. Retinal tears may also result from a blow along the axis of the eye. This is especially serious if the macula is damaged since it is likely to leave the patient with sight which is greatly impaired. Less violent blows may result in retinal haemorrhages which are serious only if they overlay the macula. Sometimes the force of the blow may be so great that the optic nerve is 'popped out' of the globe and there is no prospect of repairing this catastrophe. If the force is directed through the iris there may be a little bleeding into the anterior chamber. The blood gravitates to the lower segment forming a hyphaema which usually disperses in a few days. If the accumulated blood blocks the drainage of the anterior chamber, secondary glaucoma will ensue and surgical drainage will be required. The iris root is sometimes completely torn by the force of a blow. This is referred to as iridodialysis and the pupil becomes D-shaped. Such tears seldom heal but, on the other hand, they rarely interfere with vision.

In addition to the damage described above, any blow to the eye may cause a black eye or corneal abrasions, neither of which is serious as a rule. In addition, any perforating injury is liable to become infected and steps must be taken to prevent this from happening.

Patients with damage to the eye should be referred to an ophthalmic unit. Dislocated lenses can be removed and adequate vision restored with spectacles, much as the sight can be given back to a patient with cataracts. The prognosis for patients with retinal tears varies according to the site of the tear. Peripheral tears do not impair normal vision greatly, although there may be some loss of night vision; tears involving the macula can almost invariably be expected to leave some deficit.

Arc-eye

This condition occurs in men engaged in electric arc-welding or gas-welding using oxyacetylene torches. It comes about from the intense ultraviolet irradiation which is experienced when gazing at the welding site with the naked eye. It may occur, although less commonly, from looking at molten steel or at an unscreened arc-lamp.

There is no immediate sensation apart from a momentary glare. After a few hours, however, coloured lights may be noted around objects in vision due to oedema of the cornea epitheleum. This is followed by symptoms of pain and conjunctival irritation; the patient feels as though he has dust in his eyes and produces copious tears; he is photophobic. The eyes may become suffused and there may be marked blepharospasm.

The condition is self-limiting and simple treatment will relieve the pain. It need never occur if all those at risk wear goggles or visors which conform to the British Standards specifications.

Bursitis

Bursitis occurs whenever there is repeated mechanical trauma over a bursa. The condition arises in a variety of situations and is known by many colloquial names, for example, weavers' bottom, clergymen's or housemaid's knee and hodman's shoulder, affecting respectively the ischial, prepatellar and subacromial bursea. Bursea may be produced in connective tissues which are subject to frequent but unusual movements and these were also well recognized in the past as being associated with specific occupations. Thus came about Covent Garden lump, Billingsgate lump, humpers' lump and deal-runners' shoulder. These occurrred over the vertex in the porters in Covent Garden, over the seventh cervical vertebra in fish porters and timber porters and over the upper part of the clavicle and shoulder, also in timber porters. The increasing use of mechanization has relegated most of these conditions to the status of curiosities; fork-lift drivers' bottom remains to be described.

Patients seldom seek medical treatment for this condition unless there is a sudden increase in its fluid content as the result of a blow when the sac may become filled with blood or interstitial fluid. In either event, the sudden increase in fluid content is painful. The bursa may become secondarily infected and require surgical drainage. If the patient complains that the bursa is unsightly he should be warned that unless he changes his occupation it is likely to persist and that it is, in fact, fulfilling a protective function. As a sop to vanity, the bursal sac can be removed but will recur if the patient continues at his old job.

Beat disorders

There are three so-called beat disorders recognized for the purposes of compensation under the Industrial Injuries Act, beat knee, beat elbow and beat hand.

The first two are in effect the results of acute infection in the bursae around the knee joint and in the olecranon bursa, or acute cellulitis in the tissues around these two joints. In some cases bursitis and cellulitis co-exist. In the case of beat knee the condition is found predominantly in those whose job involves a lot of kneeling with repeated minor trauma. It occurs, as one could expect, most frequently in miners. If the skin is wet, then the disease occurs more frequently. Employees returning to work from a period of absence, or workers unaccustomed to the job, are more likely to contract it than others. In beat elbow the cause can more often be tracked down to a single injury sustained at work.

Beat hand differs from the other two conditions in that it consists only of cellulitis. It is the result of repeated minor trauma to the hand—so that miners again present frequently with it—but it occurs also in other men who work with a pick or shovel. Those with 'soft' hands are most at risk and wet working conditions also favour its appearance.

The signs are those classically associated with infection, that is to say, pain, swelling, redness and heat. In the hand, the palm of the hand and the palmar surfaces of the thumb and forefinger are most often affected and if uncontrolled the infection may spread to involve the tendon sheaths. The swelling may spread to involve adjacent tissues and if the infection is severe, may affect underlying joints.

Treatment must be prompt and thorough and have as its aim the restoration of completley normal function. This may call for surgical intervention. In uncomplicated cases, a cure should be expected within a month.

Tenosynovitis

This condition is a noninfective inflammation of the tendon sheaths in the forearm or in the musculotendinous junction. When confined to the latter site, the condition is sometimes referred to as peritendonitis crepitans. The usual cause is an unaccustomed and arduous use of the muscles of the forearm brought about either by a change of occupation or a return to a familiar job after a period of absence. Rarely is the condition bilateral.

The presenting signs and symptoms include pain, swelling and tenderness, usually with some loss of function. There are no signs of infection. Crepitus may be felt over affected tendons and is pathogonomic. The avid searcher of clinical signs will be able to hear the crackling in the tendon sheaths with the aid of a stethoscope but it is not often necessary to go to such lengths to make the diagnosis.

Rest and splinting of the wrist will cure the condition in the majority of cases. Where simple measures fail, injections of hydrocortisone may succeed.

Writer's cramp

This condition is characterized by painful spasms of the hand or forearm brought about by repetitive muscular activity. The patient loses the ability to co-ordinate the movements necessary for the performance of the task, although very often other activities requiring fine motor co-ordination, such as tying shoelaces, can be undertaken with ease.

There are no physical concomitants of the disease and there are no pathological abnormalities; the condition is usually referred to as being psychiatric in origin. This conclusion is supported by the fact that the condition invariably occurs in those patients, often of obsessional nature, whose job depends on their ability to write. The prognosis is not favourable and the patient is seldom referred for psychiatric help although this would seem to be the logical step in view of the presumptive cause. Usually the patient is advised to seek an occupation which does not call for the tasks which precipitate the attack. Before arriving at the diagnosis it is prudent to take advice from a neurologist lest some serious neurological disorder be overlooked.

Chapter 12
Control of Occupational Hazards

Since occupational diseases have specific causes which can be identified, measures can be taken to control them. Once a hazard has been identified, a number of preventive measures can be taken, including substitution, enclosure, removal at source, segregation and what may broadly be called good housekeeping.

Substitution

If one is considering a hazard from a chemical then the most certain way to eliminate the risk associated with its use is to substitute a non-toxic material for the poisonous one. There are a number of instances where this has been done successfully. For example, freon is used instead of methyl bromide as a refrigerant, phosphorus sesquiphosphide has been substituted for white phosphorus in match making, and other substances are used as insulatory materials in place of asbestos. In some instances, however, the toxic material offers so many technical and economic advantages to the industry using it that legislation is necessary to implement a substitution. In yet other cases, it is impossible to eliminate the toxic material because there is no satisfactory alternative.

When considering physical hazards such as noise and radiation, substitution is, of course, not possible, but machines can be designed to keep noise to a minimum and to prevent the escape of radiation into those areas in which people are working.

Enclosure

Processes which are particularly dangerous can be totally enclosed and then performed mechanically or by an operator using special apparatus as in the way that radioisotopes are handled.

Removal at source

The aim of this method is to prevent toxic dusts or vapours from entering the breathing zone of the operator by some form of local exhaust ventilation. The hazard from dust can also be lessened by using wet methods for drilling and grinding. In order to work effectively, exhaust ventilation systems require to be well maintained and they must be well designed. To offer adequate protection, ventilation systems must remove the airborne particles of respirable size (<5 μm diameter) and these are often the most difficult to remove.

Segregation

Where it is impractical completely to enclose a process, then exposure may be limited to a small segregated group of workers. The hazard is not eliminated, but by this means, methods of supervision and control are considerably simplified.

Good housekeeping

High standards of cleanliness in the workplace ensure that exposure to harmful materials will be kept to a minimum and also encourage workers to take due care when engaged in potentially hazardous jobs. Adequate ventilation in the workplace reduces the risk from toxic materials by assisting removal and by reducing local concentrations through a dilution effect.

Personal hygiene is an important protective measure and workers should be made fully aware of the hazards to which their occupation is exposing them. At the same time they should be made aware of appropriate safety measures which they can take to reduce the risks. These measures will often include the wearing of protective clothing and it is too often the case that employees will not make the fullest use of the protective clothing which is provided for them. Very often workers complain that protective clothing is uncomfortable to wear and to some extent this criticism is justified. In order to protect against solvents and oil splashing on the skin, for example, the aprons and other garments must obviously be impervious, but such materials are also impervious to water and so the workers become hot and sweaty. Goggles and ear-protectors may also be uncomfortable in hot working conditions if the wearer sweats under them. There is every good reason to continue working towards finding protective clothing which is both safe and comfortable, but until this ideal has been achieved, workers should be strongly urged by management and preferably by their unions that some degree of discomfort is better than a lost eye, deafness or some disability which could have been prevented.

Monitoring

Even when attention is given to all these points an element of risk still remains in many occupations which requires to be controlled by some form of monitoring, either physical or biological.

Physical monitoring

The risk from toxic materials at the workplace arises principally from the inhalation of airborne particles or vapours. The philosophy underlying physical monitoring is that if the airborne concentration of a potentially harmful substance (or substances) is kept below some predetermined level, then no harm will come to exposed workers. Predetermined exposure levels exist for a wide variety of materials and they are known as occupational exposure standards (OES). Formerly they were known as threshold limit values (TLVs) and may still be referred to as such. The list of recommended exposure standards is published by the Health and Safety Executive at regular intervals and is compiled by the Health and Safety Commission's Advisory Committee on Toxic Substances.

Table 12.1. Excursion factors permitted above OEL

OEL range mg m	Excursion factor
0–1	3
>1–10	2
>10–100	1.5
>100–1000	1.25

There are two kinds of OES, occupational exposure limits (OEL) and maximum exposure limits (MEL); the latter were called control limits and are still sometimes referred to by this name.

OELs come in two forms, as long-term and short-term exposure limits. This is because recognition is given to the fact that the untoward effects of exposure may be either immediate or apparent only after the toxic material has accumulated within the body or if the risk of disease increases with increasing contact. Short-term exposure limits are particularly applicable to materials which are irritant to the lungs or to mucous membranes or which are acutely narcotic.

Both short-term and long-term exposure limits are time-weighted average concentrations. For long-term limits the time over which the concentration is averaged is normally 8 hours. It is recognized that within this 8-hour period there may be excursions above the OEL but this is permitted so long as there are corresponding dips below it so that the average is not exceeded. The short-term limit is averaged over 10 minutes and this is such a short time that it scarcely permits of any deviation from the recommended level.

When mixtures of substances are present in the atmosphere they are generally considered to have additive effects and the sum of the ratio of observed to permitted concentrations should not exceed unity. That is to say, if

$$\frac{C_1}{L_1} + \frac{C_2}{L_2} + \frac{C_3}{L_3} \cdots \frac{C_n}{L_n} \leqslant 1$$

where C = the observed and L = the permitted concentrations, then the OEL for the mixture is considered not to have been exceeded.

For 32 substances MELs have been proposed (they are contained within the Appendix). These are exposure limits which are contained in Regulations, in Codes of Practice or in Directives of the European Community and which have been adopted by the Health and Safety Commission. They are limits which are considered to be reasonably practicable on scientific, medical and engineering grounds and they must not be exceeded at any time. The number of substances subject to MELs is steadily increasing and we can expect many more in the years to come.

Establishment of OELs

The establishment of OELs is at best empirical and no one should be under any delusion that they necessarily have a firm toxicological basis. It is, of course, much easier to establish limits for substances which have immediate effects. For example, it is relatively easy to determine the concentration of a solvent vapour which will result in unconsciousness if inhaled for more than a few moments and it is not difficult to determine what concentration of an irritant gas will bring tears to the eyes. It is a much more difficult proposition, however, to say what concentration of a toxic material such as mercury or chromium may safely be inhaled 8 hours a day, 50 weeks a year for the best part of an individual's lifetime without expecting him to come to any harm. The information on which such decisions must be made can come only from long term animal studies, with all the inherent risk of extrapolating these to humans, or from cohort studies of groups of exposed workers. In the latter case, the relevant exposures associated with ill effects are likely to have been those experienced many years in the past and may be difficult, if not impossible to quantify. Long term OELs, then, should be considered as educated guesses which will require modification as new information accumulates. The trend is generally towards lowering OELs, and although one would like to believe that this trend follows closely upon an increase in toxicological information, in fact it owes more to developments in technology and in the availability of better control measures.

There are some deficiencies in OELs which need to be borne in mind when using them as control measures in industry. For example, the size of the dust particles in the atmosphere is an important factor in determining the risk they represent since particles which are greater than about 7 μm in diameter are unlikely to penetrate to the alveoli and will not be absorbed. As a rule the OEL does not take account of particle size. Nor does it make any allowance for undue susceptibility on the part of the exposed worker even though this is well known to be a factor in, for example, exposure to lead, benzene, hydrogen sulphide and DNOC.

Although it should be obvious, it is sometimes necessary to remind occupational physicians and others that the OEL can be used only to control risks which arise from inhalation. A good many toxic substances are absorbed through the skin and although there is a 'skin' notation attached to the OEL of such materials, the degree to which uptake occurs may well be independent of the atmospheric concentration. Likewise, where the risk is primarily through ingestion, airborne concentrations may give an entirely inadequate estimate of exposure. In some parts of the lead industry, for example, the risk occurs not from the inhalation of lead dust or fume but from the transfer of lead from the hands to the mouth, and reliance on atmospheric concentrations as a measure of risk is utterly inappropriate. It must also be remembered, that once an individual has become sensitized to an allergen, there is almost no concentration to which he or she may be safely exposed and only complete removal from exposure or the most stringent personal protection will be adequate to protect health.

Finally, it is possible to be misled by the results of general air sampling on other grounds. For example, although the overall concentration of pollutants may be lower than the OEL, there may be local concentrations in excess of it and employees working in these local conditions may be subjected to an unsuspected hazard. To some extent this can be guarded against by the use of personal samplers which can be worn by an individual during the shift and which make it possible to estimate individual exposure. Personal samplers may be battery operated but for a wide range of gases and vapours, passive samplers are available. Passive samplers have a number of advantages over their pump driven counterparts. In addition to being safe to use in atmospheres which contain flammable gases or vapours, they are much less cumbersome and do not interfere with normal work practices. Many can be put directly into an automatic gas chromatogram for analysis; the analysis can be run overnight and the sampler ready for reuse in the morning. Some passive samplers contain a reagent which changes colour according to the concentration of the material which diffuses into it and these can be used rather like the film badges which workers exposed to ionizing radiation wear. Before they can be used in the field, however, a great deal of preliminary work has to be carried out in the laboratory to determine the diffusion characteristics of the gases or vapours it is proposed to monitor, and to calibrate the device. The number of applications to which passive samplers can be put is gradually increasing and they are likely to become more widely used as time goes on.

Biological monitoring

Measurements of atmospheric concentrations are a guide to a potential hazard and may serve to draw attention to the need for improved control, but, in order to assess the effects on those exposed, some form of biological monitoring is required. It may be sufficient to measure the concentration of the toxic substance (or a metabolite) in the blood or urine from which an index of the degree of absorption is obtained. On the other hand, it may be preferable to utilize a test which gives an indication of the degree of metabolic disturbance which is being produced by the absorbed material. In lead workers, for example, the blood or urine lead concentrations can be determined as measures of absorption whereas the concentrations of ALA in the urine or of protoporphyrin in the erythrocytes can be taken as indices of interference with haem synthesis. Similarly, the concentration of cadmium in the urine gives some guide to the amount of absorption, but the presence of proteinuria is the measure of the degree of interference with kidney tubular function. Exposure to physical hazards such as dust and noise is controlled by indirect methods which include radiography and pulmonary function tests for workers exposed to dusts and audiometry for those in noisy occupations.

Workers coming into contact with carcinogenic substances such as aromatic amines in the rubber industry or mineral oil in the engineering industry rely on periodical medical examinations to detect any premalignant change such as may be found, for example, in the skin of a man exposed to cutting oils. Where the changes are not visible, special techniques are employed, such as the examination of the urine of men in the rubber industry for malignant cells.

Some degree of prevention can also be achieved in certain occupations by preemployment medical examinations. These not only establish a base line against which any future change can be judged but also allow unsuitable workers to be disqualified from entering dangerous jobs. For example, one would not wish a chronic bronchitic to take up an occupation where there was a likelihood of exposure to dust or some other pulmonary irritant.

Biological thresholds

There is no legislation regulating the concentration of any toxic compound or its metabolites in blood, urine or exhaled air, but some recommended maxima are shown in Table 12.2.

Biological threshold values are based on the assumption that below some given concentration, toxic substances will not produce clinical poisoning even though there may be some degree of metabolic abnormality which is considered tolerable. The question which is constantly posed to those concerned with occupational health is, how much deviation from normal is *tolerable?*

In Russia and some of the other eastern European countries, threshold values have been established on the basis of behavioural studies with animals following the work of Pavlov. Animals are exposed to varying concentrations of the toxic substances under examination and its effect on conditioned reflex responses is noted. The levels permitted are just below those which at first produce alterations in behaviour and are generally much lower than levels permitted in this country. Studies on workers exposed to some heavy metals and solvents have reported abnormalities in behaviour as judged by their performance in a range of psychological tests and some changes in reproductive function are also said to occur in the absence of clinical signs or symptoms. There is no general agreement concerning the significance or validity of these results but nevertheless, their publication has led to a demand for a downward revision of present threshold values. Whether or not the results of the studies support such a move, it is important to remember that threshold values are not immutable but must constantly be revised in the light of new knowledge and of different expectations of those at work and of society at large.

On the basis of these results a number of authorities are pressing for a downward revision of present threshold values. Whether or not they are successful in their attempt, they have underlined the important principle that threshold values are not to be regarded as fixed and immutable, but must constantly be revised in the light of new knowledge.

Central control

Governmental control of occupational health and safety was originally placed in the hands of the Factory Inspectorate which was established in 1833. The first Medical Inspector of Factories, Sir Thomas Legge, was not appointed until 1896 with the specific duty of reducing the dreadful toll of death and disease from lead and phosphorus poisoning. Other inspectorates have been established since then, all of whom came under the aegis of the Health and Safety Executive since the passage of the Health and Safety at Work Act in 1974. The inspectorates are responsible for the health and safety of all those who work (except for domestic servants, not a numerically significant cohort these days) in well over half a million establishments, factories and farms, mines and quarries and North Sea oil rigs. To accomplish this task there is provision for

Table 12.2. Suggested maximum permissible values for use in biological monitoring

Chemical	Biological monitor	Normal value	Suggested maximum
Acetone	Blood concentration	<0.2 mg/dl	2 mg/dl
	Urinary concentration per gram creatinine*	<2 mg/g	20 mgm/g
Aniline	Methaemoglobin	<2%	5%
Arsenic	Total concentration in urine	<10 µg/g	200 µg/g
Benzene	Urinary phenol	<20 mg/g	45 mg/g
Cadmium	Blood concentration	<0.5 µg/dl	
	Urinary concentration	<2 µg/g	10 µg/g
Carbamate insecticides	Inhibition of ChE activity		
	in plasma		– 50%
	in whole blood		– 30%
	in red cells		– 30%
Carbon disulphide	Iodine-azide test		6.5 (Vasak index)
Carbon monoxide	Carboxyhaemoglobin	<1%	5% (non smokers)
Chromium (soluble compounds)	Urinary concentration	<5µg/g	30 µg/g
Cyclohexane	Exhaled air concentration	Nil	200 ppm
	Blood cyclohexanol	Nil	40 µg/dl
	Urinary cyclohexanol	Nil	3 mg/g
Dieldrin	Blood concentration	Nil	15 µg/dl
DNOC	Blood concentration	Nil	1 mg/dl
Endrin	Blood concentration	Nil	5 µg/dl
Ethylbenzene	Blood concentration	Nil	0.15 mg/dl
	Urinary mandelic acid		2g/g
Fluoride	Urinary concentration	<0.4 mg/g	4 mg/g preshift
			7 mg/g postshift
n-Hexane	Blood concentration	Nil	15 µg/dl
	Expired air concentration	Nil	50 ppm
	Urinary 2,5 hexanol	Nil	0.2 mg/g
	Urinary 2,5 hexanedione	Nil	5.5 mg/g
Halothane	Blood trifluoroacetic acid concentration	Nil	0.25 mg/dl
	Urinary trifluoracetic acid concentration	Nil	10 mg/g
Hexachlorobenzene	Blood concentration	Nil	0.3 mg/dl
Lead (inorganic)	Blood concentration	<35 µg/dl	70 µg/dl
	Urinary concentration	<50 µg/g	150 µg/g
	Urinary ALA	<4.5 mg/g	10 mg/g
	Urinary Cp	<100µg/g	250 µg/g
	Free erythrocyte	<75 µg/dl	300 µg/dl
	Protoporphyrin	RBC	RBC
	Zinc protoporphyrin	<2.5 µg/g Hb	12.5 µg/dl Hb
Lead (organic)	Urinary concentration	<50 µg/g	150 µg/g
Mercury (inorganic)	Blood concentration	<2 µg/dl	3 µg/dl
	Urinary concentration	<5 µg/g	50 µg/g
Mercury, methyl	Blood concentration	<2 µg/dl	10 µg/dl
Methanol	Urinary concentration	<2.5 mg/g	7 mg/g
Methylene chloride	Blood concentration	Nil	100 µg/dl
	Exhaled air concentration	Nil	35 ppm
	Carboxyhaemoglobin	<1%	5% (non smokers)

Table 12.2. Suggested maximum permissible values for use in biological monitoring (*Continued*)

Chemical	Biological monitor	Normal value	Suggested Maximum
Methyl ethyl ketone	Urinary concentration	Nil	2.5 µg/g
Nickel (soluble compounds)	Plasma concentration	<1 µg/dl	1 µd/dl
	Urinary concentration	<5 µg/g	70 µg/g
Nitrobenzene	Urinary p-aminophenol	Nil	5 mg/g
	Methaemoglobin	<2%	5%
Organophosphorus	Inhibition of ChE activity		
insecticides	in plasma		– 50%
	in whole blood		– 30%
	in red cells		– 30%
Parathion	Urinary p-nitrophenol	Nil	2 mg/g
Pentachlorophenol	Urinary concentration	Nil	1 mg/g
Phenol	Urinary concentration	<20 mg/g	300 mg/g
Selenium	Urinary concentration	<25 µg/g	100 µg/g
Styrene	Urinary mandelic acid	<5 mg/g	1 g/g
Tellurium	Urinary concentration	<1 g/g	1 µg/g
Tetrachloroethylene	Exhaled air concentration	Nil	4 ppm
Thallium	Urinary concentration	1 µg/g	1 g/g
1,1,1-Trichloro-ethane	Exhaled air concentration	Nil	50 ppm
	Urinary trichloroethanol	Nil	30 mg/g
	Urinary trichloroethanol + trichloroacetic acid	Nil	50 mg/g
Toluene	Blood concentration	Nil	100 µg/dl
	Exhaled air concentration	Nil	20 ppm
	Urinary hippuric acid	<1.5 g/g	2.5 g/g
	Urinary o-cresol	<0.3 mg/g	1 mg/g
Trichloroethylene	Blood concentration	Nil	0.6 mg/dl
	Exhaled air concentration	Nil	12 ppm
	Urinary trichloroethanol	Nil	125 mg/g
	Urinary trichloroacetic acid	Nil	75 mg/g
Vanadium	Urinary concentration	<1 g/g	50 µg/g
Vinyl chloride	Urinary thiodiglycolic acid	<2 mg/g	2 mg/g
Xylene	Blood concentration	Nil	0.3 mg/dl
	Urinary methylhippuric acid	Nil	1.5 g/g

*All urinary concentrations in the Table are expressed per gram creatinine

about a thousand inspectors; it takes only a few seconds on the calculator to see how frequently a work place may expect a routine visit from an inspector.

The medical arm of the Health and Safety Executive is the Employment Medical Advisory Service (EMAS) which operates on a regional basis and has provision for about 120 doctors; at the time of writing the service is about 50% understaffed. The duty of the Employment Medical Advisers is to give advice to anyone (medical or lay) on all matters to do with the effects of work on health or health on work. Again, the prospect of even a fully staffed service providing more than the most rudimentary health cover is obvious although it must be pointed out that many of the large industries have their own medical service. The chances of a factory with less than 100 employees having any medical cover, however, is less than one in 20 and only half the factories with more than

250 employees have a doctor; the majority of the work force of this country are employed in factories having fewer than 50 employees, and they are not likely to have any form of medical supervision whilst at work. Thus, there is a large potential target population for EMAS and again, it is clear that their facilities are much too limited to permit them to carry out their duties to the best effect.

Under the terms of the Health and Safety at Work Act, employers are obliged to ensure, so far as is reasonably practicable, the health, safety and welfare at work of all their employees. They must also ensure that plant and systems of work are safe and without risk to health, and that the working environment is without risk to health and provide such information, instruction, training and supervision as is necessary to ensure the health and safety of their work force. All those who manufacture or import materials must ensure that they are without risk to health if properly used. For their part, employees have a duty for their own health and safety and must co-operate with the employer so far as is necessary to fulfil that requirement. It is straining credulity to its limits to suppose that all employers—or indeed all employees—will obey the strictures of the Act without the sure and certain knowledge that any misdemeanours will be detected and punished. The Act can work effectively only if it is adequately enforced, and, as has been seen, the size of the Inspectorates and of EMAS is totally inadequate for the task. If these bodies are not considerably enlarged then some other form of control may be necessary.

There is one means by which effective local control of working conditions could be ensured; this is through the Safety Committees which the Health and Safety at Work requires to be set up at places of work. The members of the Safety Committees include representatives of the management and the Safety Representative appointed by the Trade Unions, and others who may be appointed ex officio, for instance the occupational nurse or physician, the occupational hygienist or the radiation protection officer. The Safety Representatives have wide ranging authority; they are entitled to inspect the work place and make recommendations to management, they are entitled to time off with pay in order to carry out their duties and they have a right to see the results of environmental monitoring. There is sometimes a fear in the minds of occupational physicians that the role of the safety representatives or the safety committee may conflict with their own, and there is no doubt that some safety representatives consider that the occupational physician is an ally of management rather than being an impartial adviser. With diplomacy and education, these difficulties can be overcome and the occupational physician can play an important role in feeding expert opinion into the safety committee and so help to improve local working conditions. The Safety Committee is potentially an important tool in controlling hazards at work and there seems to be no reason why it should not negotiate local exposure limits or local biological thresholds; it seems perfectly proper that those who are exposed to dangerous substances at work should have a large say in the extent to which they are prepared to take risks to their health providing that their views are based on sound toxicological or medical advice. The occupational physician should have nothing to fear from such an approach; his or her special expertise is required in order that the committee can function most satisfactorily and, in any case, all parties are ostensibly working towards the same end, that is to make the workplace as safe as it can possibly be.

Control of substances hazardous to health regulations

The Health and Safety at Work Act of 1974 was a major advance in health and safety legislation even if in recent years the Health and Safety Executive has been depleted to such an extent that its ability to carry out its functions adequately must be called into question. The HSW Act is an enabling act and from time to time the Health and Safety Commission has promulgated regulations relating to certain dangerous occupations; the Control of Lead at Work Regulations and the Control of Asbestos at Work Regulations are examples.

The most recent regulations are the Control of Substances Hazardous to Health (COSHH) Regulations which are in force as from 1 October 1989. These regulations are extremely wide ranging and effectively apply to all chemical and microbiological substances likely to be encountered in the workplace.

The core of the COSHH Regulations is Regulation 6 which states that an employer shall not carry on any work which is liable to expose employees to substances hazardous to health unless he or she has made a suitable and sufficient assessment of the risks created by that work to the health of his or her employees. Substances hazardous to health include all those with an OEL or an MEL; any micro-organism which creates a hazard to health; dust of any kind when present in a substantial concentration in air (greater than 5 mg/m^3) or any substance which creates a hazard to health comparable to that created by the substances already listed. For all practical purposes, it may be assumed that *all* chemical, microbiological and biological substances fall within the remit of the regulations.

The assessment must take into account a consideration of the substances present, their effects on the body, where and in what form they are likely to be present and the way in which employees are or may be exposed. It must also determine the steps needed to achieve adequate control of exposure and it must also make an estimate of exposure with the use of atmospheric monitoring if this is considered necessary.

The assessment must be carried out by a person (or persons) with the necessary information, instruction and training. There is no clear definition in the regulations as to what constitutes necessary instruction and training but the tenor of the regulations is to suggest that the person would normally be an industrial hygienist working in conjunction with other experts as required.

Except in the most simple cases the results of the assessments must be recorded and must be readily accessible to those who may need to know the results. This includes factory inspectors but also employees or their representatives who now have a statutory right to see the assessments.

Under Regulation 7, every employer shall ensure that exposure to toxic substances is either prevented or where this is not reasonably practicable, adequately controlled. One important novel feature of the regulations is that control must be ensured, so far as is reasonably practicable, by measures other than the provision of personal protective equipment. Where there is an MEL, exposure must be kept below this and as low as is reasonably practicable. Where there is an OEL, control to this level is considered adequate.

The incorporation of OELs into the COSHH Regulations may have some important consequences. Firstly, the wording of the regulations is such that the OELs could come to be seen as maximum allowable concentrations and employers may make no efforts to reduce exposure *below* these levels. Previously, exposure had to be below the suggested standard and as low as was reasonably practicable. Secondly, the regulations may have the effect of giving the OELs a legal status which they have not enjoyed before.

Where control measures are put into place or where personal protective equipment is provided, employers have a duty to take all reasonable steps to ensure that it is properly used and applied. There is an equally important clause in the regulations which makes it the duty of *employees* to make full and proper use of any control measure or any item of personal protective equipment which is provided for them.

Following the assessment it may be necessary to institute systems of atmospheric monitoring. This provision is contained within Regulation 10 which states that where it is requisite for ensuring the maintenance of adequate control of exposure or for protecting the health of employees, employers shall ensure that exposure is monitored in accordance with a suitable procedure. Records must be kept of any monitoring and these records, or a suitable summary of them, must be available for inspection by any employee who wishes to see them. Records of personal exposure of identifiable employees must be kept for at least 30 years and all other records must be kept for a minimum of 5 years.

Regulation 11 relates to the health surveillance of employees. Where it is appropriate for the protection of the health of employees, the regulation states, the employer shall ensure that such employees are under suitable health surveillance. 'Appropriate' in this context means where exposure is known to be associated with disease or other adverse effects and where there are valid techniques for detecting the disease or indications of adverse effects. The form which health surveillance can take will vary according to what is known of the effects; it may require measurement of lung function in those handling experimental animals; the measurement of urinary metabolites in some solvent workers; examination of the skin in those working with sensitizers and so on. The records of any health surveillance must be kept and summaries made available to those who may legitimately have access to them although medical confidentiality will be maintained. All records of health surveillance must be retained for at least 30 years after the date of the last entry; how this formidable task is to be achieved and what happens to the records when individuals move from job to job is not made clear.

The final regulation to which reference needs to be made is Regulation 12. This concerns training of employees exposed to hazardous substances and states that an employer who undertakes work which exposes employees to such substances shall provide those employees with such information, instruction and training as is suitable and sufficient for them to know the risks created by such exposure and the precautions which should be taken to avoid exposure.

The regulations apply to all employees except those covered by other regulations relating to exposure to lead, asbestos and ionizing radiation and they do not apply to work below ground in the mines nor do they apply where the risk to health arises solely in the context of medical treatment. They do apply, however, so far as is reasonably practicable, to other persons, *whether at work or not* who may be affected by the work being carried out. An employer is not responsible for the health surveillance of employees of another company who may be working on his premises but he *is* responsible for the instruction and training of such persons. Where the employees of one company work on the premises of another, both have duties under the regulations and co-operation and collaboration between them will be necessary to ensure that these duties are carried out.

The COSHH Regulations are seen by HSE as a system of health and safety management and there is no doubt that the responsibility for seeing that they are complied with lies with management. However, occupational health personnel will be looked to for an input into the assessments by providing expert advice on the toxicology of the substances encountered in the workplace and on the need for health surveillance; the occupational health department will also have the duty to carry out health surveillance and, in some cases, atmospheric monitoring and they will have to keep the required records.

These regulations are potentially the most important piece of health and safety legislation since the HSW itself. However, they have serious deficiencies which could nullify their effect. Firstly employers are not required to register with HSE to signify that they are carrying on work which falls within the remit of the regulations. Secondly there is no requirement for employers to send the results of their assessments—or at least a summary of them—to HSE and this means that interpretation will all be carried out in-house as will the decision whether or not to carry out monitoring or health surveillance. Conscientious employers will, of course, adhere strictly to the letter and spirit of the regulations but there is no doubt that some will ignore them, waiting for the inspector to call before they do anything. And with its dwindling band of inspectors (numbers in the Factory Inspectorate have fallen from 742 in 1979 to 598 in 1988), HSE has nowhere near the resources necessary adequately to police the regulations.

The EC directive on health and safety at work

The European Community framework directive on health and safety at work was adopted by the Council of Ministers in June 1989 and the United Kingdom government has until the end of 1992 to bring its health and safety laws into line with the objectives in the directive. The directive follows closely what is contained in the HSW Act but new legislation will be required when the directive is more detailed or goes further than present UK law.

In form and intent the directive resembles the Health and Safety at Work Act in assigning the primary responsibility for ensuring the health and safety of employees to the employer. In particular the employer is called upon to:

1   Develop a coherent overall policy on health and safety.

2   Evaluate risks and introduce necessary preventive measures.

3   Co-operate with other employers.

4   Designate personnel to carry out health and safety activities, or enlist competent external services.

5   Take necessary measures for first aid, fire fighting and evacuation of employees.

6   Provide health and safety information and training for employees.

7   Consult employees and their representatives.

It should not prove too difficult to comply with these requirements since those which are not covered by the Health and Safety at Work Act should be met by the COSHH Regulations.

1992 and the single European market

In 1992 the single European market comes into being and whilst the present legislators have enthusiastically exhorted employers to take advantage of it, they are somewhat less keen on the social implications which will follow. The Social Charter which is now being developed will confer equal rights on all workers throughout the member states of the European Community; the intention is to bring all rights and benefits into line with the highest standards no matter in which country these prevail. Thus, the minimum wage might be related to that which is paid in Germany, the number of holidays set at the level in Italy and the number of months for which pay is given during the year adjusted to the Portuguese norm (14). It is intended that health and safety benefits will also be equalized and this may have profound effects upon a government which has not seen this as a field in which expansion is to be encouraged. If, for example, occupational health services became mandatory, this would have the most profound consequences in the UK both in terms of training of personnel and establishment of new services. Whether this desirable state will ever be attained will presumably have to depend upon the vigour with which the UK delegation resists the proposals in the council chamber.

Chapter 13
The Effects of Health on Work

Although those who practice occupational medicine are principally concerned with the effects of work on health, they also have the important task of studying the effects which health may have on work; as the workplace becomes less dangerous and the prevalence of occupational disease decreases, this aspect of occupational medicine will assume greater importance. There are few medical conditions which are an absolute bar to work, but many may impair an individual's capacity to perform certain jobs to some degree and so a large part of the occupational physician's time is taken up in ensuring that the worker and the job are as well suited as possible. This process begins by assessing the health and capabilities of prospective employees before they are appointed. However, this does not mean to say that all new employees must necessarily be medically examined and indeed this is generally a poor use of the physician's time since the pick-up rate of abnormalities is likely to be small and by no means all those who attend for preemployment medicals will be offered a job, nor will they all accept even if one is offered them. Nevertheless, they should all be subjected to some form of screening process and this can satisfactorily be undertaken by a trained occupational nurse who will ask each prospective employee to complete a health questionnaire which has been devised by the company doctor. The precise form which the questionnaire takes will depend upon individual preferences and special local requirements, but normally such a form is simple to construct and quick to administer. In the majority of cases the questionnaire will confirm that the worker is fit and no further action need be taken, except to inform the personnel department that there are no evident medical grounds for refusing the person work. A few questionnaires will need to be referred to the doctor for an opinion when there is some doubt as to the person's fitness to work, and some physicians may wish to check all the questionnaires themselves.

Whilst this simple screening procedure will generally be sufficient there will clearly be some categories of new employee who must be seen by the doctor. Those being taken on to work in a job which entails exposure to specific hazards, heavy metals, radiation or noise, for example, will need to be examined in order to establish base line clinical data which may need to be supplemented by laboratory investigations such as a blood lead estimation, full blood count or an audiogram. Food handlers must be free of gastrointestinal infection and those who are to work in dialysis units must be hepatitis B antigen negative. Common sense dictates that those who are likely to be called upon to lift heavy loads must be free from a history of back pain, that lorry drivers or crane drivers must have good vision and no restriction of their visual fields, that those to be exposed to dust are free from lung disease, and so on. Each firm should be able to construct its own list of 'high risk' occupations which will require the special attention of the medical adviser.

Ill health which develops when the worker is in employment may require the doctor to re-assess the worker's fitness to continue in the job. The occupational physician is often asked to undertake this assessment by the management, especially if the worker in question is requiring frequent sickness absence. This is a perfectly reasonable request and should raise no problems of medical confidentiality so long as the doctor reports in general terms and does not enter into clinical details in any report to management without the written consent of the worker concerned. To assess fully fitness to work, the occupational physician may require more clinical information than is available from his own records and he may wish to supplement his knowledge of the case by writing to the general practitioner or a hospital consultant. Again, this should pose no ethical problems so long as consent is obtained from the worker and he is assured that any information which is forthcoming will remain confidential to the medical department.

In many firms all employees who are sick for a period of more than a few days or who have had a particularly severe illness are required to have a medical examination before their return to work. In some cases this is also done to encourage a employee back to work after what seems an unseemly delay! The doctor should ensure that those who return from an illness are not put into situations with which they will be unable to cope, and that their return to work is supervised and graded as required. In many cases the return to work will be achieved most satisfactorily if there is a close liaison between the worker's general practitioner and the occupational physician, but all too often lines of communication between the two are poor and each chooses to operate without reference to the other, sometimes to the detriment of their patient.

Case indexes

In any firm there will be a proportion of men and women with nonoccupational diseases of one sort or another, some serious, some trivial. Whether the physician tries to maintain a separate case index for a large number of diseases will depend upon his or her inclinations and resources. Some diseases, however, should be given special attention, the most important of which are epilepsy and diabetes mellitus.

With proper medical supervision workers with epilepsy may undertake most jobs, and may drive so long as they have been without a fit for 3 years whilst awake regardless of whether or not they are receiving treatment. Most doctors tend to be cautious in their dealings with epileptics, however, and prefer to keep them away from jobs which might involve contact with moving machinery or heights; many firms would also not allow them to drive. A *grand mal* fit is a spectacular and also a rather frightening episode for the layman to witness, and on this account alone epileptics are often not well tolerated by their work mates and so encouragement and support from the doctor is essential. A regular visit to the surgery will allow the doctor to satisfy himself that the worker is taking anticonvulsant therapy and it is prudent to keep in a small stock of anticonvulsants in case the employee forgets to bring a supply to work.

Diabetics in industry do not require the same degree of medical supervision as epileptics, but they need to be known so that they may be dealt with promptly and efficiently in an emergency. The most likely event is a hypoglycaemic coma and there should be provision for urine testing in the medical department and ideally a simple method for blood sugar estimation (such as the Ames Dextrostix). There should be no difficulty in distinguishing between hypogly-caemia and a diabetic coma; the latter is not a condition amenable to treatment in any setting other than a hospital, but the doctor should see that 50% dextrose is available for the initial treatment of the former before the patient is referred elsewhere. It is also a sensible precaution to keep in a small supply of antidiabetic drugs for those who come to work without their own.

Psychiatric illness

Neurotic disorders are a common contribution to illness of all kinds and may often masquerade as physical disease. Estimates of the number of people with some kind of neurotic illness vary widely, but it has been suggested that they may represent 40% of all general practitioner consultations. This must be reflected in the industrial setting and it has been estimated that the total number of days lost due to incapacity from 'nervous debility and headache' are rising, and are currently running at over 5 million a year. In addition to this, it is likely that between 20 and 25% of all absenteeism can be attributed to neurosis.

In general terms, it is obvious that problems of adjustment and coping will be intimately related to productivity and efficiency in the industrial setting. There is evidence that the increase in the size of companies and in automation are producing effects on the motivation of individual workers and on their sense of identity with and responsibility to the company, and that they are not encouraged to see their individual importance to the firm as a whole. It is reasonable to suppose that this sense of alienation may have a greater effect on the more vulnerable personality and help to tip the balance between being able to cope, and not able to cope with work.

In more specific terms, one of the most important responsibilities of the occupational physician in the area of psychiatric illness is to identify those who are not declaring their symptoms. This is a serious consideration in those who have repeated sickness absence for apparently trivial conditions especially after promotion or an increase in responsibilities or whose efficiency and concentra-tion are declining for no apparent reason. There are times when a change of job may be appropriate to alleviate a specific stress such as a personality clash with a supervisor, although it must always be borne in mind that the expressed cause of anxiety and depression may not reflect the true conflict which may be areas of the patient's life inaccessible to the intervention of the occupational physician. A common cause of failure to cope with work is a mismatch of the demands of the job and the worker's ability and it must be remembered that difficulties may arise equally because a man is doing a job beneath his capacity as well as when it is beyond him.

Other factors which may be predictive of the onset of psychiatric illness include an excess of zeal and over-conscientiousness in a worker who is attempting to make up for a fall in efficiency. Emotional or aggressive outbursts as a response to minor provocation in a previously stable worker should be taken seriously and the worker referred for psychiatric advice if it seems appropriate. Numerically, most illnesses of psychiatric origin in the work setting will be neurotic, but the possibility of psychotic breakdown must be considered if bizarre behaviour is reported.

The return to work after a psychiatric breakdown is complicated by two factors. Firstly, whatever the nature of the illness, a severe blow to the patient's self confidence has almost always occurred, and as a consequence he may undervalue his capacity and be unrealistically anxious about his ability to cope in future. Secondly, psychiatric illness still carries a stigma and not infrequently provokes fear and ridicule in others so that the reaction of close associates at work may have to be borne in mind. If it can be arranged it is often extremely helpful to grade the return to work in terms of time and responsibility, starting with a return of as little as one day a week with a steady increase until the full working week is achieved. Ideally the degree of support required should be estimated for each individual; it can be harmful to be too protective and liaison between industry and the psychiatrist concerned can be very helpful in handling the return to work. The Disablement Resettlement Officer may also usefully be involved in these decisions (see below).

Workers who suffer from psychotic disorders pose particular problems. Many chronic schizophrenics are able to work in open industry, perhaps as part of the quota of jobs kept for the registered disabled, but they may be peculiarly susceptible to small changes in the job iself or to their immediate environment. Although they may work steadily and accurately, they are likely to work more slowly than the fit worker and so they should not usually be placed in situations where their workmates' output depends on theirs. If it is possible, tolerance of sickness absence should be exercised; the ability to work is crucial to the mental health of the schizophrenic and so it is preferable that they keep their jobs.

It must be remembered that whilst schizophrenia can be a disease which renders the patient less able and skilled after recurrences, manic-depressive psychosis is not. Most manic-depressives are perfectly able to continue their jobs at their previous level after attacks of illness and their return to this level must be facilitated whenever possible.

Finally, many psychotic patients need to return comparatively frequently to the clinic for long acting antipsychotic medication and for routine examinations, estimating serum lithium concentrations for example, and this should be actively encouraged by the industrial physician.

Alcoholism

Dependent drinking, or drinking to a degree which regularly impairs abilities in social, family or work relationships is the most important psychiatric problem in industry. This is not only due to the numbers affected but also because alcoholics conceal their condition either from a sense of shame or by denying that they have a problem. The heavy, nondependent drinker has considerable nuisance value if he is drunk at work or hungover in bed on a Monday morning, but these activities do not pose the same problem to the occupational physician as the recognition and treatment of dependent drinking with its progressive mental and physical damage.

It is impossible to give a clear estimate of the prevalence of alcoholism, but one more reliable estimate is that there are 70 000 longstanding and 200 000 early alcoholics in England and Wales, making a prevalence of 8.5 per 1000 for the population at risk. The rate is likely to be higher than this in industry since the population at risk is comprised largely of those at work. The contribution made by the unemployed population, whilst not high in absolute terms, is unknown. Although alcoholism in women and in the young is on the increase, the most susceptible group in industry remains the middle-aged man in his fifth decade, perhaps because the increase of female alcoholics is confined largely to the group of comparatively well off, nonemployed housewives.

Recent drives to increase awareness of alcoholism in industry have had moderate success but the recognition of individuals who have become dependent upon alcohol is still inadequate. One should not have to wait until a man is suddenly found to have been admitted to an alcoholism unit, or until he has a withdrawal fit or patches of complete amnesia for events at work before the diagnosis is made. Deterioration to this degree places work colleagues at risk as well as the dependent drinker himself. There are many pointers towards the development of alcoholism which taken together should provide enough suspicion for the physician to intervene. These include persistent bad timekeeping, especially after weekends, and prolonged lunch hours. Withdrawal tremor may be marked early on in the working day or if an unusually long meeting prevents the worker from abolishing it by topping up with alcohol. Frequent absence due to 'gastritis' may also be significant especially if coupled with a decline in the standard of work and in moodiness. The carrying of alcohol on the person (except perhaps at Christmas) should immediately make one suspect dependence on alcohol.

The group which is perhaps most at risk of escaping detection is higher management; it is much easier to drink continuously during the day when alcohol is provided freely for refreshment and entertainment in the board room. Alcoholism is most prevalent in the highest and lowest social classes so company executives are greatly at risk, perhaps as a response to stress, and are encouraged by having alcohol readily available at work. The occupational physician should not shrink from his duty to protect and advise his colleagues in management despite the fact that he will be more tempted to accept the rationalizations of those who deny it is a problem whilst at the same time pointing to colleagues who apparently drink more than they do themselves. If alcoholism is suspected, the doctor should insist on the necessity for treatment which may involve psychiatric referral, or contact with Alcoholics Anonymous, or some other organization. For most alcoholics, continued abstinence is the index of successful treatment, although in some centres controlled drinking programmes have met with some success. It may therefore be seen as part of the occupational physician's duties to encourage the acceptance of abstinence in those at risk, and certainly a known interest in, and nonpejorative view of dependent drinking is likely to result in more open discussion and a more frank acknowledgement of the problem

Treatment of alcoholics is rarely totally successful, at least in the early stages, and it must be remembered that the risk of recurrence is high, and the occupational physician should not consider that his job has been completed after the initial referral. Those who use alcohol as an anxiolytic are particularly at risk of becoming dependent and so there may be a case for recommending a change of job to one which is less stressful.

Finally, it is well to remember that the absence of drunkenness is no guide to the presence of alcoholism.

The disabled

Firms over a certain size are required to keep 3% of their vacancies for the registered disabled but few comply with this regulation, especially in times of high unemployment. The tasks which a disabled person can perform will necessarily depend upon the nature of the disability but by no means all are restricted to minor clerical jobs or to answering the telephone.

The responsibility for training disabled persons, for finding them suitable employment and for maintaining the registers of disabled persons lies with the Disablement Resettlement Officer (DRO) and the Blind Persons' Resettlement Officer (BPRO). Both the DRO and BPRO are employed by the Employment Service Agency (ESA) which is one of the executive arms of the Manpower Services Commission (MSC) established in 1974. The ESA runs a number of Employment Rehabilitation Centres at which disabled persons may attend for retraining or for a re-assessment of their capacity to work.

Some larger firms have their own rehabilitation centres which they encourage employers who have suffered accidents or severe illnesses to attend but not all will choose to do so.

Some disabled persons benefit from training schemes which are organized by the Training Services Agency of the MSC at their Skillcentres or technical colleges. These courses are intensive and usually last for about 6 months and may be supplemented by further periods of training when in employment.

Here, as in many other areas of occupational medicine, the patient is best served if there is a close working relationship between all with responsibilities towards him. In this case, there is a need for liaison between the occupational health services, the personnel at the Employment Rehabilitation Centres and Skillcentres, hospital staff and the general practitioner, but such liaison is often not well developed to put it mildly.

Chapter 14
Occupational Health Services

The provision of health care for people at work varies enormously from industry to industry as may be seen in Table 14.1. From Table 14.2 it will be noted that a large proportion of the work force, most of whom work in factories employing less than 250 persons, has neither medical nor nursing cover. In general, where facilities are available the quality of the occupational health service is directly related to size. Thus, some of the largest private firms have sophisticated medical departments which employ a number of doctors and nurses, have surgeries at different points throughout the factory, provide rehabilitation, physiotherapy, laboratory and radiographic services, employ hygienists with the nessary back-up to undertake environmental surveys, and offer dental and other ancillary services free or on greatly subsidized terms. At the lower end of the scale are the large number of (usually small) firms who offer no kind of service at all beyond the provision of first aid facilities which all employers are obliged by law to provide in relation to the size of their work force. Since the most unhygienic working conditions are usually to be found in small factories, it follows that those most at risk have the least provision made for their health and safety.

Intermediate between these two extremes in an almost infinite variety of service, some run by full-time physicians, others by nurses with the supervision of part-time medical advisers, still others by nurses working with no direct medical help.

The nationalized industries are required to provide a comprehensive health service for their employees and theirs are undoubtedly amongst the best in the country. Ironically, the National Health Service, which is one of the largest of all the nationalized industries has only lately developed an awareness that it should have a health service for its own employees, largely in response to the recommendations contained within the Tonbridge report. The number of health service districts which have an effective occupational health service, however, is relatively small and the prospects for change are not great especially as there is no proper provision for the training of occupational physicians within the NHS. The DOH has a duty to provide training posts for doctors in all specialties but it has established none for occupational physicians.

There has been a general agreement since the Dale Committee reported in 1951 that

> it is desirable that there should eventually be some comprehensive provision for occupational health covering not only industrial establishments of all kinds, both large and small, but also the non-industrial occupations...

Table 14.1. Provision of types of occupational health service by size of firm
% of firms

Number of employees	Medical and nursing staff	Medical staff only	Nursing staff only	Doctor on call only	Other staff only*	No service†	Total
0–10	0.8	0.4	0.4	0.4	0.0	98.0	100.0
11–24	1.2	0.5	0.4	3.8	0.9	93.2	100.0
25–49	0.9	1.5	1.5	7.1	2.4	86.6	100.0
50–99	0.9	4.1	2.2	8.4	4.4	80.0	100.0
100–249	5.4	9.8	4.9	11.0	2.6	66.3	100.0
250–499	22.5	9.8	14.9	7.1	6.3	39.4	100.0
500–999	42.9	11.1	21.0	6.3	3.2	15.5	100.0
1000–2499	78.9	4.4	7.0	3.8	0.6	5.3	100.0
2500–4999	80.0	2.5	7.5	2.5	0.0	7.5	100.0
5000 +	76.9	3.8	7.6	7.7	0.0	4.0	100.0

*e.g. first aiders employed as such for at least 10 hours a week.
†Other than first aiders employed as such for less than 10 hours a week.
Reproduced with permission from *Occupational Health Services*, HMSO, 1977.

By contrast, there is no consensus on the means by which an occupational health service can be provided for the many smaller firms which have none at present. Governments of various shades have been urged by several medical bodies, including most notably the British Medical Association, to provide something akin to a National Occupational Health Service. Such an approach seems to me to be the only satisfactory solution. At present, occupational physicians are the only group of doctors not employed by the DOH and, amongst other things, this has a markedly adverse effect on their training. If a national occupational health service were to be established in parallel with the

Table 14.2. Frequency distribution of types of service, adjusted for sampling bias

Type of service	% firms	% workforce
Full-time medical and full-time nursing staff	0.5	16.5
Full-time medical and part-time nursing staff	0.1	0.1
Full-time medical staff; no nursing staff	0.04	0.3
Part-time medical and full-time nursing staff	1.5	25.2
Part-time medical and part-time nursing staff	0.4	2.4
Part-time medical staff; no nursing staff	1.1	5.1
Doctor on call; no nursing staff	6.8	6.1
Full-time nursing staff; no medical staff*	1.1	6.7
Part-time nursing staff; no medical staff*	0.9	1.6
No medical or nursing staff, but some other occupational health staff (e.g. first-aider employed as such for at least 10 hours a week)	2.7	1.8
No service except first-aiders employed as such for less than 10 hours a week	84.9	34.2
	100.0	100.0

*Other than a doctor on call.
Reproduced with permission from *Occupational Health Services*, HMSO, 1977.

NHS, not only would the imputation that occupational physicians are not entirely impartial disappear—no one suggests that a cardiologist or a neurologist is a tool of *his* management (the DOH)—but there would be an immediate benefit from improved contacts with other specialists in the NHS and better access to diagnostic and treatment facilities. Unfortunately, since the DOH has only a minimal interest in preventive medicine, the chances that large sums of money will be deflected into creating an effective nationwide occupational health service are remote; this should not prevent interested parties from agitating for change and improvement, however.

Some firms which have no facilities of their own make some provision for their occupational health needs by subscribing to the 7 or 8 group occupational health services which there are in the United Kingdom, but the total number of workers who are covered in this way is relatively small.

The purpose of an occupational health service

The purpose of an occupational health service is to ensure that the health of men and women at work is not adversely affected by their occupation. The first duty of any occupational physician or occupational nurse must be towards securing that end. This principle is enshrined in Recommendation 112 of the International Labour Organization, formulated in 1959. This recommendation states that an occupational health service has the functions of:

1 Protecting the worker against any health hazard which may arise out of their work or the conditions in which it is carried on.

2 Contributing towards the workers' physical and mental adjustment, in particular, by the application of the work to the workers and their assignment to jobs for which they are suited.

3 Contributing to the establishment and maintenance of the highest degree of physical and mental well-being of the workers. In this country, most occupational health services concentrate their efforts in three main areas: prevention, adjustment to work, and treatment. The emphasis given to each varies from industry to industry as would be expected. In addition, one should not forget the research which is undertaken by doctors and others working in occupational health services and upon which the future development of the specialty largely depends.

Prevention

The prevention of occupationally induced diseases is paramount to the work of an occupational health service and involves not only protecting against well-recognized hazards but also the identification and evaluation of new hazards to health. This increasingly requires some form of epidemiological study, perhaps involving co-operation between different firms and collaboration with academic depatments which have the necessary epidemiological and statistical skills to enable such a study to be carried out successfully. In the past occupational physicians and nurses have received little in the way of training in epidemiology but this deficiency is slowly becoming remedied, and future training programmes are certain to place more emphasis on this subject.

Programmes for preventing ill health in industry must, of course, contain a large educative component if they are to be successful. However, there is still too little effort given to the study of the best means whereby workers can be made aware of the potential hazards to which their job exposes them and of the steps which they can take themselves to protect their health. Likewise, management are not always made aware of their responsibilities in the preventive field as they ought to be, and it is the duty of occupational physicians and nurses to see that both sides of industry are better educated in these matters.

There is, of course, no reason why an occupational health service should restrict its health education solely to occupational disease; it can with advantage give advice on such matters as smoking and health, and on dietary habits, and can also make arrangements for services such as cervical cytology or mass radiography to be carried out within the work place.

Adjustment to work

This has been discussed in the previous chapter and will not be gone into further here.

Treatment

Occupational services do not normally offer a comprehensive treatment service except for accidents which may occur at work. Some firms will be able to offer nothing more than simple first-aid measures, but in the best case the occupational health service is equipped with a full range of resuscitation apparatus and may also have its own ambulance to ensure that accident victims are transported to hospital with the minimum delay.

The occupational health service will usually choose to udertake casualty-type work, the removal of foreign bodies from eyes, dressing of wounds, removal of sutures and so on, but it should not provide initial treatment for medical conditions since this properly falls within the province of the general practitioner or the hospital consultant.

Confidentiality

The physician in industry is sometimes in the invidious position of being viewed with mistrust by the employees because he is thought to be a tool of management, whilst management may think that he is not nearly obliging enough! If the occupational health service is to function well the doctor has to be seen to be impartial. Moreover the patients who attend the surgery must have confidence in the staff and must be assured that the doctor–patient (or nurse–patient) relationship is the same in the setting of the work place as elsewhere. Thus confidentiality must be respected and it must be made very clear to management that the medical records belong to the medical department and not the firm and that no one has the right of access to records by virtue of his or her position within the company.

The doctor in industry frequently encounters difficulties in trying to exercise impartiality, however. For example, the doctor may learn that a patient has a condition which may make him or her unfit for work, or worse, a potential danger were he to carry on, and the patient requests that management are not informed. The doctor will of course encourage the patient to change jobs or seek medical treatment, or both, if if this is unsuccessful then the patient will have to be told that the doctor's duty extends also to the other employees and to the management and that the patient cannot be allowed to continue at work. If such a decision is transmitted to management, then it must be couched in general terms and no clinical details should be included.

On the other hand, the physician may also discover instances in which the health of workers has suffered as a direct consequence of their work and he then has the duty to advise the workers affected of their statutory benefits, if they are suffering from one of the prescribed diseases, and he should also discuss frankly with them the question of compensation if he considers management to be in any way culpable. If there is no possibility of compensation, he should nevertheless see that the employees are treated as generously as possible by the company.

Perhaps the most important function of the occupational physician, however, is to ensure that all those who have a part to play in creating the safest possible working environment do so in harmony; disease is no respecter of class or political divisions, and progress will be achieved by co-operation and not conflict.

Future developments

As a society becomes more affluent its expectations increase and it will not tolerate those conditions under which its forebears lived and worked. During the present century and especially in the last 3 decades, working conditions for the majority of people have improved enormously. This has been due not only to the introduction of better control of hazards at the work place and to improved medical supervision but also to the change in the pattern of industry in the country. Many of the traditional heavy industries have contracted or disappeared altogether and a much greater proportion of the work force is employed in service industries or in light industry in which the risks to health are relatively small. No occupational physician who practices in the developed countries in the future will have personal experience of the huge numbers of cases of toxic diseases which are so elegantly described in Donald Hunter's *Diseases of Occupations*. Hunter was able to conduct ward rounds at the London Hospital in the late 1940s during which he could demonstrate a seemingly endless number of cases such as lead poisoning, mercury poisoning, toxic jaundice or silicosis, cases which formed the basis of his book, for he never was employed in industry. Today the book is read more as an important social document than as a medical text since Hunter's medical practice is beyond our experience in the same way that cholera and smallpox no longer form a part of the day to day practice of a community physician.

The corollary of this decline in the prevalence of the classic occupational diseases is that those who work in the new conditions have new expectations. And the concerns of the present generation of workers are becoming increasingly centred around smaller deviations from normality, and around behavioural and reproductive effects of exposure to potentially toxic materials and about the possible mutagenic or carcinogenic risks at the workplace. The occupational physician has necessarily to adapt to this change; much of the research into the effects of work on health is now in the hands of epidemiologists rather than clinicians, dermatologists and chest physicians investigate occupational skin diseases and chest diseases and the control of accidents, through which most lives are lost at work, is the province of the safety officer. What is the occupational physician to do? He will first of all have to concentrate increasingly on the effects of health on work and he may also find that he becomes the source of general health education; if present economic trends continue, much of his time may also be spent in preparing people to spend the large part of their life out of work.

Occupational medicine in the fully developed countries therefore seems about to enter into a subclinical period, where opinion will be given in shades of grey rather than in black and white and where there is a danger that words will come to mean whatever the speaker wishes them to mean. On the broader front, however, things are different. Occupational health in many of the developing countries has many similarities to that in the UK in the 1920s and 30s and it is the duty of fully industrialized nations to share their experience with the developing countries in order that they do not repeat the mistakes which we made.

Appendix: Occupational Exposure Standards

Some occupational exposure limits (OEL) and maximum exposure limits (MEL). OELs shown for long-term (8-hour time weighted average values) or short-term (10-minute TWA) exposures. Where the word 'skin' is shown, this denotes the fact that a significant amount of the material may be absorbed through the skin and mucous membranes.

Substances	Long term		Short term	
	ppm	mg/m^3	ppm	mg/m^3
Acetone	1000	2400	1250	3000
Acrylamide—skin	—	0.3	—	0.6
Acrylonitrile—skin MEL	2	4		
Aldrin—skin	—	0.25	—	0.75
Aluminium, metal and oxide	—	10	—	20
Ammonia	25	18	35	27
Aniline—skin	2	10	5	20
Antimony and compounds (as Sb)	—	0.5		
Arsenic and compounds (as As) MEL		0.2		
Arsine	0.05	0.2		
Azinphos-methyl—skin	—	0.2	—	0.6
Barium (soluble compounds)	—	0.5		
Benzene—skin	10	30		
Beryllium		0.002		
Bromine	0.1	0.7	0.3	2
Buta-1, 3-diene MEL	10			
2-Butoxyethanol MEL	25	120		
Cadmium and cadmium compounds (as Cd) MEL		0.05		
Cadmium oxide MEL		0.05		0.05
Cadmium sulphide	10	30		
Carbon black		3.5		7
Carbon dioxide	5000	9000	15000	27000
Carbon disulphide (skin) MEL	10	30		
Carbon monoxide	50	55	400	440
Carbon tetrachloride—skin	10	65	20	130
Chlorine	1	3	3	9
Chlorobenzene	75	350		
Chlorinated biphenyls—skin				
(42% chlorine)		1		2
(54% chlorine)		0.5		1
Chloroform	10	50		
Chromium		0.5		
Chromium (II) compounds (as Cr)		0.5		
Chromium (III) compounds (as Cr)		0.5		
Chromium (VI) compounds (as Cr)		0.05		

Substances	Long term		Short term	
	ppm	mg/m^3	ppm	mg/m^3
Coal dust containing				
<5% respirable quartz		2		
>5% respirable quartz	See section on airborne dusts			
Coal dust in mines MEL		7		
Cobalt and compounds (as Co)		0.1		
Copper fume		0.2		
Copper dusts and mists		1		2
Cotton dust (total dustless fly)		0.5		
Cresol, all isomers—skin	5	22		
Cristabolite total dust		0.15		
Cyanide, as CN—skin		5		
Cyclohexane	300	1050	375	1300
DDT		1		3
Demeton—skin	0.01	0.1	0.03	0.3
1,2-Dichlorobenzene	50	300	50	300
1,4-Dichlorobenzene	75	450	110	675
1,2-Dichloroethane	10	40	15	60
Dichloromethane MEL	100	350		
Dichloro-methylene dianiline (MbOCA) MEL		0.005		
Dichlorovos—skin	0.1	1	0.3	3
Dieldrin—skin		0.25		0.75
Di-isobutyl ketone	25	150		
Dinitrobenzene all isomers—skin	0.15	1	0.5	3
Dinitro-o-cresol—skin		0.2		0.6
Dinitrotoluene—skin		1.5		5
Dioxan (diethylene dioxide)—skin	50			
Diphenylamine		10		20
Diquat		0.5		1
Endrin—skin		0.1		0.3
Epichlorhydrin—skin	2	8	5	20
Ethyl alcohol	1000	1900		
Ethyl ether	400	1200	500	1500
Ethylene chlorohydrin—skin	1	3	1	3
Ethylene dibromide MEL	1	8		
Ethylene dinitrate—skin	0.2	2	0.2	2
Ethylene glycol monobutyl ether—skin	50	240	150	720
Ethylene glycol monoethyl ether—skin	100	370	150	560
Ethylene glycol monomethyl ether—skin	25	80	35	120
Ethylene glycol				
particulate		10		20
vapour	100	250	125	325
Ethylene oxide MEL	5	10		
2-Ethoxyethanol MEL	10	37		
2-Ethoxyethanol acetate MEL	10	54		
Fluoride (as F)		2.5		
Fluorine	1	2	2	4
Formaldehyde MEL	2	2.5	2	2.5
Formic acid	5	9		
Furfural—skin	5	20	15	60
Glutaraldehyde	0.2	0.7	0.2	0.7
Glyceryl trinitrate—skin	0.2	2	0.2	2

Substances	Long term		Short term	
	ppm	mg/m^3	ppm	mg/m^3
Graphite (synthetic)		10		
Heptachlor—skin		0.5		2
n-Hexane	100	360	125	450
Hydrogen bromide	3	10		
Hydrogen chloride	5	7	5	7
Hydrogen cyanide—skin MEL			10	10
Hydrogen fluoride (as F)	3	2.5	6	5
Hydrogen peroxide	1	1.5	2	3
Hydrogen sulphide	10	14	15	21
Hydroquinone		2		4
Iodine	0.1	1	0.1	1
Iron oxide fumes (as Fe)		5		10
Iron salts, soluble (as Fe)		1		2
Isocyantes, all (as NCO) MEL		0.02		0.07
Isophorone	2	25	2	25
Lead, all compounds except tetraethyl lead MEL		0.15		
Limestone		10		20
Lindane—skin		0.5		1.5
Magnesium oxide fume		10		
Malathion—skin		10		
Man-made mineral fibres MEL		5		
Manganese and compounds (as Mn)		5		5
Manganese fume (as Mn)		1		3
Mercury alkyls (as Hg)—skin		0.01		0.03
Mercury and compounds, except alkyls (as Hg)		0.05		0.15
Methanol—skin	200	260	250	310
1-Methoxypropan-2-ol MEL	100	360		
2-Methoxyethanol MEL	5	16		
2-Methoxyethyl acetate MEL	5	24		
Methyl alcohol—skin	200	260	250	325
Methyl bromide—skin	15	60		
Methyl butyl ketone	25	100	40	165
Methyl chloride	100	210	125	260
Methylcyclopentadienyl manganese tricarbonyl (as Mn)—skin	0.1	0.2	0.3	0.6
Methyl demeton—skin		0.5		1.5
Methyl ethyl ketone	200	590	300	885
Methyl isobutyl ketone—skin	100	410	125	510
Methyl methacrylate—skin	10	35		
Methyl parathion—skin		0.2		0.6
Mica				
total dust		10		
respirable dust		1		
Molybdenum (as Mo)				
soluble compounds		5		10
insoluble compounds		10		20
Naphthalene	10	50	15	75
Nickel carbonate (as Ni)	0.05	0.35		
Nickel carbonyl	0.001	0.007		
Nickel metal		1		

Substances	Long term		Short term	
	ppm	mg/m³	ppm	mg/m³
Nickel, soluble compounds (as Ni)		0.1		0.3
Nitric acid	2	5	4	10
Nitric oxide	25	30	35	45
Nitrobenzene—skin	1	5	2	10
Nitrogen dioxide	5	9	5	9
Nitrotoluene—skin	5	30	10	60
Oil mist		5		10
Osmium tetroxide (as Os)	0.0002	0.0002	0.0006	0.006
Ozone	0.1	0.2	0.3	0.6
Paraffin wax fume		2		6
Paraquat, respirable sizes		0.1		
Parathion—skin		0.2		0.6
Perchloroethylene—skin	100	670	150	1000
Phenol—skin	5	19	10	38
Phenylhydrazine—skin	5	20	10	45
Phosdrin (Mevinphos)—skin	0.01	0.1	0.03	0.3
Phosgene (carbonyl chloride)	0.1	0.4		
Phosphine	0.3	0.4	1	1
Phosphoric acid		1		3
Phosphorus (yellow)		0.1		0.3
Phosphorus pentachloride	0.1	1		
Phosphorus trichloride	0.5	3		
Phthalic anhydride	1	6	4	24
Platinum (soluble salts) (as Pt)		0.002		
Polyvinyl chloride				
total dust		10		
respirable dust		5		
Potassium hydroxide		2		2
Propylene glycol dinitrate—skin	0.2	2	0.2	2
Propylene glycol monomethyl ether	100	360	150	540
Pyrethrins		5		10
Quartz, crystalline				
total dust		0.3		
respirable dust		0.1		
Quinone	0.1	0.4	0.3	1
Resin core solder pyrolysis products				
(as formaldehyde)		0.1		0.3
Rubber process dust MEL		8		
Rubber fume MEL		0.75		
Selenium compounds (as Se)		0.2		
Selenium hexafluoride (as Se)	0.05	0.2		
Silica, amorphous				
total dust		0.3		
respirable dust		0.1		
Silver		0.1		
Silver, soluble compounds (as Ag)		0.01		0.03
Sodium fluoroacetate—skin		0.05		0.15
Sodium hydroxide		2		2
Stibene	0.1	0.5	0.3	1.5
Styrene MEL	100	420	250	1050
Sulphur dioxide	2	5	5	13
2,4,5-T		10		20

Substances	Long term		Short term	
	ppm	mg/m^3	ppm	mg/m^3
Sulphuric acid		1		
Talc				
total dust		10		
respirable dust		1		
Tantalum		5		10
Tellurium and compounds except				
hexafluoride (as Te)		0.1		
Tellurium hexafluoride (as Te)	0.02	0.2		
TEPP—skin	0.004	0.05	0.012	0.15
Tetrachloroethane—skin	5	35	10	70
Tetrachloroethylene	100	670	150	1000
Tetraethyl lead (as Pb)—skin MEL		0.1		
Thallium, soluble compounds				
(as T1)—skin		0.1		
Tin, inorganic compounds (as Sn)		2		4
Tin, organic compounds (as Sn)		0.1		0.2
Titanium dioxide		10		20
Toluene—skin	100	375	150	560
1,1,1-Trichloroethane MEL	350	1900	450	2450
Trichloroethylene—skin MEL	100	535	150	802
Trinitrotoluene		0.5		0.5
Tri-ortho-cresyl phosphate		0.1		0.3
Tungsten and compounds (as W)				
soluble		1		3
insoluble		5		10
Vanadium pentoxide (as V)				
dust		0.5		1.5
fume		0.05		0.05
Vinyl chloride MEL annual maximum	7			
exposure limit	3			
Vinylidene chloride MEL	10	40		
Welding fume		5		
White spirit	100	575	125	720
Wood dust (hard wood) MEL		5		
Xylene, all isomers—skin	100	435	150	650
Xylidene—skin	5	25	10	50
Zinc chloride fume		1		2
Zinc chromate (as Cr)		0.05		
Zinc oxide fume		5		10
Zinc distearate		10		20

Dusts

Asbestos

1　Dust consisting of, or containing any, crocidolite or amosite: 0.2 fibres/ml when averaged over any continuous period of 4 hours 0.6 fibres/ml when averaged over any continuous period of 10 minutes.

2　Dust consisting of, or containing other types of, asbestos but not crocidolite or amosite: 0.5 fibres/ml when averaged over any continuous period of 4 hours 1.5 fibres/ml when averaged over any continuous period of 10 minutes.

Airborne dusts

Mineral dusts containing silica
To calculate the recommended limits for mineral dusts containing crystalline silica, the following formulae should be used.
1   Total dust, respirable and non-respirable:

$$8 \text{ h TWA (mg/m}^3) = \frac{30}{\% \text{ quartz} + 3}$$

2   Respirable dust only:

$$8 \text{ h TWA (mg/m}^3) = \frac{10}{\% \text{ respirable quartz} + 2}$$

For mineral dusts which contain cristobalite or tridymite, a value equal to one half of that obtained from the above formulae should be used.

Coal dust
Permitted levels of respirable coal dust in coal mines are laid down in the Coal Mines (Respirable Dust) Regulations 1975 and the Coal Mines (Respirable Dust Amendment) Regulations 1978.

When exposure occurs to coal dust containing more than 5% quartz in workplaces other than coal mines, the formulae for mineral dust containing crystalline silica should be used.

Graphite
For natural or synthetic graphite which contains more than 1% quartz, the formulae for mineral dusts containing silica should be used.

Further Reading

Further information on the topics discussed here may be obtained from the following sources; this is by no means an exhaustive list.

Cotes J.E. & Steel J. *Work Related Lung Diseases*, Blackwell Scientific Publications, 1987.

Edwards F.E., McCallum R.I. & Taylor P.J. (eds) *Fitness for Work: The Medical Aspects*, Oxford University Press, 1988.

Howard J.K. & Tyrer F.H. *Textbook of Occupational Medicine*, Churchill Livingstone, 1987.

Levy B.S. & Wegman D.H. (eds) *Occupational Health*, 2nd edn, Little Brown & Co, 1988.

Parkes W.R. *Occupational Lung Disorders*, 3rd edn, Butterworth, 1990.

Raffle P.A.B., Lee, W.R., McCallum R.I. & Murray R. *Hunter's Diseases of Occupations*, Hodder & Stoughton, 1987.

Rom W.N. (ed) *Environmental and Occupational Medicine*, Little Brown & Co, 1983.

Waldron H.A. *Occupational Health Practice*, 3rd edn, Butterworths, 1989.

Waldron H.A. & Harrington J. (eds) *Occupational Hygiene*, Blackwell Scientific Publications, 1981.

World Health Organization *Early Detection of Occupational Diseases*, WHO, 1986.

Zenz C. *Occupational Medicine: Principals and Practical Applications*, 2nd edn, Year Book, 1988.

Index